Genetic Disorders Sourcebook,
  1st Edition
Genetic Disorders Sourcebook,
  2nd Edition
Head Trauma Sourcebook
Headache Sourcebook
Health Insurance Sourcebook
Health Reference Series Cumulative
  Index 1999
Healthy Aging Sourcebook
Healthy Children Sourcebook
Healthy Heart Sourcebook for Women
Heart Diseases & Disorders
  Sourcebook, 2nd Edition
Household Safety Sourcebook
Immune System Disorders Sourcebook
Infant & Toddler Health Sourcebook
Injury & Trauma Sourcebook
Kidney & Urinary Tract Diseases &
  Disorders Sourcebook
Learning Disabilities Sourcebook,
  1st Edition
Learning Disabilities Sourcebook,
  2nd Edition
Liver Disorders Sourcebook
Leukemia Sourcebook
Lung Disorders Sourcebook
Medical Tests Sourcebook
Men's Health Concerns Sourcebook
Mental Health Disorders Sourcebook,
  1st Edition
Mental Health Disorders Sourcebook,
  2nd Edition
Mental Retardation Sourcebook
Movement Disorders Sourcebook
Obesity Sourcebook
Ophthalmic Disorders Sourcebook,
  1st Edition
Oral Health Sourcebook
Osteoporosis Sourcebook
Pain Sourcebook, 1st Edition
Pain Sourcebook, 2nd Edition
Pediatric Cancer Sourcebook
Physical & Mental Issues in Aging
  Sourcebook

Podiatry Sourcebook
Pregnancy & Birth Sourcebook
Prostate Cancer
Public Health Sourcebook
Reconstructive & Cosmetic Surgery
  Sourcebook
Rehabilitation Sourcebook
Respiratory Diseases & Disorders
  Sourcebook
Sexually Transmitted Diseases
  Sourcebook, 1st Edition
Sexually Transmitted Diseases
  Sourcebook, 2nd Edition
Skin Disorders Sourcebook
Sleep Disorders Sourcebook
Sports Injuries Sourcebook, 1st Edition
Sports Injuries Sourcebook, 2nd Edition
Stress-Related Disorders Sourcebook
Stroke Sourcebook
Substance Abuse Sourcebook
Surgery Sourcebook
Transplantation Sourcebook
Traveler's Health Sourcebook
Vegetarian Sourcebook
Women's Health Concerns Sourcebook
Workplace Health & Safety Sourcebook
Worldwide Health Sourcebook

Teen Health Series
Diet Information for Teens
Drug Information for Teens
Mental Health Information
  for Teens
Sexual Health Information
  for Teens
Skin Health Information
  for Teens
Sports Injuries Information
  for Teens

Leukemia
SOURCEBOOK

Health Reference Series

First Edition

Leukemia
SOURCEBOOK

Basic Consumer Health Information about Adult and Childhood Leukemias, Including Acute Lymphocytic Leukemia (ALL), Chronic Lymphocytic Leukemia (CLL), Acute Myelogenous Leukemia (AML), Chronic Myelogenous Leukemia (CML), and Hairy Cell Leukemia, and Treatments Such as Chemotherapy, Radiation Therapy, Peripheral Blood Stem Cell and Marrow Transplantation, and Immunotherapy

Along with Tips for Life During and After Treatment, a Glossary, and Directories of Additional Resources

Edited by
Joyce Brennfleck Shannon

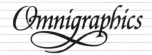

Omnigraphics

615 Griswold Street • Detroit, MI 48226

Bibliographic Note

Because this page cannot legibly accommodate all the copyright notices, the Bibliographic Note portion of the Preface constitutes an extension of the copyright notice.

Edited by Joyce Brennfleck Shannon

Health Reference Series

Karen Bellenir, *Managing Editor*
David A. Cooke, MD, *Medical Consultant*
Elizabeth Barbour, *Permissions Associate*
Dawn Matthews, *Verification Assistant*
Laura Pleva Nielsen, *Index Editor*
EdIndex, Services for Publishers, *Indexers*

* * *

Omnigraphics, Inc.

Matthew P. Barbour, *Senior Vice President*
Kay Gill, *Vice President—Directories*
Kevin Hayes, *Operations Manager*
Leif Gruenberg, *Development Manager*
David P. Bianco, *Marketing Consultant*

* * *

Peter E. Ruffner, *Publisher*

Frederick G. Ruffner, Jr., *Chairman*

Copyright © 2003 Omnigraphics, Inc.

ISBN 0-7808-0627-1

Library of Congress Cataloging-in-Publication Data

Leukemia sourcebook : basic consumer health information about adult and childhood leukemias, including acute lymphocytic leukemia (ALL), chronic lymphocytic leukemia (CLL), acute myelogenous leukemia (AML), chronic myelogenous leukemia (CML), and hairy cell leukemia, and treatments such as chemotherapy, radiation therapy, peripheral blood stem cell and marrow transplantation, and immunotherapy; along with tips for life during and after treatment, a glossary, and directories of additional resources / edited by Joyce Brennfleck Shannon. -- 1st ed.
    p. cm. -- (Health reference series)
    ISBN 0-7808-627-1 (lib. bdg.: acid-free paper)
    1. Leukemia--Popular works. I. Shannon, Joyce Brennfleck. II. Health reference series (Unnumbered)

RC643.L445 2003
616.99'419--dc21
                                                                    2003054912

Printed in the United States

Table of Contents

Part II: Childhood Leukemia

Part III: Adult Leukemia

Part IV: Leukemia Treatments

Part V: Life during and after Treatment for Leukemia

vii

Preface

About This Book

Leukemia, a cancer of the blood cells, strikes individuals of all ages and races. Each year, nearly 30,000 adults and more than 2,000 children learn that they have leukemia. Although all forms of leukemia can be treated, survival is strongly linked to age at diagnosis and the type of leukemia. Knowledge about leukemia and how to treat it continues to increase and according to the SEER (Surveillance, Epidemiology, and End Results) program of the National Cancer Institute, the overall five-year survival rate has risen from 14 percent in 1960 to 44 percent today.

This *Sourcebook* provides health information about adult and childhood leukemias—acute lymphocytic leukemia (ALL), chronic lymphocytic leukemia (CLL), acute myelogenous leukemia (AML), chronic myelogenous leukemia (CML), and hairy cell leukemia. Readers will learn about diagnosis, selection of treatment facilities, financial issues, and treatments for leukemia, including chemotherapy, radiation, drug therapy, and transplantation of peripheral blood stem cells or marrow. Also included are tips for nutrition, pain and fatigue control, and recognizing possible long-term and late effects of leukemia treatment, along with a glossary and directories of additional resources.

How to Use This Book

This book is divided into parts and chapters. Parts focus on broad areas of interest. Chapters are devoted to single topics within a part.

Part I: Leukemia Overview presents basic information about leukemia, including statistics, diagnosis, how to find a doctor and treatment facility, and facts about clinical trials. Also, included are tips for finding help through community resources and a discussion of financial issues.

Part II: Childhood Leukemia describes acute lymphoblastic leukemia and acute myeloid leukemia in children. Detailed information assists parents and children in understanding the procedures used to diagnose and treat leukemia. Guidelines give practical advice for parents seeking to help children cope with the disease, diagnostic and treatment procedures, record keeping, and interactions with friends.

Part III: Adult Leukemia explains the causes, risk factors, diagnosis, and treatment of pre-leukemia myelodysplastic syndrome (MDS), acute lymphocytic leukemia (ALL), chronic lymphocytic leukemia (CLL), acute myelogenous leukemia (AML), chronic myelogenous leukemia (CML), and hairy cell leukemia.

Part IV: Leukemia Treatments describes drug therapy, including chemotherapy, Gleevec™, and immunotherapy; radiation therapy; and peripheral blood stem cell or marrow transplantation. It describes transplant procedures, the search process, donation procedures, and success statistics. Information about alternative therapies and investigational drugs is also presented.

Part V: Life during and after Treatment for Leukemia gives practical advice for record keeping, nutrition and diet, dealing with fatigue and pain, and recognizing the long-term effects that can result from leukemia treatment. Tips for caregiver and patient support are also included.

Part VI: *Additional Help and Information* includes a glossary of important terms and directories of prescription drug assistance programs, financial assistance resources, and organizations able to provide additional information.

Bibliographic Note

This volume contains documents and excerpts from publications issued by the following U.S. government agencies: National Cancer Institute (NCI) and U.S. Food and Drug Administration (FDA).

In addition, this volume contains copyrighted documents from the following organizations and individuals: Cancer/Cancerconsultants. com; American Cancer Society; American Society of Clinical Oncology/ People Living with Cancer; Cancer Care, Inc.; Dana Farber Cancer Institute; Duke University Medical Center Adult Bone Marrow/Stem Cell

Transplant Program; Gale Group; Healthology, Inc.; Leukemia & Lymphoma Society; National Marrow Donor Program; O'Reilly and Associates; Pharmaceutical Research and Manufacturers of America; Sidney Kimmel Cancer Institute; St. Jude Children's Research Hospital; University of Minnesota Cancer Center; and Wendy Hobbie and Kathy Ruccione.

Full citation information is provided on the first page of each chapter. Every effort has been made to secure all necessary rights to reprint the copyrighted material. If any omissions have been made, please contact Omnigraphics to make corrections for future editions.

Acknowledgements

Special thanks go to the many organizations, agencies, and individuals who have contributed materials for this *Sourcebook* and to the managing editor Karen Bellenir, medical consultant Dr. David Cooke, permissions specialist Liz Barbour, verification assistant Dawn Matthews, indexer Edward J. Prucha, and document engineer Bruce Bellenir.

Note from the Editor

This book is part of Omnigraphics' *Health Reference Series*. The *Series* provides basic information about a broad range of medical concerns. It is not intended to serve as a tool for diagnosing illness, in prescribing treatments, or as a substitute for the physician/patient relationship. All persons concerned about medical symptoms or the possibility of disease are encouraged to seek professional care from an appropriate health care provider.

Our Advisory Board

The *Health Reference Series* is reviewed by an Advisory Board comprised of librarians from public, academic, and medical libraries. We would like to thank the following board members for providing guidance to the development of this series:

Dr. Lynda Baker,
Associate Professor of Library and Information Science,
Wayne State University, Detroit, MI

Nancy Bulgarelli,
William Beaumont Hospital Library, Royal Oak, MI

Karen Imarisio,
Bloomfield Township Public Library, Bloomfield Township, MI

Karen Morgan,
Mardigian Library, University of Michigan-Dearborn,
Dearborn, MI

Rosemary Orlando,
St. Clair Shores Public Library, St. Clair Shores, MI

Medical Consultant

Medical consultation services are provided to the *Health Reference Series* editors by David A. Cooke, MD. Dr. Cooke is a graduate of Brandeis University, and he received his M.D. degree from the University of Michigan. He completed residency training at the University of Wisconsin Hospital and Clinics. He is board-certified in Internal Medicine. Dr. Cooke currently works as part of the University of Michigan Health System and practices in Brighton, MI. In his free time, he enjoys writing, science fiction, and spending time with his family.

Health Reference Series *Update Policy*

The inaugural book in the *Health Reference Series* was the first edition of *Cancer Sourcebook* published in 1989. Since then, the *Series* has been enthusiastically received by librarians and in the medical community. In order to maintain the standard of providing high-quality health information for the layperson the editorial staff at Omnigraphics felt it was necessary to implement a policy of updating volumes when warranted.

Medical researchers have been making tremendous strides, and it is the purpose of the *Health Reference Series* to stay current with the most recent advances. Each decision to update a volume will be made on an individual basis. Some of the considerations will include how much new information is available and the feedback we receive from people who use the books. If there is a topic you would like to see added to the update list, or an area of medical concern you feel has not been adequately addressed, please write to:

Editor
Health Reference Series
Omnigraphics, Inc.
615 Griswold Street
Detroit, MI 48226
E-mail: editorial@omnigraphics.com

Part One

Leukemia Overview

Chapter 1

Living with Leukemia: What You Need to Know

It wasn't the flu-like symptoms that sent Neil Keller to the hospital one night in January 1995. It wasn't even the crippling back pain that left him virtually immobilized. It was the odd red stripe that Kathy Keller noticed running down the back of her husband's calf that prompted his sudden trip to the emergency room.

Following his evaluation, the physical education teacher from Frederick, MD, learned that the red stripe was a blood clot. He also learned that he had leukemia and needed immediate medical attention.

"I hastily left our two young children in the care of their grandparents because Neil was being transported quickly by ambulance to a special cancer center in Baltimore," remembers Kathy Keller. "It happened just that quickly."

According to the American Cancer Society (ACS), about 30,000 new cases of leukemia were diagnosed in the United States in 2001. And even though it is thought of primarily as a childhood disease, the ACS says that leukemia strikes more adults than children. Anyone can get it, and like many forms of cancer, its cause is unknown. Certain risk factors, such as genetic conditions or adverse environmental exposure, are believed to increase the chances of developing the disease.

Survival is strongly linked to age at diagnosis and the type of leukemia. Fortunately, the overall five-year survival rate for people with

"Living with Leukemia," by Carol Lewis, *FDA Consumer*, March-April 2002, U.S. Food and Drug Administration (FDA).

leukemia has tripled over the past 40 years. In 1960, the rate was 14 percent. By the 1970s, it had reached 35 percent. Today, the overall five-year survival rate is 44 percent.

All forms of leukemia can be treated. In the last decade, several new drugs or new uses for existing drugs have been approved by the Food and Drug Administration to treat various types of leukemia. One of the most recent of these approved drugs—Gleevec™ (imatinib mesylate)—represents a new strategy in fighting one type of leukemia. It works by blocking the rapid growth of white blood cells.

But cancer experts say the best hope of a breakthrough that will greatly improve cure rates and duration of remission lies in understanding and controlling the abnormal molecular processes that lead to the development of all types of leukemia.

More Than One Disease

Leukemia is cancer of the blood cells. It is characterized by the uncontrolled growth of developing bone marrow cells. It is not a single disease, but a group of malignancies in which the bone marrow and blood-forming organs produce excessive numbers of white blood cells. White blood cells develop from a type of cell in the bone marrow called a stem cell. When the process of white cell maturation goes awry, leukemia results. Immature white cells prevent the normal production of all blood cells, including white blood cells, which fight infection. In most leukemias, an increased number of cancerous white blood cells are produced, causing the lymph nodes, liver, or spleen to enlarge.

Leukemias are classified by the type of white blood cell that has abnormal growth and by how fast the disease is progressing. Acute leukemia can be fatal within weeks or months without aggressive treatment. Abnormal blood cells that remain very immature, called blasts, increase rapidly and the disease worsens quickly.

Chronic leukemia may produce no symptoms for years. Some immature cells may be present, but in general, these cells are more mature than those in acute leukemia and are able to carry out some normal cell functions. The number of blasts increases less rapidly than in acute leukemia, and as a result, chronic leukemia worsens gradually. Chronic leukemia can become acute leukemia.

Leukemia can arise in either of the two main types of white blood cells—lymphoid or myeloid. Leukemia that affects lymphoid cells is known as lymphocytic leukemia. When myeloid cells are affected, the disease is called myelogenous leukemia. The disease can be categorized into one of four main types, depending on whether it is acute or chronic and myelogenous or lymphocytic. While both children and adults can develop leukemia, certain types are more common in one age group than in another. However, Keller was diagnosed at age 31 with acute lymphocytic leukemia (ALL), which is most prevalent among children. Although he died less than a year later, Kathy Keller says that at the time the prognosis for people with ALL seemed good. "They said it was critical, sure—that Neil's condition was life-threatening," she remembers, "but we got lucky that the attending physician turned out to be someone who recognized the urgency in getting Neil immediate medical attention."

In addition to the four main types, there are sub-types of leukemia, such as acute promyelocytic leukemia (APL), and hairy cell—a chronic leukemia in which the abnormal white blood cells appear to be covered with tiny hairs when viewed under a microscope.

Symptoms

Some people with leukemia may not experience any symptoms at all and their first inkling of a problem could be the results of a routine blood test. Others, however, may complain of flu-like symptoms such as fatigue, fever, weight loss, and night sweats. Other signs of leukemia can include:

- easy bruising or bleeding
- lymph node enlargement
- bone pain
- swelling of the abdomen due to an enlarged liver and spleen
- increased susceptibility to infection

Diagnosis

Common blood tests, such as the complete blood cell count (CBC), as well as blood cell examination under a microscope, can provide the first evidence that a person has leukemia. Most people with acute leukemia, like Keller, will have an increased number of white blood cells, not enough red blood cells, and not enough platelets.

"Neil's white blood counts were as high as his doctor had ever seen," says Kathy Keller. "But he also indicated that Neil's type of leukemia had a 90 percent cure rate with a two-year treatment plan."

In addition to the CBC, a bone marrow test is frequently performed to confirm the diagnosis and determine the type of leukemia. Bone marrow is the soft, spongy tissue in the center of the bones that produces the white blood cells, red blood cells, and platelets. Two kinds of tissue samples are taken for examination under a microscope and for special tests such as chromosomal analysis. In a procedure known as a bone marrow aspiration, cells are withdrawn with a fine needle and syringe. A bone marrow biopsy involves taking a piece of bone with marrow inside, using a larger needle. Both samples usually are taken from the same site, generally on the back of the pelvic bone.

Other diagnostic tests could include:

- removing and testing an entire lymph node

- drawing fluid from the spinal cavity in the lower back (spinal tap)

- measuring certain chemicals in the blood (to determine liver or kidney problems caused by leukemia or certain chemotherapy drugs)

- using X-rays, computed tomography (CT) scans, magnetic resonance imaging (MRI), or ultrasound imaging, to obtain detailed images of internal organs.

Treatment

Many people died from leukemia—often within months of diagnosis—before the advent of effective treatments. Now, many more are cured (usually defined as five or more years of disease-free survival).

The goal in treating leukemia is to achieve complete remission (all signs and symptoms of leukemia have disappeared, although there still may be cancer in the body) by destroying cancerous cells so that normal cells can again grow in the bone marrow. In remission, cancerous cells cannot be seen in the blood or bone marrow, but more therapy is needed to achieve a cure. Several areas of research have yielded new approaches to treating leukemia. But the kind of treatment given and the outlook for a person with the disease vary greatly, according to the exact type of leukemia the person has, and other individual factors.

Chemotherapy refers to the use of drugs to kill cancer cells. It is the main treatment for nearly all types of leukemia. Most of these anticancer drugs are injected through a vein (IV injection or intravenously), but some can be taken by mouth. Either way, the drugs enter the bloodstream and spread throughout the body to kill cancerous cells.

Chemotherapy is given in cycles: a treatment period is followed by a recovery period. The process may be repeated. The duration of the treatment varies depending on the type of leukemia. Sometimes certain drugs are combined with others for a greater treatment effect. Unlike many people who show progress following chemotherapy, Keller periodically showed progress, but then relapsed.

"Neil responded well to chemotherapy for short periods of time," says Kathy Keller, "but he never went through a remission."

Most anticancer drugs are cytotoxic, which means they kill not only cancerous cells but also normal cells, particularly in the bone marrow. "The rationale of chemotherapy is that the normal cells are more likely to eventually survive the effects of chemotherapeutic agents than the cancer cells," says Amna Ibrahim, M.D., a medical officer in the FDA's Center for Drug Evaluation and Research.

New Treatments

Gleevec™ demonstrated in trials that it substantially reduces the level of cancerous cells in the bone marrow and blood of people with CML. A new class of drug to fight cancer, Gleevec™ is different from other cancer drugs because it specifically targets an enzyme that causes cells to become cancerous and multiply in people with CML. It works by blocking the protein product that is responsible for transforming normal cells into cancerous ones. Gleevec™ provided a new cancer treatment for chronic CML after the failure of interferon-alpha therapy, CML in blast crisis, and CML in an accelerated phase.

After two years of study, Gleevec™, manufactured by Novartis Pharmaceuticals Corp., of East Hanover, NJ, appears to offer advantages over some other leukemia treatments: oral administration, tolerable side effects, and a high response rate.

The FDA's accelerated approval of Gleevec™ was based on the response rate observed in early clinical trials. Accelerated approval allows products for serious or life-threatening illnesses to reach the market sooner, based on clinical trials that have not yet demonstrated true clinical benefit, like survival or improved disease-related symptoms, but in which early results have indicated the drug is reasonably likely to have real clinical benefit.

James Foran, M.D., a medical oncologist at the University of Nebraska Medical Center and spokesman for the Leukemia and Lymphoma Society, says that CML occurs when pieces of two different chromosomes break off and reattach on the opposite chromosome, forming what's known as the "Philadelphia chromosome." This chromosome translocation leads to the enzyme being turned on all the time. As a result, potentially life-threatening levels of both mature and immature white blood cells occur in the bone marrow and the blood. "Gleevec™ shuts down the growth signals from the Philadelphia chromosome," says Foran, and blocks the rapid growth of malignant white blood cells.

But because the information from Gleevec™ clinical trials is still early, it is not known how durable the responses to this treatment will be. In fact, relapses following initial responses to Gleevec™ are now being reported.

Another class of drugs, known as differentiating agents, is used in treating APL. These drugs promote differentiation of the very immature leukemic white blood cells into more mature functioning cells. Two drugs in this class include Vesanoid® (all-trans retinoic acid or ATRA), made by Hoffmann-La Roche Inc. of Nutley, NJ, which was approved by the FDA for first-line treatment, and Trisenox® (arsenic trioxide), made by Cell Therapeutics Inc. of Seattle and approved for second-line therapy after ATRA treatment failure. These drugs have improved the prognosis of APL.

Mylotarg® (gemtuzumab ozogamicin), another new type of leukemia drug, consists of an antibody against AML blast cells combined with a toxin to kill the cells. Mylotarg®, manufactured by Wyeth-Ayerst Pharmaceuticals of St. Davids, PA, the pharmaceutical branch of American Home Products Corp., was approved in May 2001 for treatment of elderly patients with AML who cannot tolerate more conventional chemotherapy.

Bone Marrow Transplants

Bone marrow transplants offer some people like 44-year-old Tom Kochanowicz of Omaha, NE, the best chance of survival and, in his case, a cure. Kochanowicz was diagnosed with CML at age 38 when his doctor detected a lump in his side. "Fortunately," he says, "mine was the slow-moving kind and initially was managed with medications to bring my white blood cell count under control."

However, Kochanowicz says the side effects of the radiation and chemotherapy treatments took their toll. "The aggressive treatment was wiping out my immune system," he remembers. Consequently, despite hopes that the drug treatments would conquer, or at least manage, his leukemia, Kochanowicz admits he had always known that his life ultimately would depend on a bone marrow transplant.

In this procedure, existing abnormal bone marrow is eliminated through radiation treatments or chemotherapy. Healthy marrow is then injected directly into the bloodstream in a procedure similar to a blood transfusion. The bone marrow migrates to and takes root in the recipient's bones, and the cells begin to divide. It generally takes about three weeks and sometimes longer for the transplanted bone marrow to start producing white blood cells to protect against infections, making the procedure quite risky. Healthy marrow may have been supplied either by the patient in the early stage of the disease, or by a donor. Only someone who has a compatible tissue type—ideally a close relative—can be a donor.

Both of Kochanowicz's brothers were perfect blood matches, giving him excellent odds for a full recovery. As the result of a successful transplant, Kochanowicz is now entering his sixth year of remission. Keller wasn't as fortunate.

"We were told that brothers and sisters were the best matches," says Kathy Keller. "But since Neil was an only child, we tested the kids, me, and his parents." Keller's father ended up donating the needed bone marrow.

A parent or child is able to donate needed bone marrow only about 1 percent of the time, says Edwin P. Alyea, a medical oncologist with the Dana-Farber Cancer Institute in Boston. As in Keller's rare situation, Alyea says, "When they can, that's very lucky."

He also says that unrelated donor registries make it possible for people to have blood matches outside their families. These registries increase the chances of finding donors based on ethnic background and other specific qualifications. But Alyea says that "more minorities need to contribute to the registries" and greater outreach is needed in these communities.

A major complication of bone marrow transplants is graft-versus-host disease (GVHD) in which the transplanted marrow cells react against the patient's tissues; primarily the liver, the skin, and the digestive tract.

Despite surviving leukemia, Kochanowicz's last six years haven't been easy. His transplant experience included severe GVHD—for nearly two years he was unable to swallow, and a condition called scleroderma hardened the connective tissue in his skin.

Alyea explains that although a bone marrow transplant plays a key role in the treatment for certain types of leukemia, as a whole "it is basically an exchange of one disease for another. You're trading the disease itself, for which the treatment options and the chances of cure may be limited, for the possible complications of the transplant treatment," he says.

Alyea also says doctors have learned that patients who develop acute or chronic GVHD have a lower risk of the disease returning after the bone marrow transplant. "This demonstrates that the donor's immune system may play a role in cure," says Alyea. After a long and frustrating battle with the unpleasant effects of GVHD, Kochanowicz now manages his symptoms with medications, and admits that he feels better than he has "in a very long time."

Biologic Therapy

A relatively new addition to the family of cancer treatments is biological therapy (sometimes called immunotherapy). Biological therapy uses the body's immune system, either directly or indirectly, to fight cancer or to lessen the side effects that may be caused by some cancer treatments.

Patricia Keegan, M.D., a deputy division director in the FDA's Center for Biologics Evaluation and Research, explains that the immune system is a complex network of cells and organs that work together to defend the body against foreign invaders. This network is one of the body's main defenses against cancer. For example, the immune system may recognize the difference between healthy cells and cancerous cells in the body, and work to eliminate those that become cancerous.

Biological therapies, says Keegan, are designed to repair, stimulate, or enhance the immune system's responses when cancer prevents it from functioning adequately. Some immune system substances can be produced in the laboratory for use in cancer treatments. But Keegan says that, although biological drugs can be effective in treating different types of leukemia, there are so few available because "they are labor-intensive—the development of blood products is a relatively young field that is still developing."

The Future

Scientists are finding better ways to treat leukemia, and the chances of recovery keep improving. A physician who specializes in the treatment of leukemia is in the best position to discuss a person's prognosis and to offer the best course of treatment for a particular type of leukemia.

Survival rates may indicate how long groups of people may live. However, *it's important to remember that statistics are averages based on large numbers of people.* These numbers cannot be used to predict what will happen to an individual because no two people are identical, and treatments and responses vary.

The Four Main Types of Leukemia, Common Characteristics, and Their Distribution among Children and Adults

Acute Lymphocytic Leukemia (ALL)

- Develops from cells in the bone marrow called lymphocytes
- Accounts for slightly more than half of all cases of childhood leukemia
- Most common cancer in children
- Progresses rapidly

Chronic Lymphocytic Leukemia (CLL)

- Develops from lymphocytes
- Cells look mature but their function may not be normal
- Occurs almost exclusively in adults
- Most common leukemia in adults
- Progresses slowly

Acute Myelogenous Leukemia (AML)

- Also known as acute myeloid leukemia
- Develops from either granulocytes or monocytes (types of white blood cells)
- Affects children and adults
- Accounts for just under half of childhood leukemia cases
- Progresses rapidly

Chronic Myelogenous Leukemia (CML)

- Another form of myeloid leukemia
- Develops from granulocytes or monocytes
- Affects adults
- About half as common as CLL
- Progresses slowly

Glossary

Accelerated phase. The middle phase of chronic myeloid leukemia that lasts from six to 18 months. The white blood cell count increases as the disease is harder to control with conventional treatments.

Acute leukemia. A rapidly progressing cancer of the bone marrow and other blood-forming tissues.

Biological therapy (immunotherapy). Treatment to stimulate or restore the ability of the immune system to fight infection and disease.

Blasts. Immature blood cells.

Blast crisis. The final phase of chronic myeloid leukemia, lasting about three to six months.

Bone marrow. Soft, spongy tissue in the center of the bones that produces white blood cells, red blood cells, and platelets.

Bone marrow transplant. A procedure to replace bone marrow destroyed by treatment with high doses of anticancer drugs or radiation.

Catheter. A flexible tube used to deliver fluids into, or withdraw fluids from, the body.

Chemotherapy. Treatment with anticancer drugs.

Chromosome. The carrier of hereditary characteristics found in cells.

Chronic leukemia. A slowly progressing cancer of the blood-forming tissues.

Cure. Five or more years of disease-free survival.

Differentiating agents. A type of therapy that can trigger immature cells to become more mature and functional.

Donor. A person who donates organs, tissues, cells, or other biological material.

First-line treatment. The drugs and other therapies given to a patient who is diagnosed with a disease and has not had any therapy for the disease.

Graft-versus-host disease (GVHD). A reaction of donated bone marrow against a person's tissue.

Immune system. The complex group of organs and cells that defends the body against infection or disease.

IV injection (intravenously). Injection into a vein.

Lymph node. A rounded mass of lymphatic tissue that is surrounded by a capsule of connective tissue.

Lymphoid. Refers to lymphocytes, a type of white blood cell. Also refers to tissue in which lymphocytes develop.

Malignancy. Cancer.

Myeloid. Pertaining to, derived from, or manifesting certain features of the bone marrow. Also called myelogenous.

Oncologist. A doctor who specializes in treating cancer.

Platelets (thrombocytes). A type of blood cell that helps prevent bleeding by causing blood clots to form.

Red blood cells (erythrocytes). Cells that carry oxygen to all parts of the body.

Relapse. The return of signs and symptoms of cancer after a period of improvement.

Remission. A decrease in or disappearance of signs and symptoms of cancer. In partial remission, some, but not all, signs and symptoms disappear. In complete remission, all signs and symptoms have disappeared, although there could still be cancer in the body.

Second-line treatment. The drugs and other therapies given to a patient who has a disease that has either not responded to or recurs following first-line treatment.

Spleen. An organ that is part of the lymphatic system and produces lymphocytes, filters the blood, stores blood cells, and destroys old blood cells.

White blood cells (leukocytes). A type of cell in the immune system that helps the body fight infection and disease. White blood cells include lymphocytes, granulocytes, macrophages, and others.

Additional Information

Dana-Farber Cancer Institute
44 Binney Street
Boston, MA 02115
Tel: 866-408-3324
Website: www.dana-farber.org
E-mail: dana-farbercontactus@dfci.harvard.edu

The Leukemia & Lymphoma Society, Inc.
1311 Mamaroneck Avenue
White Plains, NY 10605
Toll-Free: 800-955-4572
Tel: 914-949-5213
Fax: 914-949-6691
Website: www.leukemia.org

National Cancer Institute
NCI Public Inquiries Office
6166 Executive Boulevard, MSC 8322
Suite 3036A
Bethesda, MD 20892-8322
Toll-Free: 800-422-6237
Toll-Free TTY: 800-332-8615
Website: www.cancer.gov

American Cancer Society
P.O. Box 102454
Atlanta, GA 30368-2354
Toll-Free: 800-227-2345
Website: www.cancer.org

Chapter 2

Leukemia Facts and Figures

What Is Cancer?

Cancer is a group of diseases characterized by uncontrolled growth and spread of abnormal cells. If the spread is not controlled, it can result in death. Cancer is caused by both external factors (tobacco, chemicals, radiation, and infectious organisms) and internal factors (inherited mutations, hormones, immune conditions, and mutations that occur from metabolism). Causal factors may act together or in sequence to initiate or promote carcinogenesis. Ten or more years often pass between exposures or mutations and detectable cancer. Cancer is treated by surgery, radiation, chemotherapy, hormones, and immunotherapy.

Who Is at Risk of Developing Cancer?

Anyone. Since the occurrence of cancer increases as individuals age, most cases affect adults beginning in middle age. About 77% of all cancers are diagnosed at ages 55 and older. Cancer researchers use the word *risk* in different ways. *Lifetime risk* refers to the probability that an individual, over the course of a lifetime, will develop cancer

This chapter includes excerpts from "What Are The Key Statistics for Adult Acute Leukemia?" © 2001 American Cancer Society, Inc., reprinted by permission of the American Cancer Society, Inc.; and "Cancer Facts & Figures 2002," © 2002 American Cancer Society, Inc. Reprinted by permission of the American Cancer Society, Inc.

or die from it. In the U.S., men have a little less than 1 in 2 lifetime risk of developing cancer: for women the risk is a little more than 1 in 3.

Relative risk is a measure of the strength of the relationship between risk factors and the particular cancer. It compares the risk of developing cancer in persons with a certain exposure or trait to the risk in persons who do not have the exposure or trait. For example, male smokers have a 20-fold relative risk of developing lung cancer compared with nonsmokers. This means that they are about 20 times more likely to develop lung cancer than nonsmokers. Most relative risks are not this large. For example, women who have a first-degree (mother, sister, or daughter) family history of breast cancer have about a 2-fold increased risk of developing breast cancer compared with women who do not have a family history. This means that women with a first-degree family history are about two times more likely to develop breast cancer than women who do not have a family history of the disease.

All cancers involve the malfunction of genes that control cell growth and division. About 5% to 10% of cancers are clearly hereditary, in that an inherited faulty gene predisposes the person to a very high risk of particular cancers. The remainder of cancers are not hereditary, but the result from damage to genes (mutations) that occurs throughout our lifetime, either due to internal factors, such as hormones or the digestion of nutrients within cells, or external factors, such as tobacco, chemicals, and sunlight.

How Many People Alive Today Have Ever Had Cancer?

The National Cancer Institute estimates that approximately 8.9 million Americans with a history of cancer were alive in 1997. Some of these individuals were considered cured, while others still had evidence of cancer and may have been undergoing treatment.

How Many New Cases Are Expected to Occur This Year?

About 1,284,900 new cancer cases are expected to be diagnosed in 2002. Since 1990, about 16 million new cancer cases have been diagnosed. These estimates do not include carcinoma in situ (noninvasive cancer) of any site except urinary bladder, and do not include basal and squamous cell skin cancers. More than 1 million cases of basal and squamous cell skin cancers are expected to be diagnosed this year.

How Many People Are Expected to Die of Cancer This Year?

This year about 555,500 Americans are expect to die of cancer, more than 1,500 people a day. Cancer is the second leading cause of death in the U.S., exceeded only by heart disease. In the U.S., 1 of every 4 deaths is from cancer.

What Percentage of People Survive Cancer?

The 5-year relative survival rate for all cancers combined is 62%. After adjusting for normal life expectancy (factors such as dying of heart disease, accidents, and diseases of old age), the 5-year relative survival rate represents persons who are living five years after diagnosis, whether disease-free, in remission, or under treatment with evidence of cancer. While 5-year relative survival rates are useful in monitoring progress in the early detection and treatment of cancer, they do not represent the proportion of people who are cured permanently, since cancer can affect survival beyond five years after diagnosis.

Table 2.1. Estimated New Leukemia Cancer Cases and Deaths by Gender, US, 2002*

	Estimated New Cases			Estimated New Deaths		
Type of Leukemia	Both Sexes	Males	Female	Both Sexes	Male	Female
Leukemia	30,800	17,600	13,200	21,700	12,100	9,600
Acute lymphocytic leukemia (ALL)	3,800	2,200	1,600	1,400	800	600
Chronic lymphocytic leukemia (CLL)	7,000	4,100	2,900	4,500	2,600	1,900
Acute myeloid leukemia (AML)	10,600	5,900	4,700	7,400	4,000	3,400
Chronic Myeloid leukemia (CML)	4,400	2,500	1,900	2,000	1,100	900
Other leukemia	5,000	2,900	2,100	6,400	3,600	2,800

*Estimates of new cases are based on incidence rates from the NCI SEER program 1979-1998.

Although these rates provide some indication about the average survival experience of cancer patients in a given population, they are less informative when used to predict individual prognosis and should be interpreted with caution. First, 5-year relative survival rates are based on patients who were diagnosed and treated at least eight years ago and do not reflect recent advances in treatment. Second, information about detection methods, treatment protocols, additional illnesses, and behaviors that influence survival are not taken into account in the estimating of survival rates.

What Are the Costs of Cancer?

The National Institutes of Health estimate overall costs for cancer in the 2001 at $156.7 billion: $56.4 billion for direct medical costs (total of all health expenditures); $15.6 billion for indirect morbidity costs (cost of lost productivity due to illness); and $84.7 billion for indirect mortality costs (cost of lost productivity due to premature death). Lack of health insurance and other barriers to health care prevent many Americans from receiving optimal health care.

According to 1999 data, about 16% of Americans under age 65 have no health insurance, and about 26% of older persons have only Medicare coverage. During 1998 and 1999, almost 18% of Americans aged 18 to 64 years reported not having a regular source of health care. Also, 5.7% of 18-64 year-old adults say cost is a barrier to obtaining needed health care in the previous year.

Childhood Cancer

New Cases: An estimated 9,100 new cases are expected to occur among children aged 0-14 in 2002. Childhood cancers are rare.

Deaths: An estimated 1,400 deaths are expected to occur among children aged 0-14 in 2002, about 1/3 of them from leukemia. Despite its rarity, cancer is the chief cause of death by disease in children between ages 1 and 14. Mortality rates have declined 50% since 1973.

Early Detection: Cancers in children often are difficult to recognize. Parents should see that their children have regular medical checkups and should be alert to any unusual symptoms that persist. These include: an unusual mass or swelling; unexplained paleness and loss of energy; sudden tendency to bruise, a persistent, localized pain or limping; prolonged, unexplained fever or illness; frequent headaches,

18

often with vomiting; sudden eye or vision changes; and excessive, rapid weight loss.

Leukemia accounts for about 30% of cancer cases in children ages 0-14.

Treatment: Childhood cancers can be treated by a combination of therapies chosen based on the specific type and stage of the cancer. Treatment is coordinated by a team of experts including oncologic physicians, pediatric nurses, social workers, psychologists, and others who assist children and their families.

Survival: Five-year survival rates vary considerably depending on the site: all sites, 77%; bone cancer, 73%; neuroblastoma, 71%; brain and central nervous system, 69%; Wilms' tumor (kidney), 92%; Hodgkin's disease, 92%; and acute lymphocytic leukemia, 85%.

Leukemia

New Cases: An estimated 30,800 new cases were expected in 2002, approximately evenly divided between acute leukemia and chronic leukemia. Although often thought of as primarily a childhood disease, leukemia is diagnosed ten times more often in adults than in children. Acute lymphocytic leukemia accounts for approximately 2,000 of the leukemia cases among children. In adults, the most common types are acute myeloid leukemia (approximately 10,600 cases) and chronic lymphocytic leukemia (approximately 7,000 cases). Incidence of acute myeloid leukemia increased by 1.8% per year among males during 1992-1998, with most of the increase occurring in the elderly, possibly attributable to cigarette smoking.

Deaths: An estimated 21,700 deaths in 2002.

Signs and Symptoms: Fatigue, paleness, weight loss, repeated infections, bruising easily, and nosebleeds or other hemorrhages. In children, these signs can appear suddenly. Chronic leukemia can progress slowly with few symptoms.

Risk Factors: Leukemia affects both sexes and all ages. Causes of most leukemias are unknown. Persons with Down syndrome and certain other genetic abnormalities have higher incidence rates of leukemia. Leukemia is caused by excessive exposure to ionizing radiation

Table 2.2. Estimated New Leukemia Cases and Deaths by Leukemia by State, U.S., 2002. (*continued on next page*)

State	New Leukemia Cases	Deaths by Leukemia
Alabama	500	400
Alaska	*	*
Arizona	500	400
Arkansas	300	200
California	3,000	2,100
Colorado	400	300
Connecticut	400	300
Delaware	100	100
Dist. Of Columbia	*	*
Florida	2,200	1,600
Georgia	700	500
Hawaii	100	100
Idaho	100	100
Illinois	1,400	1,000
Indiana	700	500
Iowa	400	300
Kansas	300	200
Kentucky	400	300
Louisiana	500	300
Maine	100	100
Maryland	500	400
Massachusetts	700	500
Michigan	1,000	700
Minnesota	600	400
Mississippi	300	200
Missouri	700	500
Montana	100	100

Table 2.2. Estimated New Leukemia Cases and Deaths by Leukemia by State, U.S., 2002. (*continued from previous page*)

State	New Leukemia Cases	Deaths by Leukemia
Nebraska	200	200
Nevada	200	100
New Hampshire	100	100
New Jersey	1,100	800
New Mexico	200	100
New York	2,000	1,400
North Carolina	900	600
North Dakota	100	100
Ohio	1,400	1,000
Oklahoma	400	300
Oregon	400	300
Pennsylvania	1,600	1,100
Rhode Island	100	100
South Carolina	400	300
South Dakota	100	100
Tennessee	700	500
Texas	1,900	1,300
Utah	200	100
Vermont	100	*
Virginia	700	500
Washington	700	500
West Virginia	300	200
Wisconsin	700	500
Wyoming	100	*
United States	30,800	21,700

* Estimate is 50 or fewer cases.

and to certain chemicals such as benzene, a commercially used toxic liquid that is present in gasoline and cigarette smoke. Leukemia also may occur as a side effect of cancer treatment. Certain leukemias and lymphomas are caused by a retrovirus, human T-cell leukemia/lymphoma virus-1 (HTLV-1).

Early Detection: Because symptoms often resemble those of other, less serious conditions, leukemia can be difficult to diagnose early. When a physician does suspect leukemia, diagnosis can be made using blood tests and bone marrow biopsy.

Treatments: Chemotherapy is the most effective method of treating leukemia. Various anticancer drugs are used, either in combinations or as single agents. Transfusions of blood components and antibiotics are used as supportive treatments. Under appropriate conditions, bone marrow transplantation may be useful in treating certain leukemias.

Survival: The 1-year relative survival rate for patients with leukemia is 64%. Survival decreases to 40% five years after diagnosis, primarily due to the poor survival of patients with certain types of leukemia, such as acute myeloid leukemia. There has been a dramatic improvement in survival for patients with acute lymphocytic leukemia from a 5-year relative survival rate of 38% in the mid-1970s to 63% in the mid-1990s. Survival rates for children with acute lymphocytic leukemia have increased from 53% to 85% over the same time period.

Table 2.3. Probability of Developing Leukemia Over Selected Age Intervals, by Sex, U.S., 1996-1998*

Sex	Birth-39	40-59	60-79	Birth to Death
Male	0.16 (1 in 627)	0.21 (1 in 483)	0.81 (1 in 124)	1.43 (1 in 70)
Female	0.12 (1 in 810)	0.15 (1 in 671)	0.47 (1 in 212)	1.04 (1 in 96)

*For those free of cancer at beginning of age interval. Based on cancer cases diagnosed during 1996-1998. The 1 in statistic and the inverse of the percentage may not be equivalent due to rounding.

Source: DevCan, *Probability of Developing or Dying of Cancer Software, Version 4.1.* Feuer EJ, Wun LM, National Cancer Institute 2001.

Table 2.4. Trends in Leukemia Five-Year Relative Survival Rates by Race and Year of Diagnosis, U.S. 1974-1997

White Relative 5-Year Survival Rate (%)			Black Relative 5-Year Survival Rate (%)			All Races Relative 5-Year Survival Rate (%)		
1974-76	1983-85	1992-97	1974-76	1983-85	1992-97	1974-76	1983-85	1992-97
35	42	46˙	31	33	38	34	41	45˙

* The difference in rates between 1974-46 and 1992-27 is statistically significant (p<0.05).

Source: *Surveillance, Epidemiology, and End Results Program, 1973-1998*, Division of Cancer Control and Population Sciences, National Cancer Institute, Bethesda, MD 2001.

What Are the Key Statistics for Adult Acute Leukemia?

• About 30,800 new cases of leukemia will be diagnosed in the United States during 2002, approximately half will be acute leukemias. The most common adult leukemia is acute myelogenous leukemia with about 10,600 new cases expected.

• About 8,800 deaths from acute leukemias will occur in the United States during 2002.

• The average age of a patient with acute myelogenous leukemia (AML) is 65 years—this is a disease of older people. The chance of developing leukemia for a 50-year-old person is 1 in 50,000; for a 70-year-old, it is 1 in 7000. AML is more common among men than among women.

• Acute lymphocytic leukemia (ALL) is more common among children than adults and most patients are under 10 years of age. The chance of a 50-year-old having this disease for is 1 in 125,000; for a 70-year-old, it is 1 in 60,000.

• African-Americans are half as likely as whites to develop ALL, and have a slightly lower risk for AML.

• AML or ALL can be kept in remission for a long time or cured in about 20%-30% of adults. Depending on certain specific features of the leukemic cells, some patients with AML or ALL can be predicted to have a better or worse outlook.

Chapter 3

Risk Factors for Leukemia

What Are the Risk Factors for Adult Acute Leukemia?

A risk factor is anything that increases a person's chance of getting a disease such as cancer. Risk factors are lifestyle-related, environmental, or genetic (inherited).

Lifestyle-related risk factors for some types of cancer include such things as smoking or unprotected exposure to strong sunlight. The only proven lifestyle-related leukemia risk factor is smoking. Although many people know that smoking is responsible for most cancers of the lungs, mouth, throat, and larynx, few realize that it can affect cells that do not come into direct contact with smoke. Cancer-causing substances in tobacco smoke are absorbed by the lungs and spread through the bloodstream to many parts of the body. Scientists estimate that about one-fifth of cases of AML are caused by smoking.

Environmental risk factors are influences in our surroundings such as radiation, chemicals, and infections. Several factors in the environment are linked to acute leukemia. In the workplace, long-term exposure to high levels of benzene is a risk factor for AML. High-dose radiation exposure (such as being a survivor of an atomic bomb blast or nuclear reactor accident) increases the risk of developing AML or

This chapter includes "What Are the Risk Factors for Adult Acute Leukemia?" © 2001 American Cancer Society, Inc., reprinted by permission of the American Cancer Society, Inc.; and "Can Adult Acute Leukemia Be Prevented?" © 2001 American Cancer Society, Inc., reprinted by permission of the American Cancer Society, Inc.

ALL. Patients with other cancers who are treated with certain chemotherapy drugs are more likely to develop AML. The drugs most often associated with these secondary (post-treatment) leukemias include mechlorethamine, procarbazine, chlorambucil, etoposide, teniposide and to a lesser degree, cyclophosphamide. Combining these drugs with radiation therapy further increases the risk. Most secondary leukemias are cases of AML and occur within 9 years after treatment of Hodgkin's disease, non-Hodgkin's lymphoma, or childhood ALL. Secondary leukemias sometimes occur following treatment of breast, ovarian, or other cancers. Chemotherapy does not work as well for patients with secondary AML. Their outlook for recovery is not as good as that of typical patients with AML.

There is conflicting evidence about electromagnetic field (EMF) exposure (such as that occurring near very high-voltage power lines) as a potential risk factor for developing leukemia. The NCI has several large studies going on now to look into this question. Most studies published so far suggest either no increased risk or a very slightly increased risk. Clearly, most cases of leukemia are not related to EMF exposure.

A small percentage of patients are also at greater risk of acute leukemia because they have inherited certain very rare diseases such as Fanconi's anemia, Wiskott-Aldrich syndrome, Bloom's syndrome, Li-Fraumeni syndrome, or ataxia telangiectasia.

Infection with the human T-cell lymphoma/leukemia virus (HTLV-1) can cause a rare type of acute lymphocytic leukemia. Most cases occur in Japan and the Caribbean area and this disease is not common in the United States.

Some patients who develop acute leukemia have had a myelodysplastic syndrome (preleukemic condition). These conditions cause defects in blood cell formation and over a period of years, may evolve into acute myelogenous leukemia. Patients who develop AML after a preleukemic syndrome typically have a poor prognosis.

Can Adult Acute Leukemia Be Prevented?

Although many types of cancer can be prevented by lifestyle changes to avoid certain risk factors, there is currently no known way to prevent most cases of leukemia. Since most leukemia patients have no known risk factors, at the present time there is no way to prevent their leukemias from developing. People with a known inherited tendency to develop leukemia should receive thorough, periodic medical checkups. The risk of leukemia in these syndromes, although higher than that in the general population, is still extremely rare.

An estimated 20% of adult acute leukemia cases are related to smoking tobacco. Smoking, which doubles the risk of acute myeloid leukemia in people over 60, is by far the most significant controllable risk factor and, for now, offers the greatest opportunity to prevent leukemias. Of course, nonsmokers are also much less likely than smokers to develop many other cancers, as well as heart disease, stroke, and other diseases.

Treatment of other cancers with chemotherapy and radiation may cause secondary (post-treatment) leukemias. Doctors are now studying ways to treat cancer patients that minimize the risk of secondary leukemia. However, the obvious benefits of treating life-threatening cancers with chemotherapy and radiation therapy must be balanced against the small chance of developing leukemia several years later.

Avoiding known cancer-causing industrial chemicals, such as benzene, can lower the risk of developing acute leukemia. But most experts agree that occupational and environmental chemicals are responsible for only a small number of leukemia cases.

Chapter 4

Diagnosing Adult Acute Leukemia

Signs and Symptoms of Acute Leukemia

Acute leukemia can cause many different signs and symptoms. Most of these occur in all kinds of acute leukemia, but some are particularly common with certain subtypes.

Patients with acute leukemia often have several generalized symptoms. These can include weight loss, fever, and loss of appetite. Of course, these are not specific to acute leukemia and are more often caused by something other than cancer.

Most signs and symptoms of acute leukemia result from a shortage of normal blood cells due to crowding out of normal blood cell-producing bone marrow by the leukemia cells. As a result, people do not have enough properly functioning red blood cells, white blood cells, and blood platelets.

Anemia, a shortage of red blood cells, causes shortness of breath, excessive tiredness, and a pale color to the skin.

Not having enough normal white blood cells (called leukopenia), and, in particular, too few mature granulocytes (called neutropenia or granulocytopenia), increases the risk of infections. Although leukemia is a cancer of white blood cells and patients with leukemia may have very high white blood cell counts, acute leukemia cells do not protect against infection. Thrombocytopenia, (not having enough of the blood platelets needed for plugging holes in damaged blood vessels), can lead to excessive bruising, bleeding, frequent or severe nosebleeds, and bleeding from the gums.

Spread of leukemia cells outside the bone marrow, called extramedullary spread, may involve the central nervous system—CNS (brain and spinal cord), the testicles, ovaries, kidneys, and other organs. Symptoms of CNS leukemia include headache, weakness, seizures, vomiting, difficulty in maintaining balance, and blurred vision. Some patients have bone pain or joint pain caused by the spread of leukemic cells to the surface of the bone or into the joint from the marrow cavity.

Leukemia often causes enlargement of the liver and spleen, two organs located on the right and left side respectively, of the abdomen. Enlargement of these organs would be noticed as a fullness, or even swelling, of the belly. These organs are usually covered by the lower ribs but when enlarged, they can be felt by the doctor examining the patient.

Leukemia may spread to lymph nodes. If the affected nodes are close to the surface of the body (lymph nodes on the sides of the neck, in the groin, underarm areas, above the collarbone, etc.), the patient, or health care provider may notice the swelling. Swelling of lymph nodes inside the chest or abdomen may also occur, but can be detected only by imaging tests such as computed tomography (CT) or magnetic resonance imaging (MRI) scans.

Acute myelogenous leukemia (AML), particularly the M5 or monocytic form, may spread to the gums, causing them to swell, be painful, and bleed. Spread to the skin, it can cause small pigmented (colored) spots that can look like common rashes. A tumorous collection of AML cells under the skin or other parts of the body is called a chloroma or granulocytic sarcoma.

The T-cell type of acute lymphocytic leukemia (ALL) often involves the thymus. An enlarged thymus can press on the nearby trachea (windpipe) causing coughing, shortness of breath, or even suffocation. The superior vena cava (SVC), a large vein that carries blood from the head and arms back to the heart, passes next to the thymus. Growth of the leukemia cells may compress the SVC and cause swelling of the head and arms known as SVC syndrome. This can also affect the brain and can be life-threatening. Patients with SVC syndrome need immediate treatment.

Types of Specimens Used in Diagnosis and Evaluation of Leukemia

If signs and symptoms suggest that a patient has leukemia, the doctor will need to sample cells from the patient's blood and bone marrow to make an accurate diagnosis. Other tissue and cell samples may also be taken in order to guide treatment.

Blood cell counts and blood cell examination: Changes in the numbers of different blood cell types and the appearance of these cells under the microscope help in the diagnosis of leukemia. Most patients with acute leukemia (ALL or AML) have too many white cells in their blood, not enough red blood cells, and not enough platelets. In addition, many of these white blood cells will be blasts, a type of cell normally found in the bone marrow but not in circulating blood. These immature cells do not function normally. Even though these findings suggest leukemia, usually the disease cannot be diagnosed for sure without obtaining a sample of bone marrow cells.

Bone marrow tests: In bone marrow aspiration a thin needle and a syringe are used to remove a small amount of liquid bone marrow (about 1 teaspoon). During a bone marrow biopsy procedure, a small cylindrical piece of bone and marrow (about 1/16 inch in diameter and 1/2 inch long) is removed with a slightly larger needle. Both samples usually are taken at the same time from the back of the hipbone. These tests are used to diagnosis leukemia and later, to tell if the leukemia is responding to therapy.

Blood chemistry tests: These tests measure the amount of certain chemicals in their blood but are not used to diagnose leukemia. In patients already known to have leukemia, these tests help detect liver or kidney problems due to damage caused by the spread of leukemic cells or to the side-effects of certain chemotherapy drugs. These tests also help determine whether treatment is needed to correct abnormally low or high blood levels of certain minerals.

Excisional lymph node biopsy: A surgeon removes the entire lymph node (excisional biopsy). If the node is near the skin surface, this is a simple operation that can be done using a local anesthetic (numbing medication), but if the node is inside the chest or abdomen, general anesthesia (the patient is asleep) is used. This procedure is important in diagnosing lymphomas, but is only rarely needed with leukemias.

Lumbar puncture: A small needle is placed into the spinal cavity in the lower back (below the level of the spinal cord) to withdraw cerebrospinal fluid (CSF) to be examined for leukemia cells.

Laboratory Tests Used to Diagnose and Classify Leukemia

All of the biopsy samples (bone marrow, lymph node tissue, blood, and cerebrospinal fluid) are examined under a microscope by a doctor with special training in blood and lymphoid tissue disease. The samples are usually examined by a pathologist (doctor specializing in diagnosis of disease by laboratory tests) and are often also reviewed by the patient's hematologist/oncologist (doctor specializing in medical treatment of cancer and blood diseases). The doctors will look at the size and shape of the cells and whether their cytoplasm contains granules (microscopic collections of enzymes and other chemicals that help white blood cells fight infections).

Based on a cell's size, shape, and granules, doctors can classify bone marrow cells into specific types. An important element of this cell classification is whether the cell appears mature (resembles normal cells of circulating blood, that can fight infections and are no longer able to reproduce) or immature (lacks features of normal circulating blood cells, not effective in fighting infections, and are able to reproduce). The most immature cells are called blasts.

The percentage of cells that are blasts is a particularly important factor. Having at least 30% blasts in the marrow is generally required for a diagnosis of acute leukemia. In order for a patient to be considered to be in remission, the blast percentage must be no higher than 5%. Sometimes this examination does not provide a definite answer, and other laboratory tests are needed.

Cytochemistry: After cells from the sample are placed on glass microscope slides, they are exposed to chemical stains (dyes) that are attracted or react with or to only some types of leukemia cells. These stains cause a color change that can be seen only under a microscope. For example, one stain causes the granules of most AML cells to appear as black spots under the microscope, but it does not cause ALL cells to change colors.

Flow cytometry: This technique is sometimes used to examine the cells from bone marrow, lymph nodes, and blood samples. It is very accurate in determining the exact type of leukemia. A sample of cells is treated with special antibodies and passed in front of a laser beam. Each antibody sticks only to certain types of leukemia cells. If the sample contains those cells, the laser will cause them to give off light that is measured and analyzed by a computer. Groups of cells can be separated and counted by these methods.

Immunocytochemistry: As in flow cytometry, cells from the bone marrow aspiration or biopsy sample are treated with special antibodies. But instead of using a laser and computer for analysis, the sample is treated so that certain types of cells change color. The color change can be seen only under a microscope. Like flow cytometry, it is helpful in distinguishing different types of leukemia from one another and from other diseases.

Cytogenetics: Normal human cells contain 46 chromosomes, pieces of DNA and protein that control cell growth and metabolism. In certain types of leukemia, part of one chromosome may be attached to part of a different chromosome. This change, called a translocation, can usually be seen under a microscope. Recognizing these translocations helps in identifying certain types of ALL and AML and is important in determining the outlook for the patient. Some types of leukemia have an abnormal number of chromosomes. For example, ALL cells with over 50 chromosomes are more sensitive to chemotherapy. Those with less than 46 are more resistant to chemotherapy. The testing usually takes about 3 weeks, because the leukemic cells must grow in laboratory dishes for a couple of weeks before their chromosomes are ready to be viewed under the microscope. The results of cytogenetic testing are written in a shorthand form that describes which chromosome changes are present.

- A translocation, written as t(1:2), for example, means a part of chromosome 1 is now located on chromosome 2.

- An inversion, written as inv 16 means that part of the chromosome 16 is upside down and is now in reverse order but is still attached to the chromosome it originated from.

- A deletion, written as -7, for example indicates part of chromosome 7 has been lost.

- An addition, +8 for example, happens when all or part of a chromosome material has been duplicated, and too many copies of it are found within the cell.

Molecular genetic studies: Certain substances, called antigen receptors, occur on the surface of lymphocytes. These receptors are important in initiating a response from the immune system. Normal lymphoid cells have many different antigen receptors, which help the body respond to many types of infection.

Lymphocytic leukemias, such as ALL, however, start from a single abnormal lymphocyte, so all cells in each patient's leukemia have the same antigen receptor. Laboratory tests of the DNA, which contain information on each cell's antigen receptors, are a very sensitive way to diagnose ALL. Because different subtypes of ALL cells have different antigen receptor features, this test is sometimes helpful in ALL classification.

Tests of leukemia cell DNA can also find most translocations that are visible under a microscope in cytogenetic tests. DNA tests can also find some translocations involving parts of chromosomes too small to be seen with usual cytogenetic testing under a microscope.

This sophisticated testing is helpful in leukemia classification because many subtypes of ALL and AML have distinctive translocations. Information about these translocations may be useful in predicting response to treatment. These tests may be used after treatment to find small numbers of leukemia cells that can be missed under a microscope.

Imaging Studies

Imaging studies are ways of producing pictures of the inside of the body. There are several imaging studies that might be done in people with leukemia.

X-rays: During the course of diagnosis and evaluation of a person with leukemia, a chest x-ray and a bone scan are often obtained. These may show a mass in the chest, or evidence of leukemia in the bones or rarely in the joints.

Computed tomography (CT scan): This is a special kind of x-ray, in which the beam moves around the body, taking pictures from different angles. These images are then combined by a computer to produce a detailed cross-sectional picture of the inside of the body. CT scans are not often used in leukemia, but they can show enlargement of lymph nodes around the heart and trachea (windpipe) or in the back of the abdomen due to spread of leukemia cells. Involvement of these areas is more common in ALL than in AML.

Magnetic resonance imaging (MRI): This procedure uses powerful magnets and radio waves to produce computer-generated pictures of internal organs. The pictures look very similar to a CT scan, but are more detailed. This scan may be used when there is concern about leukemia involving the brain.

Gallium scan and bone scan: For this procedure, the radiologist injects a radioactive chemical that collects in areas of cancer or infection. This accumulation of radioactivity can then be viewed by a special camera. These tests are useful when a patient has bone pain that might be due to bone infection or cancer involving bones. This test is not used when the patient has already been diagnosed with leukemia.

Ultrasound: This test uses sound waves to produce images of internal organs. The test can distinguish solid from fluid-filled masses. It can help to show whether the kidneys, liver, or spleen have been affected by leukemia.

Chapter 5

Understanding Blood Cell Counts

What Is a Blood Test?

Blood tests help a physician to diagnose and manage a disease. In addition to examining blood cells, there are many chemicals in the blood that give important information about the functioning of bodily systems. Important chemicals that may be measured include cholesterol, thyroid hormone, potassium, and numerous others. These various chemicals are dissolved in the plasma and circulate in the blood. For a chemical blood test, blood is drawn from a patient's vein and placed in an empty tube and usually allowed to clot; the fluid portion of the blood after clotting, called serum, is then used for the various chemical analyses.

What Is a Blood Cell Count?

Counting and examining blood cells are very important in the diagnosis of blood cell diseases. Blood cell counts are used during diagnosis, treatment, and follow-up to determine the health of the patient. Blood cell counts alone cannot determine if a patient has a blood related cancer. However, blood cell counts can alert the physician if further testing is needed.

To count and/or examine blood cells, the blood must be collected in a tube that has an anticoagulant in it to prevent blood clotting. By

"Understanding Blood Cell Counts," Fact Sheet © 1/2003 The Leukemia & Lymphoma Society, reprinted with permission. Visit www.leukemia-lymphoma. org for additional information.

so doing the cells are preserved, suspended in plasma, and can be stored for several hours without impairing the accuracy of the results.

To do a blood count, a sample of blood usually is taken from a vein in the crease of the forearm, placed in a tube containing an anticoagulant, and transported to a hematology laboratory. In the laboratory, a sample of the blood is put in a machine that can count red and white cells and platelets and measure the blood hemoglobin. Also, a small drop of blood is spread into a thin film on a glass slide, dried, and dyes are applied. The dyes color the different types of blood cells so that they are readily distinguishable from one another. The slide is examined under a microscope, the different types of white cells counted, and the cells examined to see if they are normal or, if abnormal, what the nature of the changes are.

Blood is composed of several different types of cells:

- **red blood cells**, sometimes referred to as erythrocytes, pick up oxygen as blood passes through the lungs and release it to the cells in the body

- **white blood cells**, sometimes referred to as leukocytes, help fight bacteria and viruses

- **platelets** are tiny cells produced by the bone marrow to help your blood clot in response to a cut or a wound. A decreased platelet count is called thrombocytopenia.

If all three of the blood cell types are examined, the test is referred to as a complete blood count or CBC. Some refer to the results as a hemogram.

A CBC also tests hemoglobin and hematocrit.

- **Hemoglobin** is a protein used by red blood cells to distribute oxygen to other tissues and cells in the body.

- **Hematocrit** refers to the amount of your blood that is occupied by red cells.

Why Does My Physician Request Blood Cell Counts?

There are several reasons why a physician may request blood cell counts. In a periodic health examination, blood counts, like other features of the examination, should be normal. Blood cell counts are a sensitive barometer of many illnesses; their measurement is an important part of a standard periodic health examination.

The blood cells may be altered as a result of a blood cell disease, or the counts may be altered as a reaction to another illness. For example, the white cell count may be elevated if a bacterial infection is present. The red cell count may be decreased as a result of a specific vitamin deficiency. The measurement of blood cells can contribute to the diagnosis of many disorders. If you have a blood cell disorder, measurement of the blood cell counts is an important index of the response of the disease to treatment. These counts are also important to learn the effects of drug treatment or radiation therapy. A blood count helps the physician to determine if a drug is working or not, whether the amount of drug a patient is receiving should be adjusted, or if another drug is needed.

What Is a Normal Blood Count?

Normal blood counts fall within the range that has been established by testing healthy men and women of all ages. The cell counts are compared to those of healthy individuals of similar age and sex. If a cell count is higher or lower than normal, the physician will try to determine the explanation for the abnormal results. The approximate normal ranges of blood cell counts for healthy adults are as follows:

1. Red blood cell (RBC) count:
    - 4.5 to 6.0 million red cells per microliter of blood in men
    - 4.0 to 5.0 million red cells per microliter of blood in women

2. White blood cell (WBC) count:
    - 4.5 to 11 thousand white cells per microliter of blood

3. Platelet count:
    - 150 to 450 thousand platelets per microliter of blood

4. Hematocrit is the percent of the blood that is composed of red cells:
    - 42% to 50% is normal in men
    - 36% to 45% is normal in women

5. Hemoglobin is the compound in the red blood cell that carries oxygen:

- 14 to 17 grams per 100 milliliters of blood is normal for men
- 12 to 15 grams per 100 milliliters of blood is normal for women

Differential count, sometimes referred to as a *diff*, is a breakdown of the different types of white blood cells, also called leukocytes. The observer can also tell if the white cells in the blood are normal in appearance.

The five types of white cells that are counted are neutrophils, lymphocytes, monocytes, eosinophils, and basophils. Blood contains about 60% neutrophils, 30% lymphocytes, 5% monocytes, 4% eosinophils, and less than 1% basophils.

How Does Leukemia, Lymphoma, and Myeloma Affect the Blood Count?

Leukemia

Leukemia is the term used for certain diseases that affect the white blood cells or leukocytes. The different types of leukemia affect the blood count differently. Persons with acute leukemia may have a low, a normal, or a high white blood cell count. The white cell count may occasionally be many times higher than the normal average count of about 7,000 white cells per microliter of blood. In addition, the leukemic white blood cells in patients with acute leukemia do not function normally. Patients with chronic leukemia always have an increase in white blood cells.

Lymphoma

Patients with lymphoma often have disturbances in their blood cell counts as the lymphoma may suppress red blood cell production, or because the lymphoma has spread to the marrow and suppresses all blood cell types. The lymphoma cells may enter the blood and produce high white blood cell counts made up of lymphoma cells (abnormal lymphocytes).

Myeloma

Patients with myeloma usually have anemia because the myeloma cells in the marrow interfere with red blood cell production. Later, all blood cell types may be decreased by the effects of the myeloma cells in the marrow.

- Persons with a very low white blood cell count may have an increased risk of infection.

- Persons with a low red blood cell count, hematocrit, and hemoglobin are anemic. Depending on the severity of the anemia and the rate at which it develops, it may result in fatigue, shortness of breath with exertion, and other limitations.

- Persons with a very low platelet count can bruise or bleed more readily than normal.

Will Treatment Affect My Blood Count?

Chemotherapy and radiation therapy often affect a person's blood counts. To measure the effects, a complete blood count is usually done at appropriate intervals during therapy to monitor its effects. The effect depends on the drug used, the dose used, and the duration of the therapy. Red blood cells, white blood cells, and platelets originate in the bone marrow. If the type of therapy you are receiving can suppress blood cell production in the marrow, the red blood cell count, white blood count, and/or platelet count can decrease. By following your blood counts, your doctor can determine how the therapy is affecting your body and whether to continue therapy at the same dose or change the dose or timing of treatment. If the blood counts do not recover sufficiently between treatments, a transfusion may be necessary.

Your doctor may decide to administer cytokines to boost the amount of white blood cells and red blood cells you produce following chemotherapy treatments. Cytokines are drugs that resemble naturally occurring hormones that stimulate blood cell production. The following are some names of the drugs used to help increase specific types of blood cells:

- Erythropoietin (also called Procrit®), which helps stimulate red blood cell production;

- Darbepoetin Alfa (also called Aranesp™), a long-acting form of erythropoietin that also helps stimulate red blood production but requires less frequent injections;

- Granulocyte colony stimulating factor (also called G-CSF, filgrastim, or Neupogen®), which helps stimulate white blood cell production;

- Granulocyte-monocyte colony-stimulating factor (also called GM-CSF, sargramostim, Leukine®, or Prokine®), which also helps stimulate white blood cell production.

Should Patients Keep Track of Their Blood Counts?

Some patients want to know the results of their blood counts and follow the changes that occur. If anemia develops, it may explain changes in your energy levels or an inability to carry out tasks that were easy to do before the anemia. If the white blood cell count drops to very low levels and fever develops, it is important to contact the physician promptly. If the platelet count is very low, you may bleed or bruise more easily; and it may be advisable to minimize activities that involve physical contact or the risk of injury. These matters should be discussed with your physician.

Additional Information

The Leukemia & Lymphoma Society
1311 Mamaroneck Avenue
White Plains, NY 10605
Toll-Free Information Resource Center: 800-955-4572
Tel: 914-949-5213
Fax: 914-949-6691
Website: www.leukemia-lymphoma.org

Chapter 6

Bone Marrow Aspiration and Biopsy

Definition

Bone marrow aspiration, which is also called bone marrow sampling, is the removal by suction of fluid from the soft, spongy material that lines the inside of the bones. Bone marrow biopsy, or needle biopsy, is the removal of a small piece of bone marrow. The bone marrow is where blood cells are made.

Purpose

Bone marrow aspiration is used to:

• Pinpoint the cause of abnormal blood test results.

• Confirm diagnosis or status of severe anemia from an unknown cause, other abnormalities in the blood's ability to store iron, or irregularities in the way blood cells are produced or become mature.

• Diagnose infection.

Bone marrow biopsy is used to:

• Obtain intact bone marrow for laboratory analysis.

"Bone Marrow Aspiration and Biopsy," from *Gale Encyclopedia of Medicine*, by Maureen Haggerty, Gale Group © 1999, Gale Group. Reprinted by permission of The Gale Group.

- Diagnose some types of cancer or anemia and other blood disorders.

- Identify the source of an unexplained fever.

- Diagnose fibrosis of bone marrow and myeloma when bone marrow aspiration has failed to provide an appropriate specimen.

Bone marrow aspiration and bone marrow biopsy are also used to gauge the effectiveness of chemotherapy and other medical treatments. These procedures are often used together to ensure the availability of the best possible bone marrow specimen.

Description

These procedures should be performed by a physician or nurse clinician. Each procedure takes about 20-30 minutes. It is usually performed on an outpatient basis, but can be done in a hospital if necessary.

The skin covering the biopsy site is cleansed with an antiseptic, and the patient may be given a mild sedative. A local anesthetic is administered. The hematologist or nurse clinician performing the procedure will not begin until the anesthetic has numbed the area from which the specimen is to be extracted. In adults, the specimen is usually taken from the hip or sternum (breastbone). When the patient is a child, the biopsy site is generally a vertebra or long bone in the leg.

In a bone marrow aspiration, a special needle, known as a University of Illinois needle, is inserted beneath the skin and rotated until it penetrates the cortex, or outer covering of the bone. It may hurt a little at first, but the most painful part is when the marrow is being aspirated (sucked out). At least half a teaspoon of marrow is sucked out of the bone by a syringe attached to the needle. If more marrow is needed, the needle is repositioned slightly, a new syringe is attached, and a second sample is taken. The samples are transferred from the syringes to slides and sent to a laboratory for analysis.

Bone marrow biopsy may be performed immediately before or after bone marrow aspiration. The procedure is performed with a special needle, which has a hollow core, much like a leather punch. In bone marrow biopsy, the needle is inserted, rotated to the right, then to the left, withdrawn, and reinserted at a different angle. This procedure is repeated until a small chip is separated from the bone marrow. The needle is again removed, and a piece of fine wire threaded through its tip transfers the specimen onto sterile gauze. The patient may feel discomfort or pressure when the needle is inserted and experience a brief, pulling sensation when the marrow is withdrawn. Unlike aspiration specimens, which are smeared, these samples contain bone marrow whose structure has not been disturbed or destroyed. Microscopic examination can show what material its cells contain and how they are alike or different from one another. The bone must be decalcified (a process which takes place overnight) before it can be properly stained and examined.

Preparation

The physician should be told of any medication the patient is using and any heart surgery that the patient has undergone.

Aftercare

After the needle is removed, the biopsy site will be covered with a clean, dry bandage. Pressure is applied to control bleeding. The patient's pulse, breathing, blood pressure, and temperature are monitored until they return to normal, and the patient may be instructed to lie on his back for half an hour before getting dressed.

The patient should be able to leave the clinic and resume normal activities immediately. Patients who have received a sedative often feel sleepy for the rest of the day; so driving, cooking, and other activities that require clear thinking and quick reactions should be avoided in that case.

The biopsy site should be kept covered and dry for several hours. Walking or prescribed pain medications usually ease any discomfort felt at the biopsy site, and ice can be used to reduce swelling.

A doctor should be notified if the patient:

- Feels severe pain more than 24 hours after the procedure.

- Experiences persistent bleeding or notices more than a few drops of blood on the wound dressing.

- Has a temperature above 101°F (38.3°C). Inflammation and pus at the biopsy site and other signs of infection should also be reported to a doctor without delay.

Risks

Bleeding and discomfort often occur at the biopsy site. Infection and hematoma may also develop. In rare instances, the heart or a major blood vessel is pierced when marrow is extracted from the sternum during bone marrow biopsy. This can lead to severe hemorrhage.

Normal Results

Healthy adult bone marrow contains yellow fat cells, connective tissue, and red marrow that produces blood. The bone marrow of a healthy infant is primarily red, with a limited ability to make blood.

Abnormal Results

Microscopic examination of bone marrow can reveal granulomas, myelofibrosis, lymphomas, or other cancers. Analyzing specimens can help doctors diagnose iron deficiency, vitamin B12 deficiency, and folate deficiency, as well as anemia and leukemia.

Obesity can affect the ease with which a bone marrow biopsy can be done, and the results of either procedure can be affected if the patient has had radiation therapy at the biopsy site.

Key Terms

Aspiration. A procedure to withdraw fluid from the body.

Connective tissue. Material that links one part of the body with another.

Fibrosis. A condition characterized by the presence of scar tissue or fiber-containing tissues that replace normal tissues.

Hematologist. A medical specialist who treats diseases and disorders of the blood and blood-forming organs.

Hematoma. Blood that collects under the skin and causes swelling.

Hemorrhage. Heavy bleeding.

Myeloma. A tumor that originates in bone marrow and usually spreads to more than one bone.

Nurse practitioner. A registered nurse who is qualified to perform some specialized duties.

Vertebra. A bone that is part of the spinal column.

Further Reading

The Yale University Patient's Guide to Medical Tests, edited by Barry L. Zaret, et al. Boston, MA: Houghton Mifflin Company, 1997.

Additional Information

The Leukemia & Lymphoma Society
1311 Mamaroneck Ave.
White Plains, NY 10605
Toll-Free Information Resource Center: 800-955-4572
Tel: 914-949-5213
Fax: 914-949-6691
Website: www.leukemia-lymphoma.org

National Cancer Institute
Cancer Information Service
9000 Rockville Pike
Bethesda, MD 20892
Toll-Free: 800-422-6237
Toll-Free TTY: 800-332-8615
NCI website: http://www.cancer.gov
CIS website: http://cis.nci.nih.gov

National Marrow Donor Program
3001 Broadway Street NE
Suite 500
Minneapolis, MN 55413-1753
Toll-Free: 800-627-7692
Tel: 612-627-5800
Website: www.marrow.org

The Wellness Community
1320 Centre Street
Suite 305
Newton Centre, MA 02459
Tel: 617-332-1919
Website: www.wellnesscommunity.org

Chapter 7

How to Find a Doctor or Treatment Facility

Your Health Care Team: Your Doctor Is Only the Beginning

Coping with cancer is not an easy thing. The physical effects of illness and treatment can be quite severe, and the emotional and psychological impact of having cancer can be equally challenging. However, the good news is that there are many kinds of help available to you through the different members of your health care team.

This section includes a description of the health care professionals who are usually accessible to someone who has cancer. Each of these people can play a vital role in helping you obtain the best treatment possible and maintain the highest quality of life throughout your diagnosis and treatment.

First Things First: Your Own Role

It may seem obvious, but it is very important to remember that you are the most important person on your health care team. As with any type of health care you receive, you are a consumer of services, and you should not be afraid to ask questions about what you are getting and who is providing it.

This chapter includes "Your Health Care Team: Your Doctor Is Only the Beginning," Fact Sheet 8.10, National Cancer Institute (NCI), reviewed 4/19/2000; and "How to Find a Doctor or Treatment Facility if You Have Cancer," Fact Sheet 7.47, National Cancer Institute (NCI), reviewed 3/26/2002.

You might consider these tips:

- When you are going to meet with someone (a doctor, nurse, or specialist), bring someone else with you. It helps to have another person hear what is said and think of questions to ask.

- Write out your questions beforehand to make sure you don't forget to discuss anything.

- Write down the answers you get, and make sure you understand what you are hearing.

- Do not be afraid to ask your questions or ask where you can find more information about what you are discussing. Being well informed is your most important task on the health care team.

Social Workers: Lots of Help from One Place

Social workers are professionally trained in counseling and practical assistance. They provide the broadest range of help to people with cancer, and are a good place to start if you have recently been diagnosed with cancer and are unsure of what to do next. Oncology social workers specialize in cancer; most hospitals that treat cancer patients have certified oncology social workers on staff. Clinical or psychiatric social workers have an advanced degree or Ph.D. in social work and are trained to provide family therapy, marital counseling, or counseling focused on coping with chronic illness. A hospital social worker can also refer you to a clinical social worker in private practice in the community.

The hospital social worker can also provide counseling, find a support group for you, locate services in your community that can help you with home care or transportation, and guide you through the process of applying to the government for Social Service Disability or other forms of assistance. They can also help you understand your diagnosis and talk to you about treatment, side effects, and what to expect. If you need help finding a social worker in your area, start by contacting your local hospital.

Psychiatrists: If You Need Medication or Feel Depressed

A psychiatrist is a medical doctor who specializes in providing psychotherapy, or general psychological help. A psychiatrist specializes in helping people who are depressed, anxious, or otherwise unable to cope psychologically. Because they are medical doctors, psychiatrists can also prescribe medication, such as antidepressants or medication to help you sleep. To find a psychiatrist, you can ask your doctor for a referral, ask if your hospital has a psychiatric department, call your Health Maintenance Organization (HMO) or other managed care plan, or ask a social worker to help.

Psychologists: Providing Therapy and Counseling

A psychologist is also someone who can assist you if you are feeling depressed, anxious, or sad. While not medical doctors, psychologists have obtained a doctoral degree in psychology and counseling; many specialize in marital counseling or chronic illness. Some cancer centers have psychologists on staff, but if you are looking for one, ask your doctor, your HMO, your hospital, or a social worker for a referral.

Nurses: A Very Important Role in Care

Nurses are an extremely important part of your health care team. Nurses have a wide range of skills, and are usually in charge of actually implementing the plan of care your doctor has set up for you. They are trained to administer medication and monitor side effects. All major medical centers have nurses who specialize in cancer. Whether you are staying in the hospital for care or receive it on an outpatient basis (which means you go home after each treatment), you will benefit from seeking assistance, asking questions, or getting tips and advice from your nurse or nurse-practitioner. Nurses are often aware of support services in your community and can usually provide you with educational materials and pamphlets.

You may also arrange or request a registered nurse to visit you at home if needed. If the visit is approved by your doctor, it will usually be covered by insurance. Another option is to hire a private duty nurse who does not work for your hospital or health care service. This can be expensive and often is not covered by insurance, but can ease the burden of care on your family or loved ones.

Home Health Aides: Care at Home

Another form of home care is from a home health aide. Home health aides assist people who are ill and need help moving around, bathing, cooking, or doing household chores. Some state Medicaid programs will pay for home health aide care, provided it is supervised by a nurse. However, private insurance or managed care plans rarely pay for a home health aide unless there is also a need for skilled nursing care. To find home health aide care, ask your physician, nurse, or social worker, and remember to ask if the charges vary based on income. The telephone yellow pages are another source, but be sure to check credentials, find out whether the agency is bonded, and ask for references.

Rehabilitation Specialists: Help for Recovery

Rehabilitation services help people recover from physical changes caused by cancer or cancer treatment. It includes the services of physical therapists, occupational therapists, counselors, speech therapists, and other professionals who help you physically recover from cancer. For example, physical therapy can help you rebuild the muscles in your arm and shoulder if you have had chest surgery.

Most physicians will refer you to rehabilitation services if you need them; be sure to ask if you think you might want them. Also, check to see if these types of services are covered under your insurance plan (some may be, others may not). Additionally, some cancer or social service organizations may provide you with free rehabilitation services if you are not insured for them.

Dietary or Nutritional Services

Cancer and cancer treatment can cause people to lose weight. For this reason, dietary or nutritional counseling or services are commonly prescribed for people with cancer. A dietitian can suggest ways to get enough calories, vitamins, and protein to help you feel better and control your weight, and can give you tips about increasing your appetite if you experience nausea, heartburn, or fatigue from your illness or treatment.

Most hospitals have registered dietitians on staff, and you can ask your doctor about meeting with them. If you are trying to locate a dietitian in your community, be sure to ask about experience and training. Remember to check if the services of a dietitian are covered under your insurance; if not, ask your doctor, nurse, or social worker about community-based programs that offer free services.

Clergy: Spiritual Support Is Important

Prayer and spiritual counseling can be very important in coping with a serious illness such as cancer. Many people find it useful to get help from clergy or other spiritual leaders, and there is no question that a strong sense of spirituality can help people face difficult challenges with courage and a sense of hope. Some studies show that people with cancer have less anxiety and depression, even pain, when they feel spiritually connected. Even if your beliefs are challenged by your illness, don't be afraid to reach out to others for help. It is important to remember that you are not alone at this time.

Hospice Care: Help with Terminal Illness

Hospice care focuses on the special needs of people who have terminal cancer. Sometimes called palliative care, this type of care focuses on providing comfort, controlling physical symptoms like pain, and giving emotional or spiritual support. Hospice care is usually provided at home, although there are hospice centers that operate much like hospitals and provide full-time care. Your doctor or social worker can refer you for hospice care.

Home hospice care is usually coordinated through a nurse, who then sends a home health aide, social worker, occupational therapist, clergy, or the type of specialist that is appropriate for the needs of the hospice patient. Hospice care is not for everyone. It is important to discuss this option carefully and get guidance from your doctor, nurse, or social worker.

Putting the Team Together: Find Help and Hope

A diagnosis of cancer may be the most difficult challenge you or your loved ones will ever face. That is why it is important to find help and try to maintain your sense of hope no matter what your situation. Your team of health care professionals is knowledgeable about the many different aspects of cancer: medical, physical, emotional, social, and spiritual. They are available to you as much or as little as you need, but it is difficult for them to know if you need help unless you ask for it. Don't be afraid, embarrassed, or hesitant to ask questions; voice your opinion, and seek the care you feel you need and deserve.

How to Find a Doctor or Treatment Facility If You Have Cancer

If you have been diagnosed with cancer, finding a doctor and treatment facility for your cancer care is an important step to getting the best treatment possible. Although the health care delivery system is complex, resources are available to guide you in finding a doctor, getting a second opinion, and choosing a treatment facility. This section includes suggestions and information resources to help you with these important decisions.

Physician Training and Credentials

When choosing a doctor for your cancer care, you may find it helpful to know some of the terms used to describe a doctor's training and credentials. Most physicians who treat people with cancer are medical doctors (they have an M.D. degree). The basic training for a physician includes 4 years of premedical education at a college or university, 4 years of medical school to earn an M.D. degree, and a residency consisting of 3 to 7 years of postgraduate education and training. Physicians must pass an exam to become licensed (legally permitted) to practice medicine in their state. Each state or territory has its own procedures and general standards for licensing physicians.

Specialists are physicians who have completed their residency training in a specific area, such as internal medicine. Independent specialty boards certify physicians after they have fulfilled certain requirements. These requirements include meeting specific education and training criteria, being licensed to practice medicine, and passing an examination given by the specialty board. Doctors who have met all of the requirements are given the status of *Diplomate* and are board-certified as specialists. Doctors who are *board-eligible* have obtained the required education and training, but have not completed the specialty board examination.

After being trained and certified as a specialist, a physician may choose to become a subspecialist. A subspecialist has at least 1 additional year of full-time education in a particular area of a specialty. This training is designed to increase the physician's expertise in a specific field. Specialists can be board-certified in their subspecialty as well.

The following are some of the specialties and subspecialties that pertain to cancer treatment:

- **Hematology** is a subspecialty of internal medicine. Doctors who are specialists in internal medicine treat a wide range of medical problems. Doctors who subspecialize in hematology focus on diseases of the blood and related tissues, including the bone marrow, spleen, and lymph glands.

- **Medical Oncology** is a subspecialty of internal medicine. Subspecialists in medical oncology treat all types of benign (noncancerous) and malignant (cancerous) tumors.

- **Radiation Oncology** is a subspecialty of radiology. Radiology is the use of x-rays and other forms of radiation to diagnose and treat disease. Radiation oncologists are subspecialists in the use of radiation to treat cancer.

- **Surgery** is a specialty that pertains to the treatment of disease by surgical operation. General surgeons are specialists who perform operations on almost any area of the body. Physicians can also choose to specialize in a certain type of surgery; for example, thoracic surgeons are specialists who perform operations specifically in the chest area, including the lungs and the esophagus.

Almost all board-certified specialists are members of their medical specialty society. Physicians can attain Fellowship status in a specialty society, such as the American College of Surgeons (ACOS), if they demonstrate outstanding achievement in their profession. Criteria for Fellowship status may include the number of years of membership in the specialty society, years practicing in the specialty, and professional recognition by peers.

Finding a Doctor

A common way to find a doctor who specializes in cancer care is to ask for a referral from your primary care physician. Sometimes, you may know a specialist yourself, or through the experience of a family member, co-worker, or friend.

The following resources may also be able to provide you with names of doctors who specialize in treating specific diseases or conditions. However, these resources may not have information about the quality of care that the doctors provide. Additional resource information is available at the end of this chapter.

- Your local hospital or its patient referral service may be able to provide you with a list of specialists who practice at that hospital.

- Your nearest National Cancer Institute (NCI)-designated cancer center can provide information about doctors who practice at that center.

- The American Board of Medical Specialties (ABMS) publishes a list of board-certified physicians. *The Official ABMS Directory of Board Certified Medical Specialists* lists doctors' names along with their specialty and their educational background. This resource is available in most public libraries.

- The American Medical Association (AMA) provides an online service called AMA Physician Select that offers basic professional information on virtually every licensed physician in the United States and its possessions. The database can be searched by doctor's name or by medical specialty. The AMA Physician Select service is located at http://www.ama-assn.org/aps/amahg.htm on the Internet.

- The American Society of Clinical Oncologists (ASCO) provides an online list of doctors who are members of ASCO. The member database has the names and affiliations of over 15,000 oncologists worldwide. It can be searched by doctor's name, institution's name, location, and/or type of board certification.

- The American College of Surgeons (ACOS) Fellowship Database is an online list of surgeons who are Fellows of the ACOS. The list can be searched by doctor's name, geographic location, or medical specialty.

- Local medical societies may maintain lists of doctors in each specialty.

- Public and medical libraries may have print directories of doctors' names, listed geographically by specialty.

- Your local Yellow Pages may have doctors listed by specialty under Physicians.

If you are a member of a health insurance plan, your choice may be limited to doctors who participate in your plan. Your insurance company can provide you with a list of participating primary care doctors and specialists. It is important to ask your insurance company if the doctor you choose is accepting new patients through your health plan. You also have the option of seeing a doctor outside your health plan and paying the costs yourself. If you have a choice of health insurance plans, you may first wish to consider which doctor or doctors you would like to use, then choose a plan that includes your chosen physician(s).

There are many factors to consider when choosing a doctor. To make the most informed decision, you may wish to speak with several doctors before choosing one. When you meet with each doctor, you might want to consider the following:

- Does the doctor have the education and training to meet my needs?

- Does the doctor use the hospital that I have chosen?

- Does the doctor listen to me and treat me with respect?

- Does the doctor explain things clearly and encourage me to ask questions?

- What are the doctor's office hours?

- Who covers for the doctor when he or she is unavailable? Will that person have access to my medical records?

- How long does it take to get an appointment with the doctor?

If you are choosing a surgeon, you may wish to ask additional questions about the surgeon's background and experience with specific procedures. These questions may include:

- Is the surgeon board-certified?

- Has the surgeon been evaluated by a national professional association of surgeons, such as the American College of Surgeons (ACOS)?

- At which treatment facility or facilities does the surgeon practice?

- How often does the surgeon perform the type of surgery I need?

- How many of these procedures has the surgeon performed? What was the success rate?

It is important for you to feel comfortable with the specialist that you choose, because you will be working closely with that person to make decisions about your cancer treatment. Trust your own observations and feelings when deciding on a doctor for your medical care.

Getting a Second Opinion

Once you receive your doctor's opinion about the diagnosis and treatment plan, you may want to get another doctor's advice before you begin treatment. This is known as getting a second opinion. You can do this by asking another specialist to review all of the materials related to your case. A second opinion can confirm or suggest modifications to your doctor's proposed treatment plan, provide reassurance that you have explored all of your options, and answer any questions you may have.

Getting a second opinion is very common, and most physicians welcome another doctor's opinion. In fact, your doctor may be able to recommend a specialist for this consultation. However, some people find it uncomfortable to request a second opinion. When discussing this issue with your doctor, it may be helpful to express satisfaction with your doctor's decision and care, and mention that you want your decision about treatment to be as thoroughly informed as possible. You may also wish to bring a family member along for support when asking for a second opinion. It is best to involve your doctor in the process of getting a second opinion, because your doctor will need to make all of your medical records (such as your test results and x-rays) available to the specialist.

Some health care plans require a second opinion, particularly if a doctor recommends surgery. Other health care plans will pay for a second opinion if the patient requests it. If your plan does not cover a second opinion, you can still obtain one if you are willing to cover the cost.

If your doctor is unable to recommend a specialist for a second opinion, or if you prefer to choose one on your own, the resources listed at the end of this chapter can help.

Finding a Treatment Facility (for Patients Living in the United States)

Choosing a treatment facility is another important consideration for getting the best medical care possible. Although you may not be able to choose which hospital treats you in an emergency, you can choose a facility for scheduled and ongoing care. If you have already found a doctor for your cancer treatment, you may need to choose a facility based on where your doctor practices. Your doctor may be able to recommend a facility that provides quality care to meet your needs. You may wish to ask the following questions when considering a treatment facility:

- Has the facility had experience and success in treating my condition?

- Has the facility been rated by state, consumer, or other groups for its quality of care?

- How does the facility check and work to improve its quality of care?

- Has the facility been approved by a nationally recognized accrediting body, such as the American College of Surgeons (ACOS) and/or the Joint Commission on Accredited Healthcare Organizations (JCAHO)?

- Does the facility explain patients' rights and responsibilities? Are copies of this information available to patients?

- Does the treatment facility offer support services, such as social workers and resources to help me find financial assistance if I need it?

- Is the facility conveniently located?

If you are a member of a health insurance plan, your choice of treatment facilities may be limited to those that participate in your plan. Your insurance company can provide you with a list of approved facilities. Although the costs of cancer treatment can be very high, you have the option of paying out-of-pocket if you want to use a treatment facility that is not covered by your insurance plan. If you are considering paying for treatment yourself, you may wish to discuss the potential costs with your doctor beforehand. You may also want to speak with the person who does the billing for the treatment facility. In some instances, nurses and social workers can provide you with more information about coverage, eligibility, and insurance issues.

The following resources may help you find a hospital or treatment facility for your care:

- The NCI fact sheet *The National Cancer Institute Cancer Centers Program* describes and gives contact information for NCI-designated cancer treatment centers around the country.

- The ACOS accredits cancer programs at hospitals and other treatment facilities. More than 1,400 programs in the United States have been designated by the ACOS as Approved Cancer Programs. The ACOS website offers a searchable database of these programs.

- The JCAHO is an independent, not-for-profit organization that evaluates and accredits health care organizations and programs in the United States. It also offers information for the general public about choosing a treatment facility. The JCAHO offers an online Quality Check service that patients can use to determine whether a specific facility has been accredited by the JCAHO and view the organization's performance reports.

- The Agency for Healthcare Research and Quality (AHRQ) publication *Your Guide To Choosing Quality Health Care* has suggestions and checklists for choosing the treatment facility that is right for you.

Additional Information

National Cancer Institute
NCI Public Inquiries Office
6166 Executive Boulevard, MSC 8322
Suite 3036A
Bethesda, MD 20892-8322
Toll-Free: 800-4-CANCER (800-422-6237)
Toll-Free TTY: 800-332-8615
Website: www.cancer.gov

The NCI fact sheet *The National Cancer Institute Cancer Centers Program* describes and gives contact information, including websites, for NCI-designated cancer treatment centers around the country. Many of the cancer centers' websites have searchable directories of physicians who practice at each facility.

Pediatric Oncology Branch
Center for Cancer Research, NCI
Toll-Free: 877-624-4878
Tel: 301-496-4256
Website: www.dcs.nci.nih.gov/branches/pedonc

The Pediatric Oncology Branch of NCI's Center for Cancer Research is dedicated to providing the best medical care possible to children, teenagers, and young adults with cancer or HIV disease. The Pediatric Oncology Branch offers a second opinion service to physicians, patients, and their families. To request a second opinion from the Pediatric Oncology Branch, you or your physician may call between 8:30 a.m. and 5:00 p.m., Eastern Time.

American Board of Medical Specialties (ABMS)
1007 Church St., Suite 404
Evanston, IL 60201-5913
Toll-Free: 866-ASK-ABMS (275-2267); Tel: 847-491-9091
Fax: 847-328-3596
Verification of Physician's Board Certification: 866-275-2267
Website: www.abms.org/which.asp

Information about other specialties that treat cancer is available from the American Board of Medical Specialties (ABMS) in a booklet called *Which Medical Specialist For You?* The ABMS also has a website that can be used to verify whether a specific physician is board-certified. This free service is located at www.abms.org/newsearch.asp on the Internet.

Cancer Care, Inc.
275 Seventh Avenue
New York, NY 10001
Toll-Free: 800-813-HOPE
Tel: 212-712-8080
Fax: 212-712-8495
Website: www.cancercare.org
E-mail: info@cancercare.org

Agency for Healthcare Research and Quality (AHRQ)
2101 E. Jefferson
Suite 501
Rockville, MD 20852
Toll-Free: 800-358-9295
Tel: 301-594-1364
Website: www.ahrq.gov/consumer/qntool.htm

AHRQ offers *Your Guide to Choosing Quality Health Care*, which has information for consumers on choosing a health plan, a doctor, a hospital, or a long-term care provider. The Guide includes suggestions and checklists that you can use to determine which doctor or hospital is best for you.

American College of Surgeons (ACOS)
633 North Saint Clair St.
Chicago, IL 60611-3211
Tel: 312–202–5000
Fax: 312-202-5001
Website: http://web.facs.org/cpm/default.htm
E-mail: postmaster@facs.org

The ACOS accredits cancer programs at hospitals and other treatment facilities. More than 1,400 programs in the United States have been designated by the ACOS as Approved Cancer Programs. The ACOS website offers a searchable database of these programs.

Joint Commission on Accredited Healthcare Organizations (JCAHO)
One Renaissance Blvd.
Oakbrook Terrace, IL 60181-4294
Tel: 630-792-5800
Fax: 630-792-5541
Website: www.jcaho.org
E-mail: customerservice@jcaho.org

The JCAHO offers an online Quality Check service that patients can use to determine whether a specific facility has been accredited by the JCAHO and view the organization's performance reports. This service is located at www.jcaho.org/qualitycheck/directry/directry.asp on the Internet.

R.A. Bloch Cancer Foundation, Inc.
4400 Main Street
Kansas, MO 64111
Toll-Free: 800-433-0464
Tel: 816-932-8453
Fax: 816-931-7486
Website: www.blochcancer.org/articles/xtrnew.asp

The R. A. Bloch Cancer Foundation, Inc., can refer cancer patients to institutions that are willing to provide multidisciplinary second opinions.

Chapter 8

Clinical Trials:
Questions and Answers

What Are Clinical Trials, and Why Are They Important?

Clinical trials are research studies conducted with people who volunteer to take part. Each study answers scientific questions and tries to find better ways to prevent, screen for, diagnose, or treat a disease. People who take part in cancer clinical trials have an opportunity to contribute to knowledge of and progress against cancer. They also receive up-to-date care from experts.

What Are the Types of Clinical Trials?

There are several types of clinical trials:

- **Prevention trials** study ways to reduce the risk, or chance, of developing cancer. Most prevention trials are conducted with healthy people who have not had cancer. Some trials are conducted with people who have had cancer and want to prevent the return of cancer (recurrence), or reduce the chance of developing a new type of cancer.

- **Screening trials** study ways to detect cancer. They are often conducted to determine whether finding cancer before it causes symptoms decreases the chance of dying from the disease. These trials involve people who do not have any symptoms of cancer.

"Clinical Trials: Questions and Answers," Fact Sheet 2.11, National Cancer Institute (NCI), reviewed: 07/03/2002.

- **Diagnostic trials** study tests or procedures that could be used to identify cancer more accurately and at an earlier stage. Diagnostic trials usually include people who have signs or symptoms of cancer.

- **Treatment trials** are conducted with people who have cancer. They are designed to answer specific questions about, and evaluate the effectiveness of, a new treatment or a new way of using a standard treatment. These trials test many types of treatments, such as new drugs, vaccines, new approaches to surgery or radiation therapy, or new combinations of treatments.

- **Supportive care (or quality of life) trials** explore ways to improve the comfort and quality of life of cancer patients and cancer survivors. These trials may study ways to help people who are experiencing nausea, vomiting, sleep disorders, depression, or other effects from cancer or its treatment.

- **Genetics studies** are sometimes part of another cancer clinical trial. The genetics component of the trial may focus on how genetic make-up can affect detection, diagnosis, or response to cancer treatment.

Population- and family-based genetic research studies differ from traditional cancer clinical trials. In these studies, researchers look at tissue or blood samples, generally from families or large groups of people, to find genetic changes that are associated with cancer. People who participate in genetics studies may or may not have cancer, depending on the study. The goal of these studies is to help understand the role of genes in the development of cancer.

Who Sponsors Clinical Trials?

Clinical trials are sponsored by private organizations and Government agencies that are seeking better treatments for cancer or better ways to prevent, screen, or diagnose cancer.

Drug and biotechnology companies sponsor trials of their products. They may conduct these trials in collaboration with universities, the NCI, and/or doctors in private practice.

The National Cancer Institute (NCI) sponsors many clinical trials through several programs, including the following:

- The Cancer Centers Program provides support for research-oriented institutions, including those that have been designated as NCI Comprehensive or Clinical Cancer Centers for their scientific excellence.

- The Clinical Trials Cooperative Group Program brings researchers, cancer centers, and doctors together into cooperative groups. These groups work with the NCI to identify important questions in cancer research, and design and conduct clinical trials to answer these questions. Cooperative groups are located throughout the United States and in Canada and Europe.

- The Cancer Trials Support Unit (CTSU) makes NCI-sponsored phase III treatment trials available to doctors and patients in the United States and Canada. Doctors who are not affiliated with an NCI-sponsored Clinical Trials Cooperative Group must complete an application and credentialing process to become members of the CTSU's National Network of Investigators. CTSU members can enroll patients in clinical trials through the program's website.

- The Community Clinical Oncology Program (CCOP) makes clinical trials available in a large number of communities across the United States. Local hospitals throughout the country affiliate with a cancer center or a cooperative group. This affiliation allows doctors to offer people participation in clinical trials more easily, so they do not have to travel long distances or leave their usual caregivers. The Minority-Based Community Clinical Oncology Program is a CCOP that focuses on encouraging minority populations to participate in clinical trials.

- The Warren Grant Magnuson Clinical Center is a research hospital located in Bethesda, Maryland, that is part of the National Institutes of Health (NIH). Trials at the Clinical Center are conducted by the components of the NIH, including the NCI.

How Are Participants Protected?

Research with people is conducted according to strict scientific and ethical principles. Every clinical trial has a protocol, or action plan, which acts like a recipe for conducting the trial. The plan describes what will be done in the study, how it will be conducted, and why each part of the study is necessary. The same protocol is used by every doctor or research center taking part in the trial. All federally funded clinical trials and trials to evaluate a new drug or medical device subject to Food and Drug Administration regulation must be reviewed and approved by an Institutional Review Board (IRB). Many institutions require that all clinical trials, regardless of funding, be reviewed and approved by a local IRB. The Board, which includes doctors, researchers, community leaders, and other members of the community, reviews the protocol to make sure the study is conducted fairly and participants are not likely to be harmed. The IRB also decides how often to review the trial once it has begun. Based on this information, the IRB decides whether the clinical trial should continue as initially planned and, if not, what changes should be made. An IRB can stop a clinical trial if the researcher is not following the protocol or if the trial appears to be causing unexpected harm to the participants. An IRB can also stop a clinical trial if there is clear evidence that the new intervention is effective, in order to make it widely available.

The NIH-supported phase I and II clinical trials must have a data and safety monitoring plan, and all phase III clinical trials must have a Data and Safety Monitoring Board (DSMB). The DSMB is an independent committee made up of statisticians, physicians, and other expert scientists. The DSMB ensures that the risks of participation are as small as possible, makes sure the data are complete, and stops a trial if safety concerns arise or when the trial's objectives have been met.

If the participants experience severe side effects, or there is other evidence that the risks outweigh the benefits, the IRB and DSMB will recommend that the trial be stopped early. A clinical trial might also be stopped if there is clear evidence that the new approach is effective—so the approach can be made widely available.

What Are Eligibility Criteria, and Why Are They Important?

Each study's protocol has guidelines for who can or cannot participate in the study. These guidelines, called eligibility criteria, describe characteristics that must be shared by all participants. The criteria differ from study to study. They may include age, gender, medical history, and current health status. Eligibility criteria for treatment studies often require that patients have a particular type and stage of cancer.

Enrolling participants with similar characteristics ensures that the results will be due to what is under study and not other factors. In this way, eligibility criteria help researchers achieve accurate and meaningful results. These criteria also make certain that people who could be made worse by participating in the study are not exposed to the risk.

What Is Informed Consent?

Informed consent is a process by which people learn the important facts about a clinical trial to help them decide whether to participate. This information includes details about what is involved, such as the purpose of the study, the tests and other procedures used in the study, and the possible risks and benefits. In addition to talking with the doctor or nurse, people receive a written consent form explaining the study. People who agree to take part in the study are asked to sign the informed consent form. However, signing the form does not mean people must stay in the study. People can leave the study at any time— either before the study starts or at any time during the study or the follow-up period.

The informed consent process continues throughout the study. If new benefits, risks, or side effects are discovered during the study, the researchers must inform the participants. They may be asked to sign new consent forms if they want to stay in the study.

Where Do Clinical Trials Take Place?

Clinical trials take place in doctors' offices, cancer centers, other medical centers, community hospitals and clinics, and veterans' and military hospitals in cities and towns across the United States and in other countries. Clinical trials may include participants at one or two highly specialized centers, or they may involve hundreds of locations at the same time.

How Are Clinical Trials Conducted?

Clinical trials are usually conducted in a series of steps, called phases. Treatment clinical trials listed in PDQ®, the NCI's cancer information database, are always assigned a phase. However, screening, prevention, diagnostic, and supportive care studies do not always have a phase. Genetics clinical trials generally do not have a phase.

- Phase I trials are the first step in testing a new approach in humans. In these studies, researchers evaluate what dose is safe, how a new agent should be given (by mouth, injected into a vein, or injected into the muscle), and how often. Researchers watch closely for any harmful side effects. Phase I trials usually enroll a small number of patients and take place at only a few locations. The patients are divided into smaller groups, called cohorts. Each cohort is treated with an increased dose of the new therapy or technique. The highest dose with an acceptable level of side effects is determined to be appropriate for further testing.

- Phase II trials study the safety and effectiveness of an agent or intervention, and evaluate how it affects the human body. Phase II studies usually focus on a particular type of cancer, and include fewer than 100 patients.

- Phase III trials compare a new agent or intervention (or new use of a standard one) with the current standard therapy. Participants are randomly assigned to the standard group or the new group, usually by computer. This method, called randomization, helps to avoid bias and ensures that human choices or other factors do not affect the study's results. In most cases, studies move into phase III testing only after they have shown promise in phases I and II. Phase III trials may include hundreds of people across the country.

- Phase IV trials are conducted to further evaluate the long-term safety and effectiveness of a treatment. They usually take place after the treatment has been approved for standard use. Several hundred to several thousand people may take part in a phase IV study. These studies are less common than phase I, II, or III trials.

People who participate in a clinical trial work with a research team. Team members may include doctors, nurses, social workers, dietitians, and other health professionals. The health care team provides care, monitors participants' health, and offers specific instructions about the study. So that the trial results are as reliable as possible, it is important for participants to follow the research team's instructions. The instructions may include keeping logs or answering questionnaires. The research team may continue to contact participants after the trial ends.

What Happens When a Clinical Trial Is Over?

After a clinical trial is completed, the researchers look carefully at the data collected during the trial before making decisions about the meaning of the findings and further testing. After a phase I or II trial, the researchers decide whether to move on to the next phase, or stop testing the agent or intervention because it was not safe or effective. When a phase III trial is completed, the researchers look at the data and decide whether the results have medical importance.

The results of clinical trials are often published in peer-reviewed, scientific journals. Peer review is a process by which experts review the report before it is published to make sure the analysis and conclusions are sound. If the results are particularly important, they may be featured by the media and discussed at scientific meetings and by patient advocacy groups before they are published. Once a new approach has been proven safe and effective in a clinical trial, it may become standard practice. (Standard practice is a currently accepted and widely used approach.)

People can locate the published results of a study by searching for the study's official name or Protocol ID number in the National Library of Medicine's PubMed® database.

What Are Some of the Benefits of Taking Part in a Clinical Trial?

The benefits of participating in a clinical trial include:

- Participants have access to promising new approaches that are often not available outside the clinical trial setting.

- The approach being studied may be more effective than the standard approach.

- Participants receive regular and careful medical attention from a research team that includes doctors and other health professionals.

- Participants may be the first to benefit from the new method under study.

- Results from the study may help others in the future.

What Are Some of the Possible Risks Associated with Taking Part in a Clinical Trial?

The possible risks of participating in a clinical trial include:

- New drugs or procedures under study are not always better than the standard care to which they are being compared.

- New treatments may have side effects or risks that doctors do not expect or that are worse than standard care.

- Participants in randomized trials will not be able to choose the approach they receive.

- Health insurance and managed care providers may not cover all patient care costs in a study.

- Participants may be required to make more visits to the doctor than they would if they were not in the clinical trial.

Who Pays for the Patient Care Costs Associated with a Clinical Trial?

Health insurance and managed care providers often do not cover the patient care costs associated with a clinical trial. What they cover varies by health plan and by study. Some health plans do not cover clinical trials if they consider the approach being studied experimental or investigational. However, if enough data show that the approach is safe and effective, a health plan may consider the approach established and cover some or all of the costs. Participants may have difficulty obtaining coverage for costs associated with prevention and screening clinical trials; health plans are currently less likely to have review processes in place for these studies. It may, therefore, be more difficult to get coverage for the costs associated with them. In many cases, it helps to have someone from the research team talk about coverage with representatives of the health plan.

Health plans may specify other criteria a trial must meet to be covered. The trial might have to be sponsored by a specified organization, be judged medically necessary by the health plan, not be significantly more expensive than treatments the health plan considers standard, or focus on types of cancer for which no standard treatments are available. In addition, the facility and medical staff might have to meet the plan's qualifications for conducting certain procedures, such as bone marrow transplants.

Many states have passed legislation or developed policies requiring health plans to cover the costs of certain clinical trials. Federal programs that help pay the costs of care in a clinical trial include:

- Medicare reimburses patient care costs for its beneficiaries who participate in clinical trials designed to diagnose or treat cancer.

- Beneficiaries of TRICARE, the Department of Defense's health program, can be reimbursed for the medical costs of participation in NCI-sponsored phase II and phase III cancer prevention (including screening and early detection) and treatment trials.

- The Department of Veterans Affairs (VA) allows eligible veterans to participate in NCI-sponsored prevention, diagnosis, and treatment studies nationwide. All phases and types of NCI-sponsored trials are included.

What Are Some Questions People Might Ask Their Health Care Provider before Entering a Clinical Trial?

It is important for people to ask questions before deciding to enter a clinical trial. Following are some questions people might want to ask their doctor or nurse.

The Study

- What is the purpose of the study?
- Why do the researchers think the approach being tested may be effective? Has it been tested before?
- Who is sponsoring the study?
- Who has reviewed and approved the study?
- What are the medical credentials and experience of the researchers and other study personnel?
- How are the study results and safety of participants being monitored?
- How long will the study last?
- How will the results be shared?

Possible Risks and Benefits

- What are the possible short-term benefits?
- What are the possible long-term benefits?
- What are the short-term risks, such as side effects?
- What are the possible long-term risks?
- What other treatment options are available?
- How do the possible risks and benefits of the trial compare with those of other options?

Participation and Care

- What kinds of treatment, medical tests, or procedures will the participants have during the study? How often will they receive the treatments, tests, or procedures?

- Will treatments, tests, or procedures be painful? If so, how can the pain be controlled?

- How do the tests in the study compare with what people might receive outside the study?

- Will participants be able to take their regular medications while in the clinical trial?

- Where will the participants receive their medical care? Will they be in a hospital? If so, for how long?

- Who will be in charge of the participants' care? Will they be able to see their own doctors?

- How long will participants need to stay in the study? Will there be follow-up visits after the study?

Personal Issues

- How could being in the study affect the participants' daily lives?

- What support is available for participants and their families?

- Can potential participants talk with people already enrolled in the study?

Cost Issues

- Will participants have to pay for any treatment, tests, or other charges? If so, what will the approximate charges be?

- What is health insurance likely to cover?

- Who can help answer questions from the insurance company or health plan?

Where Can People Find More Information about Clinical Trials?

People interested in taking part in a clinical trial should talk with their health care provider. Information about clinical trials is also available from the Cancer Information Service (CIS).

Additional Information

Cancer Trials Support Unit (CTSU)
CTSU Data Operations Center
1441 W. Montgomery Ave.
Rockville, MD 20850-2062
Toll-Free: 888-823-5923
Toll-Free Fax: 888-691-8039
Website: www.ctsu.org
E-mail: CTSUcontact@westat.com

Medicare
Toll-Free: 800-633-4227
Toll-Free TTY: 877-486-2048
Website: www.medicare.gov

National Library of Medicine
PubMed® database
Website: www.ncbi.nlm.nih.gov/PubMed

PubMed is an easy-to-use search tool for finding journal articles in the health and medical sciences.

National Cancer Institute Information
Cancer Information Service
6166 Executive Blvd. MSC 8322
Suite 3036A
Bethesda, MD 20892-8322
Toll-Free: 800-4-CANCER (800-422-6237)
Toll-Free TTY: 800-332-8615
Toll-Free Fax on Demand: 800-624-2511 (Follow the voice prompt instructions)
Fax: 301-402-5874
Website: www.cancer.gov
Clinical Trials Website: http://cancer.gov/clinicaltrials

NCI Fact Sheets:

- *More Choices in Cancer Care: Information for Beneficiaries on Medicare Coverage of Cancer Clinical Trials* is available at http://cis.nci.nih.gov/fact/8_14.htm

- *TRICARE Beneficiaries Can Enter Clinical Trials for Cancer Prevention and Treatment Through Department of Defense and*

National Cancer Institute Agreement available at http://cis.nci.nih.gov/fact/1_13.htm

- *NCI and VA Make It Easier for Veterans to Enter Studies, Get Advanced Care for Cancer* available at http://cis.nci.nih.gov/fact/1_17.htm

- *The National Cancer Institute Cancer Centers Program*, which is available at http://cis.nci.nih.gov/fact/1_2.htm

- *NCI's Clinical Trials Cooperative Group Program* available at http://cis.nci.nih.gov/fact/1_4.htm

- *Questions and Answers: Cancer Studies at the Warren Grant Magnuson Clinical Center* available at http://cis.nci.nih.gov/fact/1_22.htm

- NCI's State Initiatives and Legislation Digest Page available at http://cancer.gov/clinicaltrials/insurancelaws

Chapter 9

Moving Toward a New Understanding of Leukemia

This chapter includes excerpts from a speech given by Richard Klausner, MD, Director of the National Cancer Institute, before the Senate Subcommittee on Labor, Health and Human Services, Education, and Related Agencies about research on hematologic cancers.

Despite advances in diagnosis and treatment and improvements in patient survival, hematologic cancers continue to have a significant impact on the lives of Americans. Right now, almost 700,000 Americans arc living with leukemia, lymphoma, or myeloma (LLM), and an estimated 100,000 new cases occur each year. Although mortality has declined and 5-year survival rates have increased among adults and children with certain forms of these diseases, an estimated 60,000 Americans will die of them in 2001. For all forms of leukemia, the five-year survival rate is only 46%, for non-Hodgkin's lymphoma it is 54.2%, and for multiple myeloma it is only 28%. Despite the significant decline in the death rate for children with leukemia, this disease still causes more deaths in children in the U.S. than any other disease. Furthermore, the death rates for non-Hodgkin's lymphoma and multiple myeloma are increasing at a time when death rates for other cancers are dropping. Since the 1970s, incidence rates for non-Hodgkin's lymphoma have nearly doubled, although during the 1990s the rate of increase appeared to slow. Hematologic cancers strike individuals of all ages, from children to the elderly, men and women, and all races.

"Leukemia, Lymphoma, and Multiple Myeloma: Toward a New Understanding," National Cancer Institute (NCI), June 21, 2001.

What Are Leukemia, Lymphoma, and Multiple Myeloma?

To understand these diseases, we must first understand the normal development of the cells they affect. Hematopoiesis is the process by which blood cells form and mature. All the different types of blood cells arise in the bone marrow from a common pluripotent hematopoietic stem cell, and undergo a series of developmental steps to differentiate into mature cells and assume specific roles in the body. New, immature blood cells may stay in the marrow to mature or may travel to other parts of the body to mature. Normally, blood cells are produced in an orderly, controlled way, as the body needs them. Some circulate throughout our bodies via blood vessels and lymph vessels. Some reside in the lymphatic tissues that are primarily concentrated in lymph nodes, thymus, spleen, and in most of our major organ systems.

Leukemia, lymphoma, and multiple myeloma are all cancers of the blood-forming organs, or hematopoietic neoplasms. They arise due to errors in the genetic information of an immature blood cell. As a consequence of these errors, the cell's development is arrested so that it does not mature further, but is instead replicated over and over again, resulting in a proliferation of abnormal blood cells. Nearly every stage of the hematopoietic process can give rise to a distinct type of cancer.

Historically, scientists and physicians have classified these diseases by their locations in the body, the appearance of affected cells under the microscope, and the natural progression of the diseases. In leukemia, the cancerous cells are discovered circulating in the blood and bone marrow, while in lymphoma, the cells tend to aggregate and form masses, or tumors, in lymphatic tissues. Myeloma is a tumor of the bone marrow, and involves a specific subset of white blood cells that produce a distinctive protein.

Leukemia can arise in either of two main groups of white blood cell types—lymphocytes or myelocytes. Either type of leukemia can be acute, a rapidly progressing form of the disease in which the affected cells are very immature and unable to serve their proper purpose, or chronic, which progresses more slowly and is distinguished by cells that are relatively well differentiated but still function poorly.

Leukemias, lymphomas, and myelomas share some common features, but there are major differences among them—and there are similarities and differences within each disease group. These cancers actually represent a large number of diseases that vary significantly in their causes, molecular profiles, and natural progression. In the past decade we have a experienced a revolution in the field of molecular biology that has brought new tools that are helping us refine cancer classification in terms of the molecular changes that distinguish a normal cell from a cancerous one, and draw differences between cancerous cells of different types.

Moving Toward a New Understanding of LLM

A major NCI initiative, the Cancer Genome Anatomy Project (CGAP), has resulted in the cataloging of tens of thousands of human and mouse genes. The CGAP database is a unique resource that allows scientists to develop tools to perform large-scale genomic analyses to characterize tumors genetically. This genetic characterization can help explain why patients diagnosed with the same cancer differ dramatically in their responses to treatment. For example, a collaboration of scientists (including NCI scientists) genetically analyzed diffuse large B-cell lymphoma, an aggressive cancer that is the most common type of non-Hodgkin's lymphoma. For 40 percent of patients with this diagnosis, standard multi-agent chemotherapy is curative. A compelling clinical problem is to understand why the remaining 60 percent of patients succumb to this disease despite chemotherapy. Reasoning that the varying therapeutic responses of patients with diffuse large B-cell lymphoma are due to undefined molecular differences in their tumors, researchers used DNA microarray technology to define the gene expression profiles of diffuse large B-cell lymphoma samples on a genomic scale. This new technology is capable of measuring the activity of tens of thousands of genes at the same time, thus creating a molecular portrait of the cells being studied.

This powerful new technology is now being used to study many different types of cancers, including leukemia and multiple myeloma, in an attempt to identify disease subgroups. For example, a new project, "Molecular Taxonomy of Pediatric and Adult Acute Leukemia," will attempt to correlate the expression pattern of over 30,000 genes with treatment outcome and with cytogenetic abnormalities for both acute lymphocytic leukemia and acute myeloid leukemia. In the future, such gene expression profiling of cancer cells will be used to guide patients towards therapies that are tailored for their particular diseases.

Causes, Risk Factors, and Epidemiology of LLM

Our understanding of the causes of these diseases is extremely limited, perhaps in part due to extreme heterogeneity of the diseases and the inadequacy of the traditional classification schemes to adequately address this heterogeneity. As our knowledge base about molecular subtypes grows, we hope that we will be better able to understand the relationships between causative factors and the development of LLM.

Leukemia

The leukemias are very heterogeneous, with patterns of occurrence differing by age, sex, and racial and ethnic group. For example, highest incidence of acute lymphoblastic leukemia (ALL) is in children, ages 2-4, while chronic lymphocytic leukemia (CLL) is rare before age 30, and has the highest incidence among the elderly. Chronic myeloid leukemia (CML) has a higher incidence among African-Americans than Caucasians, while the incidence of CLL is highest among Caucasians and extremely rare in Asians.

The causes of leukemia in children and adults are largely unknown, but increased or decreased risks for developing leukemia have been associated with several factors. In an ongoing, collaborative follow-up study with Japanese investigators, NCI scientists have found strong evidence of radiation-induced risks for the acute leukemias and CML among Japanese atomic bomb survivors. NCI investigators and others have shown that radiotherapy and chemotherapy for a wide variety of diseases have been linked with moderately increased risks of acute myeloid leukemia (AML), although the benefits of treatment far outweigh the risks.

Occupational exposures to ionizing radiation and certain chemicals such as benzene have also been linked with increased risk of acute leukemia. NCI is conducting an epidemiologic study of workers in China exposed to benzene at levels lower than previously studied, to characterize leukemia rates and to determine mechanisms of action and factors affecting carcinogenicity of benzene. In addition, cigarette smoking has been associated with modest increases in acute leukemia, but the evidence is not yet conclusive.

The first known human retrovirus, T-lymphotropic virus type 1 (HTLV-1), discovered at NCI in 1981, is the primary cause of adult leukemia and lymphoma arising from lymphocytes known as T cells. Certain genetic conditions can increase the risk for acute leukemia, including Li-Fraumeni syndrome, Down's syndrome, Bloom's syndrome, and several other rare conditions.

New Strategies for Treatment of LLM

Therapeutic research in the treatment of patients with hematologic malignancies has made enormous progress over the past 50 years, and the NCI has shepherded this important work. Many years ago, NCI established the National Service Center to enable basic scientists to design and test chemical agents for evidence of anti-tumor activity. In addition to pioneering cancer drug screening, the NCI funded an entire pre-clinical drug discovery and development program. The NCI has continuously supported investigators to pursue all phases of clinical evaluation of products emanating from their own discovery and developmental efforts, and interacts with the pharmaceutical industry and academic institutions to explore their novel agents.

In the last decade, there has been an enormous investment in defining molecularly targeted agents in cancer chemotherapy. Recently we have seen some inspiring success stories, all of them direct results of this new approach. The first evidence of a consistent gene mutation associated with a particular cancer was provided about 40 years ago by the recognition of the Philadelphia chromosome, an abnormally small chromosome 22, in chronic myeloid leukemia (CML). Some years later, researchers noted that while chromosome 22 was shortened, chromosome 9 was lengthened in CML patients, which suggested that the pieces of each chromosome were exchanged, or translocated. This observation was followed by the identification of a unique fusion gene, called bcr-abl, resulting from the translocation, and the eventual development 5 years ago of one of the first oncogene-targeted drugs, STI571 or Gleevec™. This compound, which was recently approved by the United States Food and Drug Administration (FDA), is directed at the bcr-abl gene product, which is expressed in about 95% of CML patients, and in some patients with other types of cancers. Gleevec™ has shown remarkable promise in the treatment of chronic-phase CML, and NCI is partnering with Novartis, the drug manufacturer, to facilitate a profusion of clinical trials evaluating Gleevec™ in other cancers, including Philadelphia chromosome-positive ALL in adults and children. Additional trials are assessing the potential benefits of combining Gleevec™ with other chemotherapeutic agents. Molecular analyses of other types of leukemia have now produced the identification of more than 100 additional oncogene targets that may be accessible to similar drug development strategies.

In addition, NCI-sponsored studies are evaluating several new antibodies. Generally, leukemias, lymphomas, and multiple myelomas are derived from cells of the immune system and therefore frequently express antigens that are present on normal immune cells such as B-cells or T-cells. Since these proteins are not present on other human cells and are not present on the stem cells that give rise to normal

B-cells and the T-cells, the antigens are excellent targets for cancer therapy. NCI researchers have devised a cancer treatment strategy that kills cells containing B-cell or T-cell specific antigens. When this occurs the normal cells are regenerated, but the cancer cells are not. One strategy is to fuse the portions of antibodies that bind to CD22 (a B-cell antigen) or CD25 (a T-cell antigen) to a potent bacterial toxin termed Pseudomonas exotoxin A. The genetically modified toxin then specifically binds to and kills cells expressing CD22 or CD25. Since many lymphomas and leukemias express CD22 or CD25, these tumor cells are killed.

A promising ongoing NCI study is using this approach to combat B-cell malignancies. The antigen CD22 is expressed on about 70% of lymphomas and leukemias. A recombinant immunotoxin termed BL22 has been designed and produced to kill tumor cells expressing CD22, and patients with hairy cell leukemia, chronic lymphocytic leukemia (CLL), and some lymphomas have been treated in a Phase I trial. Remarkable anti-tumor activity has been observed in patients with hairy cell leukemia. Several patients with CLL have responded as well. Enrollment into this trial is continuing, and once the maximum tolerated dose is established, Phase II trials in hairy cell leukemia, CLL, and lymphomas (in a post-transplant setting) will be opened for enrollment.

Other antibodies under investigation are coupled to other potent anti-tumor substances, like radioactive molecules or anti-tumor antibiotics, and have the potential advantage of being able to deliver this tumor killing substance directly to the tumor site, where they attack antigen-positive tumor cells that other therapeutic agents might not penetrate well.

Anti-cancer vaccines are a high priority research area for NCI. Unlike conventional vaccines, which are used to prevent illness, the anti-cancer vaccines represent a therapeutic approach, which seeks to strengthen the body's natural defenses against diseases, such as cancer, that have already developed.

The NCI is involved in the development of a large number of new therapeutic agents with a wide array of unique mechanisms of action. We now know that cancer arises from the disruption of fundamental cell processes. Basic research findings have identified a plethora of potential therapeutic targets for further exploitation. There is an ever-lengthening list of promising agents that affect cell cycle regulation, gene expression, apoptosis (programmed cell death), and other cell functions, currently undergoing or awaiting investigation in clinical trials.

A striking example of the benefit of this kind of molecularly targeted therapy is all-trans retinoic acid (ATRA) for the treatment of acute promyelocytic leukemia (APL). ATRA works essentially by reversing the effects of a specific chromosomal translocation that disables both differentiation and apoptotic processes in affected cells. The introduction of this agent has increased the cure rate for APL from 40 percent to over 70 percent in just 10 years. Some patients who have been treated successfully with ATRA experience relapse, and recently, arsenicals, a group of rediscovered compounds that induce apoptosis via a different, more broadly applicable mechanism, have shown great utility as a second line of defense against APL. Arsenic trioxide is now being evaluated for use in a variety of lymphoid malignancies, as well as other cancers, and for use in childhood APL, and also for use as a first line treatment.

Bone marrow transplantation and peripheral blood stem cell transplantation techniques continue to be tested in clinical trials for certain LLM patients. Sometimes cancers become resistant to treatment with radiation therapy or chemotherapy. Very high doses of chemotherapy may then be used to treat the cancer. Because the high doses of chemotherapy can destroy the bone marrow, marrow is taken from the bones before treatment. The marrow is then frozen, and the patient is given high-dose chemotherapy with or without radiation therapy to treat the cancer. The marrow is then thawed and given back to the patient to replace the marrow that was destroyed. This type of transplant is called an autologous transplant. If the marrow is taken from another person, the transplant is called an allogeneic transplant. Another type of autologous transplant is called a peripheral blood stem cell transplant. The patient's circulating stem cells are collected, treated with drugs to kill any cancer cells, and frozen until they are returned to the patient. This procedure may be done alone or with an autologous bone marrow transplant.

The role of stem cell transplantation in caring for patients with LLM varies with tumor type. Autologous stem cell transplantation clearly benefits patients in a chemotherapy-sensitive relapse of their disease, but its role as initial treatment is undefined. A national trial is comparing the efficacy of initial transplantation with transplantation at the time of first relapse. Other studies are evaluating the role of biological therapies such as interleukin-2, immune response stimulator, and rituximab for their effectiveness in enhancing the benefit of transplantation.

Many patients do not benefit from stem cell transplantation, and major efforts are directed at identifying the reasons and to develop methods to improve on these results. Some investigators are developing methods to harness patients' own immune responses. Alternatively, other researchers are using a technique called donor leukocyte infusion (DLI) that introduces T cells capable of generating a graft-versus-tumor effect (in which the donor cells attack the patient's cancerous cells). However, they are also capable of generating a potent graft-versus-host disease (GVHD, in which the donor cells attack the healthy tissues of the patient) that could be fatal to the patient. Studies of the array of T cells that are present post DLI are being conducted to better understand which T cell populations are necessary to achieve the desired result while minimizing GVHD.

Allogeneic bone marrow transplant may cure patients who do not respond to standard chemotherapy, but the mortality of this procedure in patients with LLM has been very high. Moreover, age restrictions limit the number of patients who might be eligible for this procedure. There has now been an expanded information base on the use, for non-Hodgkin's lymphoma, of non-myeloablative transplants (in which the bone marrow is not completely destroyed) with DLI. Recently, investigators have described their experience with patients over the age of 55 years. GVHD occurred less frequently than expected and many patients were able to go through the procedure without requiring hospitalization. As a consequence, the notion that more intensive treatment is better is being challenged, and the role of the immune system in cancer progression is being better delineated.

The NCI sponsors the International Bone Marrow Transplant Registry, which is the world's largest body of data on outcomes following transplantation for LLM and other cancers. Data are provided from more than 400 centers and there are now data for more than 65,000 transplants worldwide. The information collected is used for determining transplant regimens for specific clinical situations, identifying prognostic factors, comparing transplant regimens, comparing transplant with non-transplant approaches, evaluating cost and cost-effectiveness, planning clinical trials, and developing approaches to evaluate outcomes.

Clinical trials for LLM treatment have demonstrated remarkable success and are a vital component of the NCI's research program. Currently, our clinical trials database contains descriptions of 177 NCI-sponsored leukemia treatment trials, 170 for lymphoma, and 67 for multiple myeloma. Our clinical trials program is the place where promising new strategies discovered at the laboratory bench are applied to real human problems at the bedside. Clinical trials offer cancer patients access to state-of-the-art care, and provide us the opportunity to learn something from every patient that may help someone else. Our rapid pace of discovery in the basic biology of cancer is refining our knowledge of how to intervene in cancer development, and clinical trials are the crucial final step in bringing these discoveries to people who are battling cancer.

Conclusion

Progress in our understanding of cancer and our ability to detect and treat it have led to a real and continuing decline in the cancer incidence and death rates. However, our excitement over important scientific progress and the very real human gains that result is tempered by the knowledge that far too many Americans continue to suffer and die from cancer each day. Moreover, all groups of people are not benefiting equally from our advances against cancer. NCI is embracing the challenge of understanding the causes of health disparities in cancer and developing effective interventions to reduce them. Plans call for increasing fundamental research into the social causes of health disparities, the psychosocial factors that mediate them, and the biologic pathways that can explain their impact. In addition, we will expand our cancer control intervention and population research on disparities, better define and monitor cancer-related health disparities, and strengthen training and education in this research area. Effective communication empowers people to make informed cancer-related decisions and to engage in behaviors that will improve their health. Few other initiatives have the potential to simultaneously improve health outcomes, decrease health care costs, and enhance community satisfaction. Our intent is to learn how to help people distinguish important from insignificant health risks and deal with contradictory or inaccurate health messages so they can make informed choices.

Too many Americans, for a host of reasons, lack access to high quality, cutting-edge cancer treatment and care. NCI is launching research to improve the quality of cancer care by strengthening the information base for cancer care decision-making. Researchers seek to better understand what constitutes quality cancer care, with an emphasis on the patient's perspective; identify geographic, racial/ ethnic, and other disparities in who receives quality care; and strengthen the scientific basis for selecting appropriate interventions. Our goal is to enhance the state of the science for defining, monitoring, and improving the quality of cancer care and inform Federal decision making on cancer care delivery, coverage, and regulation.

Chapter 10

How to Find Resources in Your Own Community If You Have Leukemia

If you have cancer or are undergoing cancer treatment, there are places in your community to turn to for help. There are many local organizations throughout the country that offer a variety of practical and support services to people with cancer. However, people often don't know about these services or are unable to find them. National cancer organizations can assist you in finding these resources, and there are a number of things you can do for yourself.

Whether you are looking for a support group, counseling, advice, financial assistance, transportation to and from treatment, or information about cancer, most neighborhood organizations, local health care providers, or area hospitals are a good place to start. Often, the hardest part of looking for help is knowing the right questions to ask.

What Kind of Help Can I Get?

Until now, you probably never thought about the many issues and difficulties that arise with a diagnosis of cancer. There are support services to help you deal with almost any type of problem that might occur. The first step in finding the help you need is finding what types of services are available. The following pages describe some of these services and how to find them.

"How to Find Resources in Your Own Community If You Have Cancer," Fact Sheet 8.9, National Cancer Institute (NCI), reviewed 12/18/2000.

Information on Cancer

Most national cancer organizations provide a range of information services, including materials on different types of cancer, treatments, and treatment-related issues.

Counseling

While some people are reluctant to seek counseling, studies show that having someone to talk to reduces stress and helps people both mentally and physically. Counseling can also provide emotional support to cancer patients and help them better understand their illness. Different types of counseling include individual, group, family, self-help (sometimes called peer counseling), bereavement, patient-to-patient, and sexuality.

Medical Treatment Decisions

Often, people with cancer need to make complicated medical decisions. Many organizations provide hospital and physician referrals for second opinions and information on clinical trials (research studies with people), which may expand treatment options.

Prevention and Early Detection

While cancer prevention may never be 100 percent effective, many things (such as quitting smoking and eating healthy foods) can greatly reduce a person's risk for developing cancer. Prevention services usually focus on smoking cessation and nutrition. Early detection services, which are designed to detect cancer when a person has no symptoms of disease, can include referrals for screening mammograms, Pap tests, or prostate exams.

Home Health Care

Home health care assists patients who no longer need to stay in a hospital or nursing home, but still require professional medical help. Skilled nursing care, physical therapy, social work services, and nutrition counseling are all available at home.

Hospice Care

Hospice is care focused on the special needs of terminally ill cancer patients. Sometimes called palliative care, it centers around providing comfort, controlling physical symptoms, and giving emotional support to patients who can no longer benefit from curative treatment. Hospice programs provide services in various settings, including the patient's home, hospice centers, hospitals, or skilled nursing facilities. Your doctor or social worker can provide a referral for these services.

Rehabilitation

Rehabilitation services help people adjust to the effects of cancer and its treatment. Physical rehabilitation focuses on recovery from the physical effects of surgery or the side effects associated with chemotherapy. Occupational or vocational therapy helps people readjust to everyday routines, get back to work, or find employment.

Advocacy

Advocacy is a general term that refers to promoting or protecting the rights and interests of a certain group, such as cancer patients. Advocacy groups may offer services to assist with legal, ethical, medical, employment, legislative, or insurance issues, among others. For instance, if you feel your insurance company has not handled your claim fairly, you may want to advocate for a review of its decision.

Financial

Having cancer can be a tremendous financial burden to cancer patients and their families. There are programs sponsored by the Government and nonprofit organizations to help cancer patients with problems related to medical billing, insurance coverage, and reimbursement issues. There are also sources for financial assistance, and ways to get help collecting entitlements from Medicaid, Medicare, and the Social Security Administration.

Housing/Lodging

Some organizations provide lodging for the family of a patient undergoing treatment, especially if it is a child who is ill and the parents are required to accompany the child to treatment.

Children's Services

A number of organizations provide services for children with cancer, including summer camps, make-a-wish programs, and help for parents seeking child care.

How to Find These Services

Often, the services that people with cancer are looking for are right in their own neighborhood or city. The following is a list of places where you can begin your search for help.

- The hospital, clinic, or medical center where you see your doctor, received your diagnosis, or where you undergo treatment should be able to give you information. Your doctor or nurse may be able to tell you about your specific medical condition, pain management, rehabilitation services, home nursing, or hospice care.

- Most hospitals also have a social work, home care, or discharge planning department. This department may be able to help you find a support group, a nonprofit agency that helps people who have cancer, or the government agencies that oversee Social Security, Medicare, and Medicaid. While you are undergoing treatment, be sure to ask the hospital about transportation, practical assistance, or even temporary childcare. Talk to a hospital financial counselor in the business office about developing a monthly payment plan if you need help with hospital expenses.

- The public library is an excellent source of information, as are patient libraries at many cancer centers. A librarian can help you find books and articles through a literature search.

- A local church, synagogue, YMCA or YWCA, or fraternal order may provide financial assistance, or may have volunteers who can help with transportation and home care. Catholic Charities, the United Way, or the American Red Cross may also operate local offices. Some of these organizations may provide home care, and the United Way's information and referral service can refer you to an agency that provides financial help. To find the United Way serving your community, visit their online directory at http://www.unitedway.org on the Internet or look in the White Pages of your local telephone book.

- Local or county government agencies may offer low-cost transportation (sometimes called para-transit) to individuals unable to use public transportation. Most states also have an Area Agency on Aging that offers low-cost services to people over 60. Your hospital or community social worker can direct you to government agencies for entitlements, including Social Security, state disability, Medicaid, income maintenance, and food stamps. (Keep in mind that most applications to entitlement programs take some time to process.) The Federal government also runs the Hill-Burton program (800-638-0742), which funds certain medical facilities and hospitals to provide cancer patients with free or low-cost care if they are in financial need.

Getting the Most from a Service: What to Ask

No matter what type of help you are looking for, the only way to find resources to fit your needs is to ask the right questions. When you are calling an organization for information, it is important to think about what questions you are going to ask before you call. Many people find it helpful to write out their questions in advance, and to take notes during the call. Another good tip is to ask the name of the person with whom you are speaking in case you have follow-up questions. Below are some of the questions you may want to consider if you are calling or visiting a new agency and want to learn about how they can help:

- How do I apply [for this service]?
- Are there eligibility requirements? What are they?
- Is there an application process? How long will it take? What information will I need to complete the application process? Will I need anything else to get the service?
- Do you have any other suggestions or ideas about where I can find help?

The most important thing to remember is that you will rarely receive help unless you ask for it. In fact, asking can be the hardest part of getting help. Don't be afraid or ashamed to ask for assistance. Cancer is a very difficult disease, but there are people and services that can ease your burdens and help you focus on your treatment and recovery.

Additional Information

Cancer Care, Inc.
275 Seventh Avenue
New York, NY 1001
Toll-Free: 800-813-HOPE (4673)
Tel: 212-712-8080
Fax: 212-712-8495
Website: www.cancercare.org
E-mail: info@cancercare.org

The National Cancer Institute and Cancer Care, Inc., are in partnership to increase awareness of the psychosocial issues faced by cancer patients and to provide resources to cancer patients and their families.

National Cancer Institute Information
Cancer Information Service
6166 Executive Blvd., MSC 8322
Suite 3036A
Bethesda, MD 20892-8322
Toll-free: 800-4-CANCER (800-422-6237)
Toll-Free TTY: 800-332-8615
Website: www.cancer.gov

Chapter 11

Financial Issues for People with Cancer

Chapter Contents

Section 11.1

Ways to Advocate for Yourself or Someone Else Who Has Cancer

This first part of this section is from "Non-Medical Expenses Related to Cancer," © 5/18/2002 American Society of Clinical Oncology (ASCO), www.asco.org for more information, reprinted with permission; and the remaining text in this section is from "Ways to Advocate for Yourself or Someone Else Who Has Cancer: Health Insurance and Financial Issues," © 2001 Cancer Care, Inc., www.cancercare.org for more information, reprinted with permission.

Be Aware of Non-Medical Expenses Related to Cancer

The financial impact of cancer extends beyond doctor visits and treatment-related costs. These additional expenses can become a great financial burden if you don't seek help from the start.

The non-medical costs associated with cancer can be divided into six basic categories:

- **Clinic visits** which include costs for meals, child or elder care, and transportation to and from treatments and appointments.

- **Symptoms and side effects** including medication, equipment, supplies, clothing, and accessories (wigs, comfortable clothing, and special foods). Not all drugs are covered by insurance, and many patients try a variety of over-the-counter medications in an effort to relieve treatment side effects.

- **Support or assistance** including childcare, housekeeping, and meals ordered out due to fatigue.

- **Administrative costs** such as increases in telephone bills and insurance premiums.

- **Counseling, supportive therapies, special gifts, vacations, and other quality of life items.** When some people are very ill, they do things they normally wouldn't have done, including buying things to make them feel better. These expenses should be considered costs related to being seriously ill.

- **Lost income**, whether through taking time off work for treatment, or losing one's job altogether because of illness.

Advocating Health Insurance and Financial Issues for People with Cancer

Today, the health care system in our country is undergoing dramatic changes. While some people still have their care covered by private insurance, the majority of people are now covered by managed care, which usually involves getting medical services from a health maintenance organization, or HMO. Learning about what choices you have, what types of insurance exist, what your rights are, and what to do if you are not insured, will help you be a more effective advocate in this arena.

Choosing an Insurance Plan

If you or someone you love has cancer, it is especially important for you to understand how your insurance plan actually works. If you are purchasing insurance/health care on your own, or are considering whether to join under a coverage offered by an employer, you should definitely shop around to find the best fit for your particular needs. If you now have a regular doctor and/or oncologist, it is probably a good idea to ask what managed care plans they belong to, or which ones they recommend.

If you are considering a new plan, or are now covered, make sure the plan provides at least most of these services:

- Access to high quality cancer screening and other diagnostic tests;

- In-network access to board-certified oncologists, oncology nurses, oncology social workers, and experts in cancer pain;

- Other forms of supplemental care such as home care, prescription drugs, rehabilitative services, prosthetic devices, and durable medical equipment;

- Timely referral for treatments such as radiation and chemotherapy;

- Access to state-of-the-art cancer treatments such as off-label drug usage, effective symptom management, and clinical trials; and

- Palliative (supportive) care and/or hospice care.

Types of Insurance

The two main types of insurance now available are HMO/managed care plans, and fee-for-service (or indemnity) plans. This section includes some basic information on both, and on a few other, less common types of plans.

HMO/Managed Care

An HMO/Managed Care plan is a type of health care plan created in an effort to lower health care costs both for the consumer (you) and whoever helps you pay (your employer or the government). If you join an HMO or managed care plan, you get health care services at a very low cost, far less than if you went to a doctor and paid for it yourself. As a consumer of health care, this works in your favor. HMOs and other forms of managed care can offer some very real advantages to you, depending on your medical condition. However, they are far from perfect, and there are disadvantages, too. Most often, HMOs and other managed care plans require that you use only doctors and care providers that are part of their plan. If your regular doctor is part of that plan, you have no problem. If not, you may be required to find a new doctor, who can act as your primary care physician.

Fee-for-Service, or Indemnity Plans

Fee-for-service (or indemnity) policies are what people think of as the traditional type of insurance. These plans pay doctors and hospitals for services you receive, or reimburse you for services you have paid for. Fee-for-service plans have two parts: a basic policy, that covers minimum expenses, and a major medical policy, which provides coverage where your basic leaves off (for instance, if you are hospitalized). These types of policies have a deductible—an amount that you have to pay yourself before they will begin paying for anything—and a lifetime maximum benefit, or cap. Once you have met your deductible, they will usually pay 75%-80% of what they consider usual, reasonable, and customary, and you pay the rest.

Other Types of Insurance

There are also other types of financial planning vehicles and insurance that may assist you depending on your situation. These include catastrophic medical insurance, medical savings accounts, disability insurance, insurance for long-term care such as in a nursing home, and supplemental Medicare insurance.

Medicare and Medicaid

There are also two health insurance plans paid for by the government, Medicare and Medicaid. Medicare is health insurance paid by the federal government and funded through the Social Security program. You are eligible for Medicare if you meet any of the following criteria:

- 65 years or older and entitled to Social Security, Widow's, or Railroad Retirement benefits

- Totally disabled and collecting social security, regardless of age

- Legally blind

- On renal dialysis, regardless of age

Medicare is now being administered mostly through a system of managed care. There are also new health reforms that continually update the coverage you get under Medicare.

Medicaid is a health insurance program that is funded jointly by the federal and state governments. On the federal level, it is administered through Centers for Medicare and Medicaid Services. On the state level, it is administered through the Department of Social Services, Department of Public Welfare or equivalent. In order to be eligible for Medicaid, you must meet certain income requirements. These vary from state to state. If you have Medicare, you also can have Medicaid to supplement your Medicare policy. To determine if you are eligible for any of these benefits, you must apply through your local department of social services.

What to Do If You Aren't Insured or Are about to Lose Your Insurance

If you aren't insured through Medicare or Medicaid, and are not able to get insurance through an employer, finding health insurance for yourself and/or your dependents can be difficult. The good news is that many states have now passed laws helping individuals to purchase health insurance when they have been blocked from getting it due to preexisting conditions (like cancer).

Check with your state insurance department to find out all of your options.

Other Options

- If you have been covered under the Consolidated Omnibus Budget Reconciliation Act (COBRA), check to see if there is an individual conversion clause, which would allow you to convert the plan to an individual policy when the COBRA period ends. While this would allow you to remain covered, the cost can be very high, and the converted policy may provide fewer benefits than the group policy. Make certain to ask about the coverage carefully, and follow all the rules for conversion properly.

- Some states have *high-risk pools*, meaning they require one or several insurance companies to provide a special type of insurance for those people who cannot get coverage elsewhere. Although the premiums for these types of plans are almost always higher, most states have a maximum that the insurance companies can charge. There may also be a waiting period for a preexisting condition such as cancer, meaning some of your bills may not immediately be paid.

- Some states have laws that require insurance companies to have open enrollment periods. During these periods, individuals can purchase health insurance regardless of their health status or claims history. These laws vary from state to state. Check with your state insurance department.

- Sometimes professional societies, religious organizations, and/or credit card companies will let you join their group insurance coverage plan. Check your local area organizations to find out if such programs exist.

- If you are unable to get insurance, and need medications and/or chemotherapy, you can check to see if the pharmaceutical company that makes the drug you are taking has a patient assistance program. Often companies will provide the drug for you if you cannot afford it. Your doctor will have to request the drug, but you can get the application forms and information.

- If you are disabled due to your cancer (and are unable to maintain employment), you may be eligible for Social Security Disability (SSD). After two years on SSD you are eligible for Medicare benefits. If you are determined under Social Security to have been disabled at the time of a termination of employment or reduction in hours of employment and you notify the plan administrator of this disability determination, the 18-month period of your COBRA is expanded to 29 months. This expansion of benefits will cover you until Medicare coverage begins. Applying for and/or receiving disability does not mean you can never work again. In fact, you are encouraged to return to work if you can and Social Security Disability allows for this.

- If you have not paid enough money into the Social Security system and are disabled, you may be eligible for Supplemental Security Income (SSI). The application you file with Social Security for disability will determine eligibility for this program. If you are approved for SSI then you will be insured through Medicaid.

- If you are unable to pay your hospital bills, check to see if the hospital you are being treated at is eligible for Hill-Burton funds. The Hill-Burton Free Medical Care Program provides free or reduced cost medical services through obligated facilities to those persons who are uninsured or underinsured and meet eligibility criteria.

What Rights Do You Have Regarding Health Insurance?

Unfortunately, there is no federal law that guarantees health care insurance to people in the United States. Under our system, your rights for getting and keeping health care coverage depend on one or all of the following:

- federal laws that help protect certain rights
- state insurance laws (which regulate insurance sales)
- the terms of your specific insurance policy

Federal Laws

Currently, while there are no federal laws that guarantee you can get insurance, there are two laws that afford you some protection in keeping your health insurance if you already have it. If you lose or change jobs, you may be eligible for continued coverage under the first of these two laws, commonly referred to as COBRA.

COBRA does the following:

- Requires employers with more than 20 employees to offer group medical coverage to employees and their dependents that have lost or changed their jobs.
- Allows for 18 months coverage of employee, 36 months for spouse and dependents.

- Requires coverage to be offered, regardless of preexisting condition.

- Offers special rules for disabled individuals that may extend the maximum periods of coverage. If you are determined under Social Security to have been disabled at the time of a termination of employment or reduction in hours of employment and you notify the plan administrator of this disability determination, the 18-month period is expanded to 29 months. For details about COBRA, talk to your department of human resources.

The second important federal law is one that was recently enacted, called the **Health Insurance Portability and Accountability Act (HIPAA)** and known as the Kennedy-Kassebaum Act.

HIPAA does the following:

- Limits who can be excluded for preexisting conditions;

- Forbids discrimination against employees and dependents based on their health status;

- Guarantees availability and renewal of health coverage to certain employers and individuals;

- Protects many workers who would otherwise lose health coverage by providing better access to individual health insurance coverage.

Because HIPPA is very recent, it is difficult to gauge the impact it will have. One benefit is that it was designed to alleviate job lock. Often, people with cancer and other illnesses have felt forced to stay in an unsatisfying job in order to maintain their health benefits. HIPPA allows you to take your benefits with you to another job (called portability). It also requires most plans to renew your coverage regardless of any illness that may occur.

However, it is not a cure-all for insurance problems for people with cancer. It does not require all employers to provide health insurance, and it has no provision for cost containment, meaning you can be charged a high amount for coverage.

State Insurance Laws

State insurance laws generally help regulate the companies that sell insurance in each state; however, they vary dramatically. You will have to do some of your own homework to find out what the laws are for your state. For example, some states have passed comprehensive laws that regulate managed care companies, as New York did with its Managed Care Bill of Rights. To find out which laws are active in your state, contact your state insurance department.

The Terms of Your Own Insurance Policy

The terms of your particular insurance policy spell out the details of your benefits. It is important that you try to read and understand those benefits, particularly if you are trying to appeal any claims that have been denied. Your health insurance policy is a contract between you and the insurance company. Since medical care is very complex, there are times when something may not be covered in your plan. However, you may be able to appeal and get it paid for. Also, managed care plans sometimes deny benefits for treatments that your doctor has prescribed. Often, you can turn these decisions around. Although it takes some energy, it can be worth fighting for coverage. Don't take the first, or even the second *no* for an answer!

Appealing Claims That Have Been Denied

If you have been turned down for coverage for a medical procedure, or your insurance company has informed you that they do not intend to reimburse you for something you require medically, don't be afraid to appeal that decision. Sometimes a claim is denied for a simple reason, like information was missing from the claim form. As they say, the squeaky wheel gets the grease.

Included are some helpful hints if you find yourself in a situation where you are fighting for a treatment to be covered. In the meantime, if you have decided that you want to appeal a claim, you should take the following steps:

- Read your entire insurance contract. This can be obtained from your employer or the insurance company. Make copies of the sections that apply to your situation and send them with your appeal.

- Follow the appeal guidelines for your insurance closely. You do not want a bureaucratic snag to harm your appeal.

- Record the name of anyone you speak to along with the date, and ask them to send a confirmation in writing. A phone conversation on an unknown day with a no-name person is probably of no use. Your plan's customer service line is the place to start. However, be aware that the customer representative probably does not have the power to change the situation. Ask for a supervisor if you are not satisfied with their response. Record notes about the call, including quotes from what they say. Ask whom to send a letter to, and write up your grievance after the initial phone conversation in a letter and send it as a follow-up step.

- Keep thorough records. Make photocopies of everything you send your insurance company.

- Get a second medical opinion about the procedure in question. Your insurance may pay for this. If you are enrolled in an HMO, however, it is often better to go outside the network in order to get an objective opinion about the treatment in question. This second opinion (which should be in writing) may be crucial, especially when trying to get the insurance company to pay for a costly or experimental treatment.

- Get help from your doctor. Your doctor can also be helpful in advocating for a treatment or service for you. On the other hand, if your doctor is part of a managed care plan and disagrees with you, you may want to consider first changing doctors within the plan itself, or going outside the plan as mentioned above.

- Ask your doctor to write a letter of support for your treatment and explain what you want the letter to say. A letter like this should state: why the doctor believes that the treatment is necessary, why there are no reasonable alternatives, and what the outcome would be if you do not receive the prescribed treatment. Ask your doctor to attach medical articles supporting the treatment.

- Look for help from others. Your employer can sometimes advocate for you with the managed care plan, or perhaps reimburse for uncovered expenses.

- Establishing a friendly relationship with one representative within the managed care plan can often help you get a quicker response. If you find someone who is helpful, get a full name and extension. Try to talk with that person each time you call.

- Your hospital may also have someone on staff that helps facilitate insurance claims. Check with the insurance department or hospital social worker.

- Get the specifics about what action the managed care plan will take and when it will happen. What is the time frame in which a response should be forthcoming?

- Call your state insurance department and elected representatives. Each state has a department of insurance that can help. Many states have enacted legislation around managed care issues that affords you some protection. In addition, some elected officials might take up your cause. Sometimes all you need to do is let the HMO representative know your intentions to seek outside help. Be sure to copy all letters sent to your insurer.

- To find out about the state insurance department in your state, go to the Health Insurance Association of America website.

- If all else fails, get legal help. Lawyers can be very powerful advocates. If you have been put off once or twice after carefully following the appeals process, find an attorney who specializes in insurance. Contact your local city or state bar associations.

- Organizations that advocate for your particular diagnosis may provide support.

- Whatever your level of frustration, remember: don't change insurance plans without having somewhere else to get coverage. Be careful not to cancel your plan until you have been approved by a new insurance company, HMO, or other managed care plan. Also, be sure to investigate how a new policy handles pre-existing conditions such as cancer. Health care reform has made it easier to change plans with the Health Insurance Portability and Accountability Act (HIPAA).

Websites about Insurance and Managed Care

The Alliance of Community Health Plans
Website: www.achp.org

A website designed to provide information about ACHP member plans. ACHP is a national alliance (formerly known as the HMO Group) of 26 not-for-profit and provider based health plans serving 7 million Americans in 27 states.

Blood and Bone Marrow Transplant Newsletter/Insurance Help Form
Website: www.bmtnews.org/attorney.html

The BMT Newsletter will help you locate an attorney to help you pursue denial of claims for blood and bone marrow transplants.

Centers for Medicare & Medicaid Services (CMS)
Website: www.cms.hhs.gov

In addition to information on Medicare and Medicaid, information is available on child health care initiatives and reforms.

National Committee for Quality Assurance
Website: www.ncqa.org

Has interesting and useful information about rating managed care plans and determining quality. Lists plans and their ratings, and provides a search mechanism by plan, city, and state.

Health Insurance Association of America (HIAA)
Website: www.hiaa.org

A trade organization that provides useful consumer information on health insurance issues.

U.S. Department of Labor Employee Benefits Security Administration
Website: www.dol.gov/ebsa/welcome.html

The website offers information on benefits such as COBRA, consumer information on saving for retirement and pension plans.

Patient Access Coalition
Website: http://home.patientaccess.com/pac

The Patient Access Coalition is a group of 130 national patient and medical service provider organizations dedicated to ensuring that the focus of health care be on patients and the quality of their medical care. The website contains information about specialty care and insurance coverage.

Families USA
Website: www.familiesusa.org

Families USA, a national nonprofit organization, advocates high quality, affordable health and long-term care for all Americans. Their website posts reports and analyses of health insurance issues and provides education to the public, opinion leaders, and policymakers about problems consumers experience in the health care marketplace and what should be done to solve them.

Section 11.2

Clinical Trials and Insurance Coverage

"Clinical Trials and Insurance Coverage–A Resource Guide: Basics," National Cancer Institute (NCI), updated: 01/30/2002; and "Clinical Trials and Insurance Coverage–A Resource Guide: Strategies," National Cancer Institute (NCI), updated: 01/30/2002.

What Costs Do Trials Involve, and Who Is Usually Responsible for Paying Them?

There are two types of costs associated with a trial: patient care costs and research costs.

Patient care costs fall into two categories:

- *Usual care costs*, such as doctor visits, hospital stays, clinical laboratory tests, x-rays, etc., which occur whether you are participating in a trial or receiving standard treatment. These costs have usually been covered by a third-party health plan, such as Medicare or private insurance.

- *Extra care costs* associated with clinical trial participation, such as the additional tests that may or may not be fully covered by the clinical trial sponsor and/or research institution. The sponsor and the participant's health plan need to resolve coverage of these costs for particular trials.

Research costs are those associated with conducting the trial, such as data collection and management, research physician and nurse time, analysis of results, and tests purely performed for research purposes. Such costs are usually covered by the sponsoring organization, such as NCI or a pharmaceutical company.

What Criteria Do Health Plans Use to Make Decisions about Reimbursement for Trials?

Health insurance companies and managed care companies decide which health care services they will pay for by developing coverage policy regarding the specific services. In general, the most important factor determining whether something is covered is a health plan's judgment as to whether the service is established or investigational. Health plans usually designate a service as established if there is a certain amount of scientific data to show that it is safe and effective. If the health plan does not think that such data exist in sufficient quantity, the plan may label the service as investigational.

Health care services delivered within the setting of a clinical trial are very often categorized as investigational and not covered. This is because the health plan thinks that the major reason to perform the clinical trial is that there is not enough data to establish the safety and effectiveness of the service being studied. Thus, for some health plans, any mention of the fact that the patient is involved in a clinical trial results in a denial of payment.

Your health plan may define specific criteria that a trial must meet before extending coverage, such as:

- *Sponsorship*: Some plans may only cover costs of trials sponsored by organizations whose review and oversight of the trial is careful and scientifically rigorous, according to standards set by the health plan.

- *Trial phase and type*: Some plans may cover patient care costs only for the clinical trials they judge to be *medically necessary* on a case-by-case basis. Trial phase may also affect coverage; for example, while a plan may be willing to cover costs associated with Phase III trials, which include treatments that have already been successful with a certain number of people, the plan may require some documentation of effectiveness before covering a Phase I or II trial. While health plans are interested in efforts to improve prevention and screening, they currently seem less likely to have a review process in place for these trials. Therefore, it may be more difficult to get coverage for the care costs associated with them.

Some plans, especially smaller ones, will not cover any costs associated with a clinical trial. Policies vary widely, but in most cases your best bet is to have your doctor initiate discussions with the health plan.

- *Cost neutrality*: Some health plans may limit coverage to trials they consider cost-neutral (i.e., not significantly more expensive than the treatments considered standard).

- *Lack of standard therapy*: Some plans limit coverage of trials to situations in which no standard therapy is available.

- *Facility and personnel qualifications*: A health plan may require that the facility and medical staff meet specific qualifications to conduct a trial involving unique services, especially intensive therapy such as a bone marrow transplant (high-dose chemotherapy with bone marrow/stem cell rescue).

Medicare Coverage

For up-to-date information about Medicare coverage of clinical trials, go to the website for the Centers for Medicare and Medicaid (formerly the Health Care Financing Administration).

If I Am in a Clinical Trial, What Will Medicare Pay?

- Anything normally covered is still covered when it is part of a clinical trial. This includes tests, procedures, and doctor visits that are ordinarily covered.

- Anything normally covered even if it is a service or item associated with the experimental treatment. For example, Medicare will pay for the intravenous administration of a new chemotherapy drug being tested in a trial, including any therapy to prevent side effects from the new drug.

- Anything normally covered even if it resulted from your being in the clinical trial. For example, a test or hospitalization resulting from a side effect of the new treatment that Medicare would ordinarily cover.

What Costs Are Not Covered?

- Investigational items or services being tested in a trial. Sponsors of clinical trials often provide the new drug free, but make sure you ask your doctor before you begin.

- Items or services used solely for the data collection needs of the trial.

- Anything being provided free by the sponsor of the trial.

What Kinds of Clinical Trials Are Covered?

Generally, Medicare covers cancer treatment and diagnosis trials if:

- They are funded by the National Cancer Institute (NCI), NCI-Designated Cancer Centers, NCI-Sponsored Clinical Trials

105

Cooperative Groups, and all other Federal agencies that fund cancer research. Other trials may be eligible for coverage and doctors can ask Medicare to pay the patients' costs. Ask your doctor about this before you begin.

- They are designed to treat or diagnose your cancer.

- The purpose or subject of the trial is within a Medicare benefit category. For example, cancer diagnosis and treatment are Medicare benefits, so these trials are covered. Cancer prevention trials are not currently covered.

What Can I Do to Increase the Likelihood of Coverage?

There are several steps you can follow to deal with coverage issues up front when deciding to enter a clinical trial. Along the way, enlist the help of family members and your doctor or other health professionals. You may find the following checklist useful:

- *Understand the costs associated with the trial.* Ask your doctor or the trial's contact person about the costs that must be covered by you or your health plan. Are these costs significantly higher than those associated with standard care? Also, inquire about the experience of other patients in the trial. Have their plans paid for their care? Have there been any persistent problems with coverage? How often have the trial administrators been successful in getting plans to cover patient care costs?

- *Understand your health plan.* Be sure you know what's in your policy; request and carefully review the actual contract language. If there's a specific exclusion for *experimental treatment*, look closely at the policy to see how the plan defines such treatment and under what conditions it might be covered. If it is not clearly defined, call the plan's customer service line, consult their website, and/or write to them. Ask for specific information about clinical trials coverage.

- *Work closely with your doctor.* Talk with your doctor about the paperwork he or she submits to your health plan. If there have been problems with coverage in the past, you might ask your doctor or the hospital to send an information package to the plan that includes studies supporting the procedure's safety, benefits, and medical appropriateness. This package might include:

106

- publications from peer-reviewed literature about the proposed therapy that demonstrate patient benefits;

- a letter that uses the insurance contract's own language to explain why the treatment, screening method, or preventive measure should be covered;

- letters from researchers that explain the clinical trial;

- support letters from patient advocacy groups.

Be sure to keep your own copy of any materials that the doctor sends to your health plan for future reference.

- *Work closely with your company's benefits manager.* This person may be helpful in enlisting the support of your employer to request coverage by the health plan.

- *Give your health plan a deadline.* Ask the hospital or cancer center to set a target date for the therapy. This will help to ensure that coverage decisions are made promptly.

- *Take advantage of all information resources available to you.*

What If My Claim Is Denied after I Begin Participating in a Trial?

If a claim is denied, read your policy to find out what steps you can follow to make an appeal. In *What Cancer Survivors Need to Know about Health Insurance*, the National Coalition for Cancer Survivorship suggests that you and your doctor demonstrate to the health plan that:

- the therapy is not just a research study, but also a valid procedure that benefits patients;

- your situation is similar to that of other patients who are participating in clinical trials as part of a covered benefit;

- possible complications have been anticipated and can be handled effectively.

You also may wish to contact your state insurance counseling hotline or insurance department for more help, or write your state insurance commissioner describing the problem.

Where Else Can I Turn for Assistance?

It's never easy to deal with financial issues when you or a loved one faces cancer. Unfortunately, costs can present a significant barrier to clinical trials participation.

The range of insurance issues and health plan contracts makes it impossible to deal with all of them here.

Additional Information

National Coalition of Cancer Survivorship
1010 Wayne Avenue, Suite 770
Silver Spring, MD 20910
Tel: 301-650-9127
Fax: 301-565-9670
Website: www.canceradvocacy.org
E-mail: info@cansearch.org

Publishes *What Cancer Survivors Need to Know about Health Insurance.*

The Association of Community Cancer Centers
11600 Nebel Street, Suite 201
Rockville, MD 20852
Tel: 301-984-9496
Fax: 301-770-1949
Website: www.accc-cancer.org/main2001.shtml

Publishes *Cancer Treatments Your Insurance Should Cover.*

Patient Advocate Foundation
700 Thimble Shoals Blvd., Suite 200
Newport News, VA 23608
Toll-Free: 800-532-5274
Fax: 757-873-8999
Website: www.patientadvocate.org
E-mail: help@patientadvocate.org

Publishes *The Managed Care Answer Guide.*

Part Two

Childhood Leukemia

Chapter 12

Childhood Acute Lymphoblastic Leukemia

Disease Information Overview

Definition

Acute lymphoblastic leukemia (ALL), also referred to as acute lymphocytic leukemia and acute lymphoid leukemia, is the most common form of childhood cancer. It affects lymphocytes, a type of white blood cells. Leukemic cells accumulate in the bone marrow, replace normal blood cells, and spread to other organs including liver, spleen, lymph nodes, central nervous system, kidneys, and gonads.

Incidence

In the United States, about 3,000 children each year are found to have ALL. Peak incidence occurs from 3 to 5 years of age.

This chapter begins with text from "Acute Lymphoblastic Leukemia," © 2002 St. Jude Children's Research Hospital, reprinted with permission; text following "What Is Childhood Acute Lymphoblastic Leukemia?" is from PDQ® Cancer Information Summary, National Cancer Institute; Bethesda, MD, "Childhood Acute Lymphoblastic Leukemia (PDQ®): Treatment–Patient," updated 06/2002, available at: http://cancer.gov., accessed 03/31/03; and text following "Statistics, Risk Factors, and Survival," is excerpted from PDQ® Cancer Information Summary, National Cancer Institute; Bethesda, MD; "Childhood Acute Lymphoblastic Leukemia (PDQ®): Treatment–Health Professional," updated 09/2002, available at: http://cancer.gov, accessed 03/31/03.

Treatment Strategies

Chemotherapy is used to kill leukemia cells. All chemotherapy is stopped after two to three years of treatment. Hematopoietic stem cell transplantation is an option for very high-risk cases (e.g., Philadelphia chromosome-positive ALL) or those who develop an early relapse in the bone marrow.

Survival Rates

About 99 percent of children with newly diagnosed ALL attain initial complete remissions (absence of detectable leukemic cells by microscopic examination) in four to six weeks. About 80 percent of children may be cured. If a child does not have a relapse within three years after therapy is stopped, the likelihood of cure is excellent.

Influencing Factors

ALL affects slightly more boys than girls. It occurs more frequently among whites than blacks. Although siblings of leukemic children have a slightly higher risk of developing the disease, the incidence is relatively low (no more than one in 500).

Current Research

- Research aims to improve treatment outcome by optimizing dosage and scheduling of antileukemic agents based on the individual patient's leukemic cell genetic features and host normal cell pharmacogenomic characteristics.

- Molecular genetic abnormalities and the measurement of the level of minimal residual leukemia after remission induction therapy are used to help direct the type of treatment. Research on the profile of gene expression in leukemia cells using microarray technology and bioinformatics is providing new insights to the genomics of leukemia and the effects of treatment; this research may lead to unique molecular targets for developing new therapies that are more specific and effective. Pharmacogenomic studies are providing new insights to inherited differences in drug response and molecular diagnostics to further individualize treatment.

- Methods are under study to improve the efficacy and safety of stem cell transplantation and to increase the pool of donors.

What Is Childhood Acute Lymphoblastic Leukemia?

Childhood acute lymphoblastic leukemia (also called acute lympho-cytic leukemia or ALL) is a disease in which too many underdevel-oped infection-fighting white blood cells, called lymphocytes, are found in a child's blood and bone marrow. ALL is the most common form of leukemia in children, and the most common kind of childhood can-cer.

Lymphocytes are made by the bone marrow and by other organs of the lymph system. The bone marrow is the spongy tissue inside the large bones in the body. The bone marrow makes red blood cells (which carry oxygen and other materials to all tissues of the body), white blood cells (which fight infection), and platelets (which make the blood clot). Normally, the bone marrow makes cells called blasts that de-velop (mature) into several different types of blood cells that have specific jobs to do in the body.

The lymph system is made up of thin tubes that branch, like blood vessels, into all parts of the body. Lymph vessels carry lymph, a col-orless, watery fluid that contains lymphocytes. Along the network of vessels are groups of small, bean-shaped organs called lymph nodes. Clusters of lymph nodes are found in the underarm, pelvis, neck, and abdomen. The spleen (an organ in the upper abdomen that makes lymphocytes and filters old blood cells from the blood), the thymus (a small organ beneath the breastbone), and the tonsils (an organ in the throat) are also part of the lymph system.

Lymphocytes fight infection by making substances called anti-bodies, which attack germs and other harmful bacteria in the body. In ALL, the developing lymphocytes become too numerous and do not mature. These immature lymphocytes are then found in the blood and the bone marrow. They also collect in the lymph tissues and make them swell. Lymphocytes may crowd out other blood cells in the blood and bone marrow. If your child's bone marrow cannot make enough red blood cells to carry oxygen, your child may have anemia. If your child's bone marrow cannot make enough platelets to make the blood clot normally, your child may bleed or bruise easily. The cancerous lymphocytes can also invade other organs, the spinal cord, and the brain.

Leukemia can be acute (progressing quickly with many immature cancer cells) or chronic (progressing slowly with more mature-looking leukemia cells). Acute lymphoblastic leukemia progresses quickly, and can occur in both children and adults. Treatment is different for adults than it is for children.

113

Early signs of ALL may be similar to those of the flu or other common diseases, such as a fever that won't go away, feeling weak or tired all the time, aching bones or joints, or swollen lymph nodes. If your child has symptoms of leukemia, his or her doctor may order blood tests to count the number of each of the different kinds of blood cells. If the results of the blood tests are not normal, a bone marrow biopsy may be performed. During this test, a needle is inserted into a bone in the hip and a small amount of bone marrow is removed and examined under the microscope, enabling the doctor to determine what kind of leukemia your child has and plan the best treatment.

Your child's doctor may also do a spinal tap, in which a needle is inserted through the back to remove a sample of the fluid that surrounds the brain and spine. The fluid is then examined under a microscope to see if leukemia cells are present.

Your child's chance of recovery (prognosis) depends on your child's age at diagnosis, the number of white blood cells in the blood (the white blood cell count) at diagnosis, how far the disease has spread, the biologic characteristics of the leukemia cells, and how well the leukemia cells respond to treatment.

Stages of Childhood Acute Lymphoblastic Leukemia

There is no staging for childhood acute lymphoblastic leukemia. The treatment depends on age, the results of laboratory tests, and whether or not the patient has been previously treated for leukemia.

Untreated

Untreated acute lymphoblastic leukemia (ALL) means that no treatment has been given except to reduce symptoms. There are too many white blood cells in the blood and bone marrow, and there may be other signs and symptoms of leukemia.

In Remission

Remission means that treatment has been given and the number of white blood cells and other blood cells in the blood and bone marrow is normal. There are no signs or symptoms of leukemia.

Recurrent/Refractory

Recurrent disease means that the leukemia has come back (recurred) after going into remission. Refractory disease means that the leukemia failed to go into remission following treatment.

Treatment Option Overview

There are treatments for all patients with childhood acute lympho-blastic leukemia (ALL). The primary treatment for ALL is chemo-therapy. Radiation therapy may be used in certain cases. Bone marrow transplantation is being studied in clinical trials.

Chemotherapy uses drugs to kill cancer cells. Chemotherapy drugs may be taken by mouth, or may be put into the body by a needle in a vein or muscle. Chemotherapy is called a systemic treatment because the drug enters the blood stream, travels through the body, and can kill cancer cells throughout the body. For ALL, chemotherapy drugs may sometimes be injected (usually through the spine) into the fluid that surrounds the brain and spinal cord; this is known as in-trathecal chemotherapy.

Radiation therapy uses x-rays or other high-energy rays to kill cancer cells and shrink tumors. Radiation for ALL usually comes from a machine outside the body (external beam radiation therapy).

Bone marrow transplantation is a newer type of treatment. First, high doses of chemotherapy with or without radiation therapy are given to destroy all of the bone marrow in the body. Healthy marrow is then taken from another person (a donor) whose tissue is the same as or al-most the same as the patient's. The donor may be a twin (the best match), a brother or sister, or another person not related to the patient. The healthy marrow from the donor is given to the patient through a needle in a vein, and the marrow replaces the marrow that was destroyed. A bone marrow transplant using marrow from a relative or person not re-lated to the patient is called an allogeneic bone marrow transplant.

An even newer type of bone marrow transplant, called autologous bone marrow transplant, is being studied in clinical trials. During this procedure, bone marrow is taken from the patient and may be treated with drugs to kill any cancer cells. The marrow is frozen to save it. The patient is then given high-dose chemotherapy with or without radiation therapy to destroy all of the remaining marrow. The frozen marrow that was saved is thawed and given through a needle in a vein to replace the marrow that was destroyed.

Phases of Treatment

There are generally 4 phases of treatment for ALL. The first phase, remission induction therapy, uses chemotherapy to kill as many of the leukemia cells as possible to cause the cancer to go into remission.

The second phase, called central nervous system (CNS) prophylaxis, is preventive therapy using intrathecal and/or high-dose systemic chemotherapy to the CNS to kill any leukemia cells present there, or to prevent the spread of cancer cells to the brain and spinal cord even if no cancer has been detected there. Radiation therapy to the brain may also be given, in addition to chemotherapy, for this purpose. CNS prophylaxis is often given in conjunction with consolidation/intensification therapy.

Once a child goes into remission and there are no signs of leukemia, a third phase of treatment called consolidation or intensification therapy, is given. Consolidation therapy uses high-dose chemotherapy to attempt to kill any remaining leukemia cells. The fourth phase of treatment, called maintenance therapy, uses chemotherapy for several years to maintain the remission.

Treatment by Stage

Treatment for childhood acute lymphoblastic leukemia depends on the prognostic group to which your child is assigned based primarily on your child's age and white blood cell count at diagnosis.

Your child may receive treatment that is considered standard based on its effectiveness in a number of patients in past studies, or you may choose to have your child take part in a clinical trial. Not all patients are cured with standard therapy and some standard treatments may have more side effects than are desired. For these reasons, clinical trials are designed to test new treatments and to find better ways to treat cancer patients. Clinical trials are ongoing in most parts of the country for most stages of childhood ALL.

Untreated Childhood Acute Lymphoblastic Leukemia

Your child's treatment will probably be remission induction chemotherapy to kill cancer cells and cause the leukemia to go into remission. Induction chemotherapy is almost always successful in inducing remission. Intrathecal and/or high-dose systemic chemotherapy, with or without radiation therapy to the brain, may also be given to prevent the spread of cancer cells to the brain and spinal cord. Clinical trials are testing new ways of inducing remission.

Childhood Acute Lymphoblastic Leukemia in Remission

Your child's treatment will probably be intensive chemotherapy to kill any remaining cancer cells. Intrathecal and/or high doses of systemic chemotherapy, with or without radiation therapy to the brain, may also be given during this phase of treatment to prevent the spread of cancer cells to the brain and spinal cord. Following intensification therapy, chemotherapy generally continues until the child has been in continuous remission for several years.

Recurrent Childhood Acute Lymphoblastic Leukemia

Treatment depends on the type of treatment your child received before, how soon the cancer came back following treatment, and whether the leukemia cells are found outside the bone marrow. Your child's treatment will probably be systemic or intrathecal chemotherapy, radiation therapy, or bone marrow transplantation. You may want to consider entering your child into a clinical trial of new chemotherapy drugs or bone marrow transplantation.

Statistics, Risk Factors, and Survival

Cancer in children and adolescents is rare. Children and adolescents with cancer should be referred to medical centers that have a multidisciplinary team of cancer specialists with experience treating the cancers that occur during childhood and adolescence. This multidisciplinary team incorporates the skills of the primary care physician, pediatric surgical subspecialists, radiation oncologists, pediatric medical oncologists/hematologists, rehabilitation specialists, pediatric nurse specialists, social workers, and others in order to ensure that children receive treatment, supportive care, and rehabilitation that will achieve optimal survival and quality of life. Guidelines for pediatric cancer centers and their role in the treatment of pediatric patients with cancer have been outlined by the American Academy of Pediatrics.[1] Since treatment of children with ALL entails many potential complications and requires aggressive supportive care (transfusions; management of infectious complications; and emotional, financial, and developmental support), this treatment is best coordinated by pediatric oncologists and performed in cancer centers or hospitals with all of the necessary pediatric supportive care facilities. Specialized care is essential for all children with ALL, including those in whom specific clinical and laboratory features might confer a favorable prognosis. At the same time, it is equally important that the clinical centers and the specialists directing the patient's care maintain contact with the referring physician in the community. Strong lines of communication optimize any urgent or interim care required when the child is at home.

ALL is the most common cancer occurring in children, representing 23% of cancer diagnoses among children younger than 15 years of age and occurring at an annual rate of approximately 31 per million.[2] There are approximately 2,400 children and adolescents younger than 20 years of age diagnosed with ALL each year in the United States.[3] There is a sharp peak in ALL incidence among children ages 2 to 3 years (greater than 80 per million per year), with rates decreasing to 20 per million for ages 8 to 10 years. The incidence of ALL among children ages 2 to 3 years is approximately four-fold greater than that for infants and is nearly 10-fold greater than that for children who are 19 years old. For unexplained reasons, the incidence of ALL is substantially higher for white children than for black children, with a nearly three-fold higher incidence at 2 to 3 years of age for white children compared to black children.[3]

There are few identified factors associated with increased risk of ALL.[3] The primary accepted nongenetic risk factors for ALL are prenatal exposure to x-rays and postnatal exposure to high doses of radiation (e.g., therapeutic radiation as previously used for conditions such as tinea capitis and thymus enlargement).[4] Children with Down syndrome have increased risk for developing both ALL and acute myeloid leukemia,[5] with a cumulative risk for developing leukemia of approximately 2.1% by aged 5 years and 2.7% by aged 30 years.[6] Approximately two-thirds of the cases of acute leukemia in children with Down syndrome are ALL.[6] Increased occurrence of ALL is also associated with certain genetic conditions, including neurofibromatosis,[7] Shwachman syndrome,[8,9] Bloom syndrome,[10] and ataxia telangiectasia.[11]

Seventy-five percent to 80% of children with ALL survive at least 5 years from diagnosis with current treatments that incorporate systemic therapy (e.g., combination chemotherapy) and specific central nervous system (CNS) preventive therapy (i.e., intrathecal chemotherapy with or without cranial irradiation).[2,3,12,13] Ten-year event-free survival of multiple large prospective trials conducted in different countries for children treated primarily in the 1980s is approximately 70%.[14-20] Since nearly all children with ALL achieve an initial remission, the major obstacle to cure is bone marrow and/or extramedullary (e.g., CNS, testicular) relapse. Relapse from remission can occur during therapy or after completion of treatment. While the majority of children with recurrent ALL attain a second remission, the likelihood of cure is generally poor, particularly for those with bone marrow relapse following a short initial remission duration.[21]

Lymphoblasts from a particular patient carry antigen receptors unique to that patient. There is evidence to suggest that the specific antigen receptor may be present at birth in some patients with ALL, suggesting a prenatal origin for the leukemic clone. Similarly, some patients with ALL characterized by specific translocations have been shown to have cells showing the translocation at the time of birth.[22,23]

Despite the treatment advances noted in childhood ALL, numerous important biologic and therapeutic questions remain to be answered in order to achieve the goal of curing every child with ALL. The systematic investigation of these issues requires large clinical trials, and the opportunity to participate in these trials is offered to most patients/families. Clinical trials for children and adolescents with ALL are generally designed to compare potentially better therapy with therapy that is currently accepted as standard. Much of the progress made in identifying curative therapies for childhood ALL and other childhood cancers has been achieved through clinical trials.[24,25]

References

1. Sanders J, Glader B, Cairo M, et al.: Guidelines for the pediatric cancer center and role of such centers in diagnosis and treatment. American Academy of Pediatrics Section Statement Section on Hematology/Oncology. *Pediatrics* 99(1): 139-141, 1997.

2. Ries LA, Kosary CL, Hankey BF, et al., eds.: *SEER Cancer Statistics Review, 1973-1996*. Bethesda, Md: National Cancer Institute, 1999. Also available at: http://seer.cancer.gov/csr/1973_1996. Accessed April 25, 2002.

3. Smith MA, Ries LA, Gurney JG, et al.: Leukemia. In: Ries LA, Smith MA, Gurney JG, et al., eds.: *Cancer Incidence and Survival Among Children and Adolescents: United* States SEER Program 1975-1995. Bethesda, Md: National Cancer Institute, SEER Program, NIH Pub. No. 99-4649, 1999, pp 17-34.

4. Ross JA, Davies SM, Potter JD, et al.: Epidemiology of childhood leukemia, with a focus on infants. *Epidemiologic Reviews* 16(2): 243-272, 1994.

5. Avet-Loiseau H, Mechinaud F, Harousseau L: Clonal hematologic disorders in Down syndrome. *Journal of Pediatric Hematology/Oncology* 17(1): 19-24, 1995.

6. Hasle H, Clemmensen H, Mikkelsen M: Risks of leukemia and solid tumours in individuals with Down's syndrome. *Lancet* 355(9199): 165-169, 2000.

7. Stiller CA, Chessells JM, Fitchett M: Neurofibromatosis and childhood leukaemia/lymphoma: a population-based UKCCSG study. *British Journal of Cancer* 70(5): 969-972, 1994.

8. Strevens MJ, Lilleyman JS, Williams RB: Shwachman's syndrome and acute lymphoblastic leukaemia. *British Medical Journal* 2(6129): 18, 1978.

9. Woods WG, Roloff JS, Lukens JN, et al.: The occurrence of leukemia in patients with the Shwachman syndrome. *The Journal of Pediatrics* 99(3): 425-428, 1981.

10. Passarge E: Bloom's syndrome: the German experience. *Annales de Genetique* 34(3-4): 179-197, 1991.

11. Taylor AM, Metcalfe JA, Thick J, et al.: Leukemia and lymphoma in ataxia telangiectasia. *Blood* 87(2): 423-438, 1996.

12. Pui CH, Evans WE: Acute lymphoblastic leukemia. *New England Journal of Medicine* 339(9): 605-615, 1998.

13. Pui CH: Acute lymphoblastic leukemia in children. *Current Opinion in Oncology* 12(1): 3-12, 2000.

14. Gaynon PS, Trigg ME, Heerema NA, et al.: Children's Cancer Group trials in childhood acute lymphoblastic leukemia: 1983-1995. *Leukemia* 14(12): 2223-2233, 2000.

15. Schrappe M, Reiter A, Zimmermann M, et al.: Long-term results of four consecutive trials in childhood ALL performed by the ALL-BFM study group from 1981 to 1995. *Leukemia* 14(12): 2205-2222, 2000.

16. Harms DO, Janka-Schaub GE: Co-operative study group for childhood acute lymphoblastic leukemia (COALL): long-term follow-up of trials 82, 85, 89 and 92 on behalf of the COALL study group. *Leukemia* 14(12): 2234-2239, 2000.

17. Silverman LB, Declerck L, Gelber RD, et al.: Results of Dana-Farber Cancer Institute consortium protocols for children with newly diagnosed acute lymphoblastic leukemia (1981-1995). *Leukemia* 14(12): 2247-2256, 2000.

18. Maloney KW, Shuster JJ, Murphy S, et al.: Long-term results of treatment studies for childhood acute lymphoblastic leukemia: Pediatric Oncology Group studies from 1986-1994. *Leukemia* 14(12): 2276-2285, 2000.

19. Pui C-H, Boyett JM, Rivera GK, et al.: Long-term results of Total Therapy studies 11, 12 and 13A for childhood acute lymphoblastic leukemia at St. Jude Children's Research Hospital. *Leukemia* 14(12): 2286-2294, 2000.

20. Eden OB, Harrison G, Richards S, et al.: Long-term follow-up of the United Kingdom Medical Research Council protocols for childhood acute lymphoblastic leukaemia, 1980-1997. *Leukemia* 14(12): 2307-2320, 2000.

21. Gaynon PS, Qu RP, Chappell RJ, et al.: Survival after relapse in childhood acute lymphoblastic leukemia: impact of site and time to first relapse—the Children's Cancer Group Experience. *Cancer* 82(7): 1387-1395, 1998.

22. Yagi T, Hibi S, Tabata Y, et al.: Detection of clonotypic IGH and TCR rearrangements in the neonatal blood spots of infants and children with B-cell precursor acute lymphoblastic leukemia. *Blood* 96(1): 264-268, 2000.

23. Fasching K, Panzer S, Haas OA, et al.: Presence of clone-specific antigen receptor gene rearrangements at birth indicates an in utero origin of diverse types of early childhood acute lymphoblastic leukemia. *Blood* 95(8): 2722-2724, 2000.

24. Vietti TJ, Land V, et al, for the Pediatric Oncology Group: Progress against childhood cancer: the Pediatric Oncology Group experience. *Pediatrics* 89(4 pt 1): 597-600, 1992.

25. Bleyer WA: The U.S. pediatric cancer clinical trials programmes: international implications and the way forward. *European Journal of Cancer* 33(9): 1439-1447, 1997.

Cellular Classification

Children with acute lymphoblastic leukemia (ALL) are usually treated according to risk groups defined by both clinical and laboratory features. The intensity of treatment required for favorable outcome varies substantially among subsets of children with ALL. Risk-based treatment assignment is utilized for children with ALL so that those children who have a very good outcome with modest therapy can be spared more intensive and toxic treatment, while a more aggressive (and thus more toxic) therapeutic approach can be provided for patients who have a lower probability of long-term survival.[1]

Clinical and laboratory features at diagnosis which are associated with outcome include the following:

1. **Age at diagnosis**: Age at diagnosis has strong prognostic significance, reflecting the different underlying biology of ALL in different age groups.

   - Infants with ALL have a particularly high risk of treatment failure, with the risk of treatment failure being greatest for young infants (less than 6 months) compared to older infants (greater than or equal to 6-9 months).[2-5] Rearrangement of the MLL gene at chromosome band 11q23 can be detected in the leukemia cells of a large percentage of infants with ALL,[6] and the poor outcome for infants with ALL is strongly associated with the presence of the t(4;11) translocation involving the MLL gene.[7,8] ALL in infants is also associated with a constellation of other characteristics associated with poor outcome, including elevated white blood cell (WBC) count, central nervous system leukemia, lack of CD10 (cALLa antigen) expression, and poor response to initial treatment.[2,4]

   - Young children (1-9 years) have a favorable outcome in comparison to either older children and adolescents or in comparison to infants.[1,9,10]

   - Older children and adolescents (greater than or equal to 10 years) have a less favorable outcome than young children, and more aggressive treatments are generally employed in order to improve outcome for these patients.

2. **WBC count at diagnosis:** Patients with higher WBC counts at diagnosis have a higher risk for treatment failure than do patients with lower WBC counts. A WBC count of $50,000/mm^3$ is generally used as an operational cut point between better and poorer prognosis,[1] although the relationship between WBC count and prognosis is a continuous rather than a step function.[10,11] Elevated WBC count is associated with other high-risk prognostic factors, including unfavorable chromosomal translocations such as t(4;11) and t(9;22).

3. **Gender:** The prognosis for girls with ALL is slightly better than that for boys with ALL.[12-14] One reason for the superior prognosis for girls is the occurrence of testicular relapses among boys, but boys also appear to be at increased risk for

bone marrow relapse for reasons that are not well understood.[14]

4. **Race:** Survival rates for black children with ALL are somewhat lower than those for white children with ALL.[9,15-17] The reason for the better outcome for white children compared to black children is not known, but it cannot be completely explained based on known prognostic factors.[16]

5. **Cellular Morphology**: In the past ALL lymphoblasts were classified using the French-American-British (FAB) criteria as having L1 morphology, L2 morphology, or L3 morphology.[18] Due to the lack of independent prognostic significance and the subjective nature of this classification system, it is no longer used in the United States. The FAB L3 morphology is morphologically and cytogenetically identical to that of Burkitt's lymphoma. B-cell ALL (surface immunoglobulin (Ig) expression, generally with FAB L3 morphology and c-myc gene translocation) is a systemic manifestation of Burkitt's and Burkitt's-like non-Hodgkin's lymphoma, and its treatment is completely different from that for other forms of childhood ALL. (NOTE: Rare cases of FAB L3 ALL with c-myc gene translocations lack surface immunoglobulin expression, and these cases are appropriately treated as B-cell ALL).[19] Conversely, rare cases of ALL that express surface Ig but that lack L3 morphology and lack c-myc gene translocations are appropriately treated as B-precursor ALL rather than B-cell ALL.[20]

Evaluating Leukemia Cell Response to Treatment

The rapidity with which leukemia cells are eliminated following onset of treatment is also associated with outcome. Various ways of evaluating the leukemia cell response to treatment have been utilized, including:

1. **Day 7 and day 14 bone marrow responses**: Patients who have a rapid reduction in the leukemia cells in their bone marrow within 7 or 14 days following initiation of multiagent chemotherapy have a more favorable prognosis than do patients who have slower clearance of leukemia cells from the bone marrow.[21,23-25] This "response to treatment" prognostic factor is used by the Children's Cancer Group to stratify patients into prognostic categories for treatment assignment.

2. **Peripheral blood response to steroid prephase**: Patients with a reduction in peripheral blast count to less than 1000/ mm³ after a 7-day induction prephase with prednisone and one dose of intrathecal methotrexate (good prednisone response) have a more favorable prognosis than patients whose peripheral blast counts remain above 1000/mm³ (poor prednisone response).[3,22,26] Treatment stratification for protocols of the German BFM clinical trials group is based on early response to the prednisone 7-day induction prephase.

3. **Peripheral blood response to multiagent induction therapy**: Patients with persistent circulating leukemia cells at 7 to 10 days after the initiation of multiagent chemotherapy are at increased risk of relapse compared to patients who have clearance of peripheral blasts within 1 week of therapy initiation.[27,28] Rate of clearance of peripheral blasts has been found to be of prognostic significance in T-lineage as well as B-lineage ALL.[29]

4. **Minimal residual disease**: Patients in clinical remission after induction therapy may have minimal residual disease, i.e., leukemia cells that can only be detected by highly sensitive techniques such as polymerase chain reaction (PCR) or specialized flow cytometry. Numerous groups have reported an association between minimal residual disease and outcome with early absence of minimal residual disease being associated with better outcome and presence of minimal residual disease being associated with poor outcome.[30-35]

References

1. Smith M, Arthur D, Camitta B, et al.: Uniform approach to risk classification and treatment assignment for children with acute lymphoblastic leukemia. *Journal of Clinical Oncology* 14(1): 18-24, 1996.

2. Reaman GH, Sposto R, Sensel MG, et al.: Treatment outcome and prognostic factors for infants with acute lymphoblastic leukemia treated on two consecutive trials of the Children's Cancer Group. *Journal of Clinical Oncology* 17(2): 445-455, 1999.

3. Frankel LS, Ochs J, Shuster JJ, et al.: Therapeutic trial for infant acute lymphoblastic leukemia: the Pediatric Oncology

Group experience (POG 8493). *Journal of Pediatric Hematology/Oncology* 19(1): 35-42, 1997.

4. Dordelmann M, Reiter A, et al, for the ALL-BFM Group: Prednisone response is the strongest predictor of treatment outcome in infant acute lymphoblastic leukemia. *Blood* 94(4): 1209-1217, 1999.

5. Biondi A, Cimino G, Pieters R, et al.: Biological and therapeutic aspects of infant leukemia. *Blood* 96(1): 24-33, 2000.

6. Rubnitz JE, Link MP, Shuster JJ, et al.: Frequency and prognostic significance of HRX rearrangements in infant acute lymphoblastic leukemia: a Pediatric Oncology Group study. *Blood* 84(2): 570-573, 1994.

7. Felix CA, Lange BJ: Leukemia in infants. *Oncologist* 4(3): 225-240, 1999.

8. Heerema NA, Sather HN, Ge J, et al.: Cytogenetic studies of infant acute lymphoblastic leukemia: poor prognosis of infants with t(4;11)—a report of the Children's Cancer Group. *Leukemia* 13(5): 679-686, 1999.

9. Trueworthy R, Shuster J, Look T, et al.: Ploidy of lymphoblasts is the strongest predictor of treatment outcome in B-progenitor cell acute lymphoblastic leukemia of childhood: a Pediatric Oncology Group study. *Journal of Clinical Oncology* 10(4): 606-613, 1992.

10. Reiter A, Schrappe M, Ludwig W, et al.: Chemotherapy in 998 unselected childhood acute lymphoblastic leukemia patients: results and conclusions of the multicenter trial ALL-BFM 86. *Blood* 84(9): 3122-3133, 1994.

11. Chessells JM, Bailey C, Richards SM, et al.: Intensification of treatment and survival in all children with lymphoblastic leukaemia: results of UK Medical Research Council trial UKALL X. Medical Research Council Working Party on Childhood Leukaemia. *Lancet* 345(8943): 143-148, 1995.

12. Pui CH, Boyett JM, Relling MV, et al.: Sex differences in prognosis for children with acute lymphoblastic leukemia. *Journal of Clinical Oncology* 17(3): 818-824, 1999.

13. Shuster JJ, Wacker P, Pullen J, et al.: Prognostic significance of sex in childhood B-precursor acute lymphoblastic leukemia:

a Pediatric Oncology Group study. *Journal of Clinical Oncology* 16(8): 2854-2863, 1998.

14. Chessells JM, Richards SM, Bailey CC, et al.: Gender and treatment outcome in childhood lymphoblastic leukaemia: report from the MRC UKALL trials. *British Journal of Haematology* 89(2): 364-372, 1995.

15. Pui CH, Boyett JM, Hancock ML, et al.: Outcome of treatment for childhood cancer in black as compared with white children: the St. Jude Children's Research Hospital experience, 1962 through 1992. *JAMA: Journal of the American Medical Association* 273(8): 633-637, 1995.

16. Bhatia S, Sather H, Zhang J, et al.: *Ethnicity and survival following childhood acute lymphoblastic leukemia (ALL): follow-up of the Children's Cancer Group (CCG) cohort.* Proceedings of the American Society of Clinical Oncology 18: A2190, 568a, 1999.

17. Pollock BH, DeBaun MR, Camitta BM, et al.: Racial differences in the survival of childhood B-precursor acute lymphoblastic leukemia: a pediatric oncology group study. *Journal of Clinical Oncology* 18(4): 813-823, 2000.

18. Bennett JM, Catovsky D, Daniel MT, et al.: The morphological classification of acute lymphoblastic leukemia: concordance among observers and clinical correlations. *British Journal of Haematology* 47(4): 553-561, 1981.

19. Navid F, Mosijczuk AD, Head D, et al.: Acute lymphoblastic leukemia with (8:14)(q24:q32) translocation and FAB L3 morphology associated with a B-precursor immunophenotype: the Pediatric Oncology Group experience. *Leukemia* 13(1): 135-141, 1999.

20. Behm FG, Head DR, Pui CH, et al.: B-precursor ALL with unexpected expression of surface immunoglobulin (sig) mu and lambda. *Laboratory Investigation* 72: A-613, 106a, 1995.

21. Hann I, Vora A, Harrison G, et al.: Determinants of outcome after intensified therapy of childhood lymphoblastic leukaemia: results from Medical Research Council United Kingdom acute lymphoblastic leukaemia XI protocol. *British Journal of Haematology* 113(1): 103-114, 2001.

22. Schrappe M, Arico M, Harbott J, et al.: Philadelphia chromosome-positive (Ph+) childhood acute lymphoblastic leukemia: good initial steroid response allows early prediction of a favorable treatment outcome. *Blood* 92(8): 2730-2741, 1998.

23. Gaynon PS, Bleyer WA, Steinherz PG, et al.: Day 7 marrow response and outcome for children with acute lymphoblastic leukemia and unfavorable presenting features. *Medical and Pediatric Oncology* 18(4): 273-279, 1990.

24. Gaynon PS, Desai AA, Bostrom BC, et al.: Early response to therapy and outcome in childhood acute lymphoblastic leukemia: a review. *Cancer* 80(9): 1717-1726, 1997.

25. Steinherz PG, Gaynon PS, Breneman JC, et al.: Cytoreduction and prognosis in acute lymphoblastic leukemia - the importance of early marrow response: report from the Childrens Cancer Group. *Journal of Clinical Oncology* 14(2): 389-398, 1996.

26. Arico M, Basso G, et al, for the Associazione Italiana Ematologia Oncologia Pediatrica (AIEOP): Good steroid response in vivo predicts a favorable outcome in children with T-cell acute lymphoblastic leukemia. *Cancer* 75(7): 1684-1693, 1995.

27. Gajjar A, Ribeiro R, Hancock ML, et al.: Persistence of circulating blasts after 1 week of multiagent chemotherapy confers a poor prognosis in childhood acute lymphoblastic leukemia. *Blood* 86(4): 1292-1295, 1995.

28. Rautonen J, Hovi L, Siimes MA: Slow disappearance of peripheral blast cells: an independent risk factor indicating poor prognosis in children with acute lymphoblastic leukemia. *Blood* 71(4): 989-991, 1988.

29. Griffin TC, Shuster JJ, Buchanan GR et al.: Slow disappearance of peripheral blood blasts is an adverse prognostic factor in childhood T cell acute lymphoblastic leukemia: a Pediatric Oncology Group study. *Leukemia* 14(5): 792-795, 2000.

30. Cave H, van der Werff ten Bosch J, Suciu S, et al.: Clinical significance of minimal residual disease in childhood acute lymphoblastic leukemia. European Organization for Research and Treatment of Cancer—Childhood Leukemia Cooperative

Group. *New England Journal of Medicine* 339(9): 591-598, 1998.

31. Dibenedetto SP, Lo Nigro L, Mayer SP, et al.: Detectable molecular residual disease at the beginning of maintenance therapy indicates poor outcome in children with T-cell acute lymphoblastic leukemia. *Blood* 90(3): 1226-1232, 1997.

32. Roberts WM, Estrov Z, Ouspenskaia MV, et al.: Measurement of residual leukemia during remission in childhood acute lymphoblastic leukemia. *New England Journal of Medicine* 336(5): 317-323, 1997.

33. van Dongen JJ, Seriu T, Panzer-Grumayer ER, et al.: Prognostic value of minimal residual disease in acute lymphoblastic leukaemia in childhood. *Lancet* 352(9142): 1731-1738, 1998.

34. Panzer-Grumayer ER, Schneider M, Panzer S, et al.: Rapid molecular response during early induction chemotherapy predicts a good outcome in childhood acute lymphoblastic leukemia. *Blood* 95(3): 790-794, 2000.

35. Coustan-Smith E, Sancho J, Hancock ML, et al.: Clinical importance of minimal residual disease in childhood acute lymphoblastic leukemia. *Blood* 96(8): 2691-2696, 2000.

Additional Information

National Cancer Institute
Cancer Information Service
6166 Executive Blvd., MSC 8322
Suite 3036A
Bethesda, MD 20892-8322
Toll-Free: 800-4-CANCER (422-6237)
Toll-Free TTY: 800-332-8615
Website: www.cancer.gov

Chapter 13

Childhood Acute Myeloid Leukemia and Acute Promyelocytic Leukemia

Acute Myeloid Leukemia

Acute myeloid leukemia is also referred to as non-lymphoid, myeloblastic, granulocytic, or myelocytic leukemia.

Definition

Acute myeloid leukemia (AML) affects various white blood cells including granulocytes, monocytes, and platelets. Leukemic cells accumulate in the bone marrow, replace normal blood cells, and spread to the liver, spleen, lymph nodes, central nervous system, kidneys, and gonads.

This chapter begins with information from "Disease Information: Acute Myeloid Leukemia," © 2002 St. Jude Children's Research Hospital, reprinted with permission; and "Disease Information: Acute Promyelocytic Leukemia," © 2002 St. Jude Children's Research Hospital, reprinted with permission. Text beginning with "What Is Childhood Acute Myeloid Leukemia?" is from PDQ® Cancer Information Summary. National Cancer Institute; Bethesda, MD. "Childhood Acute Myeloid Leukemia/Other Myeloid Malignancies (PDQ®): Treatment–Patient," updated 08/2002, available at: http://cancer.gov, accessed 03/31/2003; and text following "Statistics, Factors, and Risks of Childhood Acute Myelogenous Leukemia" is excerpted from PDQ® Cancer Information Summary, National Cancer Institute, Bethesda, MD, "Childhood Acute Myeloid Leukemia/Other Myeloid Malignancies (PDQ®): Treatment–Health Professional," available at http://cancer.gov, updated 12/2002, accessed 03/31/2003.

Incidence

- Approximately 500 children are diagnosed with AML in the United States each year.

- AML is diagnosed in about 20 percent of children with leukemia.

- It usually occurs in people older than 25, but sometimes is found in teenagers, toddlers, and infants.

- AML is the most common second malignancy (a different or second cancer found in a patient previously treated for cancer) in children treated for malignancies.

Influencing Factors

There is a greater incidence of leukemia among people exposed to large amounts of radiation and certain chemicals (e.g. benzene).

Treatment Strategies

- Chemotherapy is the most common form of therapy for children with AML.

- Autologous blood stem cell (harvested from bone marrow or peripheral blood) transplantation may be performed as part of treatment. Autologous transplants use the patient's own stem cells.

- Allogeneic blood stem cell (harvested from bone marrow, cord blood or peripheral blood) transplantation is preferred treatment for those patients with AML who at a high-risk of relapse or who have disease that is resistant to other treatments. Allogeneic transplants use stem cells from a donor.

Survival Rates

- Although approximately 80 to 90 percent of children with AML attain remissions (absence of leukemic cells), some of those patients have later recurrences. Between 40 to 50 percent of children with AML achieve long-term remissions with chemotherapy.

Current Research

St. Jude Children's Research Hospital has committed a substantial share of its resources to determining the genetic changes that cause AML. Current clinical trials include:

- intensive use of chemotherapy plus stem cell transplantation;

- the use of biological response modifiers to help eliminate leukemia through the body's own immune system;

- development of a treatment strategy to reduce graft-versus-host disease, a serious complication of bone marrow transplantation.

Acute Promyelocytic Leukemia

Acute Promyelocytic Leukemia is also known as acute myeloid leukemia M3 under French-American-British classification.

Definition

Acute promyelocytic leukemia (APL) is a subtype of the cancer acute myeloid leukemia (AML). APL is characterized by abnormal, heavily granulated promyelocytes, a form of white blood cells. APL results in the accumulation of these atypical promyelocytes in the bone marrow and peripheral blood, and replaces normal blood cells.

Incidence

- Approximately 50 children are diagnosed with APL, out of the estimated 500 children diagnosed each year with AML in the United States.

- APL represents about one percent of childhood leukemia.

- APL is found more often in children between the ages of two and three, and in adults over 40; however, it has also been found in older children and teenagers. APL is found more frequently in children of Hispanic and Mediterranean origin.

Treatment Strategies

- Chemotherapy is used in combination with all trans retinoic acid (ATRA).

- Some centers, including St. Jude Children's Research Hospital, are testing forms of arsenic trioxide for treating APL.

Survival Rates

With the combination treatment of chemotherapy and ATRA about 75-80 percent of young patients are expected to be long-term survivors.

What Is Childhood Acute Myeloid Leukemia?

Childhood acute myeloid leukemia (AML) is a cancer of the blood-forming tissue, primarily the bone marrow and lymph nodes. AML is also called acute nonlymphocytic leukemia or acute myelogenous leukemia, and is divided into several subtypes. It is less common than acute lymphocytic leukemia (also called acute lymphoblastic leukemia or ALL), another form of leukemia that occurs in children. Children with Down syndrome have an increased risk of AML during the first 3 years of life.

All types of blood cells are produced by the bone marrow. The bone marrow is the spongy tissue inside the large bones of the body. The bone marrow makes red blood cells (which carry oxygen and other materials to all tissues of the body), white blood cells (which fight infection), and platelets (which help make the blood clot).

The bone marrow produces new blood cells. In leukemia the bone marrow starts producing large numbers of abnormal blood cells usually white blood cells. These abnormal, immature white blood cells are called blasts. These cells flood the blood stream and lymph system, and may invade vital organs such as the brain, testes, ovaries, or skin. Acute promyelocytic leukemia is a rare type of AML that prevents blood from clotting normally. In rare cases, AML tumor cells form a solid tumor called an isolated granulocytic sarcoma or chloroma.

Leukemia can be acute (progressing quickly with many immature blasts) or chronic (progressing slowly with more mature-looking cancer cells). Acute myeloid leukemia can occur in both children and adults. Treatment is different for adults than it is for children.

Early signs of AML may be fever, chills, bleeding or bruising easily, swollen lymph nodes, and other symptoms similar to those of the flu, such as feeling weak or tired all the time, with aching bones or joints. If your child has symptoms of leukemia, his or her doctor may order a blood test to count the number of cells and examine them under a microscope. If the results of the blood tests are not normal, a bone marrow biopsy may be performed. During this test, a needle is inserted into a bone in the hip and a small amount of bone marrow is removed and examined under a microscope, enabling the doctor to determine what kind of leukemia your child has and plan the best treatment. Chromosomal analysis may also be performed. These additional tests can help distinguish AML from ALL and other leukemias and allow doctors to better plan treatment.

Other Childhood Myeloid Malignancies

Myelodysplastic syndromes (MDS) are disorders of the blood-forming cells. Myelodysplastic syndromes usually cause a deficiency in white blood cells, red blood cells, and platelets and may lead to AML.

Juvenile myelomonocytic leukemia (JMML) is an extremely rare cancer of the blood-forming cells. Children with neurofibromatosis 1 (NF1) are at an increased risk for developing JMML.

Stages of Childhood Acute Myeloid Leukemia

There is no staging for acute myeloid leukemia (AML). AML is always spread throughout the bloodstream at the time of diagnosis, and sometimes invades other body tissue. Patients are often grouped according to whether or not they have been previously treated for leukemia.

Untreated

Untreated AML means that no treatment has yet been given except to alleviate or treat symptoms of the disease. There are too many white blood cells in the blood and bone marrow, and there may be other signs and symptoms of leukemia. In rare cases, AML tumor cells appear as a solid tumor called an isolated granulocytic sarcoma or chloroma.

In Remission

Remission means that the numbers of white blood cells and other cells in the blood and bone marrow are approaching normal following initial treatment with chemotherapy and that there are no signs or symptoms of leukemia.

Recurrent/Refractory

Recurrent means that the leukemia has come back (recurred) after going into remission. Refractory means that the leukemia failed to go into remission following treatment.

Treatment Option Overview

There are treatments for all patients with childhood acute myeloid leukemia (AML). Experienced doctors working together may provide the best treatment for children with AML. Your child's treatment will often be planned by a team of childhood cancer specialists with experience and expertise in treating leukemias of childhood.

The primary treatment for AML is chemotherapy, sometimes followed by bone marrow transplantation. Radiation therapy may be used in certain cases. Biological therapy is also being studied in clinical trials.

Chemotherapy is the use of drugs to kill cancer cells. Chemotherapy drugs may be taken by mouth or injected into a vein (intravenous injection) or a muscle. Chemotherapy is called a systemic treatment because the drug enters the blood stream, travels through the body, and can kill cancer cells throughout the body. Chemotherapy may sometimes be injected into the fluid that surrounds the brain and spinal cord (intrathecal chemotherapy).

Radiation therapy uses x-rays or other high-energy rays to kill cancer cells and shrink tumors. Radiation for AML usually comes from a machine outside the body (external radiation therapy).

Bone marrow transplantation, a newer type of treatment, is used to replace the patient's bone marrow with healthy bone marrow. First, high doses of chemotherapy with or without radiation therapy are given to destroy all of the bone marrow in the body. Healthy marrow is then taken from another person (a donor) whose tissue is the same as or almost the same as the patient's. The donor may be a twin (the best match), a brother or sister, or another person not related. The healthy marrow from the donor is given to the patient through a needle in a vein, and the healthy marrow replaces the marrow that was destroyed. A bone marrow transplant using marrow from a relative or person not related is called an allogeneic bone marrow transplant.

Another type of bone marrow transplant, called autologous bone marrow transplant, may be used. During this procedure, bone marrow is taken from the patient and may be treated with drugs to kill any cancer cells. The marrow is then frozen to save it. Next, the patient is given high-dose chemotherapy, with or without radiation therapy, to destroy all of the remaining marrow. The frozen marrow that was saved is then thawed and returned to the patient to replace the marrow that was destroyed.

Biological therapy attempts to stimulate or restore the ability of the patient's immune system to fight cancer. It uses substances produced by the patient's own body or made in a laboratory to boost, direct, or restore the body's natural defenses against disease. Biological therapy is sometimes called biological response modifier therapy or immunotherapy.

Treatment for AML is ordinarily divided into 2 phases: induction and consolidation. A third phase, intensification, may also be used. During induction therapy, chemotherapy is used to kill as many of the leukemia cells as possible and cause the leukemia to go into remission. Once the leukemia goes into remission and there are no signs of leukemia, consolidation therapy is given. The purpose of post-remission therapy (consolidation and intensification) is to kill any remaining leukemia cells. Your child may receive either or both phases of post-remission therapy.

As **preventive therapy**, your child may also receive central nervous system (CNS) prophylaxis, which consists of intrathecal and/or high-dose systemic chemotherapy to the central nervous system (CNS) to kill any leukemia cells present there, or to prevent the spread of cancer cells to the brain and spinal cord even if no cancer has been detected there. Radiation therapy to the brain may also be given, in addition to chemotherapy, for this purpose.

Unwanted side-effects can result from treatment long after it ends, so it is important that your child continue to be seen by his or her doctor. Chemotherapy can lead to heart, kidney, and hearing problems after treatment is finished. Radiation therapy may cause problems with growth and development.

Treatment by Stage

Treatment for childhood AML depends on whether or not the patient has been previously treated for leukemia and the type of leukemia. The best treatment is given by cancer doctors with experience in treating children with leukemia, and is given at hospitals where leukemia patients are often treated.

Your child may receive treatment that is considered standard based on its effectiveness in a number of patients in past studies, or you may choose to have your child take part in a clinical trial. Not all patients are cured with standard therapy, and some standard treatments may have more side effects than are desired. For these reasons, clinical trials are designed to test new treatments and to find better ways to treat cancer patients, and are based on the most up-to-date information. Clinical trials are ongoing in most parts of the country for most types of childhood AML.

Untreated Childhood Acute Myeloid Leukemia

Your child's treatment will probably be induction chemotherapy using 2 or more chemotherapy drugs to kill cancer cells and cause the leukemia to go into remission. Induction chemotherapy is usually successful in inducing remission. Intrathecal chemotherapy with or without radiation therapy to the brain may be given to prevent the spread of cancer cells to the brain and spinal cord. Biological therapy may be added to treatment to help your child recover more quickly from the side effects of induction therapy.

Acute Promyelocytic Leukemia

Treatment for acute promyelocytic leukemia (APL) may include all-trans retinoic acid (ATRA) combined with chemotherapy. Arsenic trioxide is also being studied in children with APL.

Children with Down syndrome

Treatment for children with Down syndrome who have AML is chemotherapy.

Myelodysplastic Syndrome

Treatment for myelodysplastic syndromes may include chemotherapy followed by bone marrow or peripheral stem cell transplantation.

Juvenile Myelomonocytic Leukemia

Treatment for children with juvenile myelomonocytic leukemia may be peripheral stem cell transplantation, cis-retinoic acid, and chemotherapy.

Childhood Acute Myeloid Leukemia in Remission

Treatment will consist of additional chemotherapy or bone marrow transplantation. Central nervous system prophylaxis and/or maintenance chemotherapy may also be given in some cases.

Recurrent Childhood Acute Myeloid Leukemia

Treatment depends on the type of treatment your child received before. You may want to consider entering your child into a clinical trial. Treatments currently being studied in clinical trials include new chemotherapy drugs, bone marrow transplantation, and biological therapy. Treatment for recurrent acute promyelocytic leukemia (APL) may consist of arsenic trioxide or regimens including all-trans retinoic acid.

Unwanted side effects can result from treatment long after it ends, so it is important that your child continue to be seen by his or her doctor. Chemotherapy can later lead to heart problems, as well as kidney and hearing problems. Radiation therapy may interfere with a child's growth and may increase the risk of hormonal dysfunction and cataract formation.

Editor's Note: The following sections contain information written mainly for doctors and other health care professionals, but which may be helpful to your situation. If you have questions about these topics, you can ask your doctor or call the Cancer Information Service at 800-422-6237.

Statistics, Factors, and Risks of Childhood Acute Myelogenous Leukemia

Acute myelogenous leukemia (AML) is the most common type of myeloid malignancy of childhood. Between 75% and 85% of children with AML can achieve a complete remission following appropriate induction chemotherapy. Children with newly diagnosed AML have an event-free 5-year survival rate of approximately 50%.[2-4] The most consistent prognostic factor across studies of AML in children is white blood cell (WBC) count at diagnosis. Children who have a WBC count greater than 100,000 per cubic milliliter have a poor prognosis. Additional factors that have been associated with a poor prognosis are: secondary AML and monosomy 7 karyotype. Children with leukemia cell chromosomal abnormalities t(8;21) and inv 16 have a high likelihood of achieving remission [5-9] and a decreased likelihood of relapse.[8,9] Translocations of chromosomal band 11q23, including most AML secondary to epipodophyllotoxin,[10] are unfavorable in some studies. One exception to the poor prognostic significance of translocations at chromosome band 11q23 may be the t(9;11). In some reports, outcome has been relatively favorable for patients whose leukemia cells have t(9;11),[11,12] although favorable outcome has not been observed in other series.[9] In several studies, M4 and M5 FAB type, WBC greater than 20,000 per cubic milliliter, and requiring more than 1 cycle to achieve remission, predicted for a short duration of remission.[6,8] Presence of a FLT-3 internal tandem duplication has been demonstrated to be a poor prognostic factor.[13,14]

Acute promyelocytic leukemia (APL) is a distinct subtype of AML and is treated differently than other types of AML. The characteristic chromosomal abnormality associated with APL is t(15;17). This translocation involves a breakpoint that includes the retinoid acid receptor and that leads to production of the PML-RARalpha fusion protein.[15] Clinically, APL is characterized by a severe coagulopathy often present at the time of diagnosis.[16] Mortality during induction due to bleeding complications is more common in this subtype than other FAB classifications.

Children with Down syndrome have an increased risk of leukemia with a ratio of ALL to AML typical for childhood acute leukemia, except during the first 3 years of life when AML (especially M7) predominates.[17] Neonates with Down syndrome may manifest a transient myeloproliferative syndrome (TMS). This disorder mimics congenital AML but improves spontaneously within 4 to 6 weeks. Retrospective surveys indicate that as many as 30% of infants with Down syndrome and TMS will develop AML before 3 years of age.[18] Interestingly, the majority of children with Down syndrome and AML can be cured of their leukemia.[19] Appropriate therapy for these children is less intensive than current AML therapy and bone marrow transplant (BMT) is not indicated in first remission.

The myelodysplastic syndromes (MDS) represent a heterogeneous group of disorders of hematopoiesis leading to variable degrees of pancytopenia and often acute myeloid leukemia (AML). In adults, MDS have been classified by the French-American-British (FAB) group into distinct categories.[20] The FAB MDS classification is not an adequate classification for the syndromes that occur in children. The optimal management of MDS in children has not been well-studied in prospective trials.

Juvenile myelomonocytic leukemia (JMML), formerly termed juvenile chronic myeloid leukemia (JCML), is a rare hematopoietic malignancy of childhood accounting for less than 1% of all childhood leukemias.[21] A number of clinical and laboratory features distinguish JMML from adult-type chronic myeloid leukemia, a disease noted only occasionally in children. Few approaches other than hematopoietic stem cell transplantation have resulted in long-term survival for this disease.[22,23] Children with neurofibromatosis 1(NF1) are at increased risk for developing JMML [24] and up to 14% of cases of JMML occur in children with NF1.[25]

References

1. Guidelines for the pediatric cancer center and role of such centers in diagnosis and treatment. American Academy of Pediatrics Section Statement Section on Hematology/Oncology. *Pediatrics* 99 (1): 139-41, 1997.

2. Woods WG, Neudorf S, Gold S, et al.: Children's Cancer Group: A comparison of allogeneic bone marrow transplantation, autologous bone marrow transplantation, and aggressive chemotherapy in children with acute myeloid leukemia in remission. *Blood* 97 (1): 56-62, 2001.

3. Creutzig U, Ritter J, Zimmermann M, et al.: Improved treatment results in high-risk pediatric acute myeloid leukemia patients after intensification with high-dose cytarabine and mitoxantrone: results of Study Acute Myeloid Leukemia-Berlin-Frankfurt-Münster 93. *J Clin Oncol* 19 (10): 2705-13, 2001.

4. Stevens RF, Hann IM, Wheatley K, et al.: Marked improvements in outcome with chemotherapy alone in paediatric acute myeloid leukemia: results of the United Kingdom Medical Research Council's 10th AML trial. MRC Childhood Leukaemia Working Party. *Br J Haematol* 101 (1): 130-40, 1998.

5. Kalwinsky DK, Raimondi SC, Schell MJ, et al.: Prognostic importance of cytogenetic subgroups in de novo pediatric acute nonlymphocytic leukemia. *J Clin Oncol* 8 (1): 75-83, 1990.

6. Grier HE, Gelber RD, Camitta BM, et al.: Prognostic factors in childhood acute myelogenous leukemia. *J Clin Oncol* 5 (7): 1026-32, 1987.

7. Creutzig U, Zimmermann M, Ritter J, et al.: Definition of a standard-risk group in children with AML. *Br J Haematol* 104 (3): 630-9, 1999.

8. Grimwade D, Walker H, Oliver F, et al.: The importance of diagnostic cytogenetics on outcome in AML: analysis of 1,612 patients entered into the MRC AML 10 trial. The Medical Research Council Adult and Children's Leukaemia Working Parties. *Blood* 92 (7): 2322-33, 1998.

9. Raimondi SC, Chang MN, Ravindranath Y, et al.: Chromosomal abnormalities in 478 children with acute myeloid

leukemia: clinical characteristics and treatment outcome in a cooperative pediatric oncology group study-POG 8821. *Blood* 94 (11): 3707-16, 1999.

10. Pui CH, Relling MV, Rivera GK, et al.: Epipodophyllotoxin-related acute myeloid leukemia: a study of 35 cases. *Leukemia* 9 (12): 1990-6, 1995.

11. Martinez-Climent JA, Espinosa R, Thirman MJ, et al.: Abnormalities of chromosome band 11q23 and the MLL gene in pediatric myelomonocytic and monoblastic leukemias. Identification of the t(9;11) as an indicator of long survival. *J Pediatr Hematol Oncol* 17 (4): 277-83, 1995.

12. Rubnitz JE, Raimondi SC, Tong X, et al.: Favorable impact of the t(9;11) in childhood acute myeloid leukemia. *J Clin Oncol* 20 (9): 2302-9, 2002.

13. Kottaridis PD, Gale RE, Frew ME, et al.: The presence of a FLT3 internal tandem duplication in patients with acute myeloid leukemia (AML) adds important prognostic information to cytogenetic risk group and response to the first cycle of chemotherapy: analysis of 854 patients from the United Kingdom Medical Research Council AML 10 and 12 trials. *Blood* 98 (6): 1752-9, 2001.

14. Meshinchi S, Woods WG, Stirewalt DL, et al.: Prevalence and prognostic significance of Flt3 internal tandem duplication in pediatric acute myeloid leukemia. *Blood* 97 (1): 89-94, 2001.

15. Melnick A, Licht JD: Deconstructing a disease: RARalpha, its fusion partners, and their roles in the pathogenesis of acute promyelocytic leukemia. *Blood* 93 (10): 3167-215, 1999.

16. Tallman MS, Hakimian D, Kwaan HC, et al.: New insights into the pathogenesis of coagulation dysfunction in acute promyelocytic leukemia. *Leuk Lymphoma* 11 (1-2): 27-36, 1993.

17. Zipursky A, Poon A, Doyle J: Leukemia in Down syndrome: a review. *Pediatr Hematol Oncol* 9 (2): 139-49, 1992 Apr-Jun.

18. Homans AC, Verissimo AM, Vlacha V: Transient abnormal myelopoiesis of infancy associated with trisomy 21. *Am J Pediatr Hematol Oncol* 15 (4): 392-9, 1993.

19. Lange BJ, Kobrinsky N, Barnard DR, et al.: Distinctive demography, biology, and outcome of acute myeloid leukemia and myelodysplastic syndrome in children with Down syndrome: Children's Cancer Group Studies 2861 and 2891. *Blood* 91 (2): 608-15, 1998.

20. Bennett JM, Catovsky D, Daniel MT, et al.: Proposals for the classification of the myelodysplastic syndromes. *Br J Haematol* 51 (2): 189-99, 1982.

21. Aricò M, Biondi A, Pui CH: Juvenile myelomonocytic leukemia. *Blood* 90 (2): 479-88, 1997.

22. Sanders JE, Buckner CD, Thomas ED, et al.: Allogeneic marrow transplantation for children with juvenile chronic myelogenous leukemia. *Blood* 71 (4): 1144-6, 1988.

23. Bunin N, Saunders F, Leahey A, et al.: Alternative donor bone marrow transplantation for children with juvenile myelomonocytic leukemia. *J Pediatr Hematol Oncol* 21 (6): 479-85, 1999 Nov-Dec.

24. Stiller CA, Chessells JM, Fitchett M: Neurofibromatosis and childhood leukaemia/lymphoma: a population-based UKCCSG study. *Br J Cancer* 70 (5): 969-72, 1994.

25. Niemeyer CM, Aricò M, Basso G, et al.: Chronic myelomonocytic leukemia in childhood: a retrospective analysis of 110 cases. European Working Group on Myelodysplastic Syndromes in Childhood (EWOG-MDS) *Blood* 89 (10): 3534-43, 1997.

Untreated Childhood Acute Myeloid Leukemia and Other Myeloid Malignancies

Induction Chemotherapy for Acute Myelogenous Leukemia

Contemporary effective pediatric AML protocols result in 75% to 90% complete remission (CR) rates.[1-3] Of those patients who do not go into remission, about one-half have resistant leukemia and one-half die from the complications of the disease or its treatment. To achieve a complete remission, inducing profound bone marrow aplasia (with the exception of the M3 APL variant) is usually necessary. Because induction chemotherapy produces severe myelosuppression, morbidity and mortality from infection or hemorrhage during the induction period may be significant.

The two most effective drugs used to induce remission in children with acute myeloid leukemia (AML) are cytarabine and an anthracycline. Commonly used pediatric induction therapy regimens use cytarabine and an anthracycline in combination with other agents such as etoposide and/or thioguanine.[1-3] For example, the CCG [Children's Cancer Group] DCTER [dexamethasone, cytosine arabinoside, 6-thioguanine, etoposide, rubidamycin] regimen utilizes cytarabine, daunorubicin, dexamethasone, etoposide, and thioguanine and is given as two 4-day treatments separated by 6 days.[3] The German Berlin-Frankfurt-Munster (BFM) Group has studied cytarabine and daunorubicin plus etoposide (ADE) given over 8 days,[2] and the United Kingdom Medical Research Council (MRC) has studied a similar ADE regimen given over 10 days.[1] The MRC has also studied cytarabine and daunorubicin given with thioguanine (DAT).[1] A randomized trial that included both children and adults comparing either etoposide or thioguanine given with cytarabine and daunorubicin (i.e., ADE versus DAT) showed no difference between the thioguanine and etoposide arms in remission rate or disease-free survival.[4]

The anthracycline that has been most used in induction regimens for children with AML is daunorubicin,[1-3] although idarubicin has also been used.[5] A randomized study in children with newly diagnosed AML comparing daunorubicin and idarubicin (each given with cytarabine and etoposide) observed a trend favoring idarubicin, but the small benefit for idarubicin in terms of remission rate and event-free survival was not statistically significant.[5] Similarly, studies comparing idarubicin and daunorubicin in adults with AML have not produced compelling evidence that idarubicin is more efficacious than daunorubicin.[6] In the absence of convincing data that another anthracycline produces superior outcome to daunorubicin when given at an equitoxic dose, daunorubicin remains the anthracycline most commonly used during induction therapy for children with AML.

The intensity of induction therapy influences the overall outcome of therapy. The CCG 2891 study demonstrated that intensively-timed induction therapy (4-day treatment courses separated by only 6 days) produced better event-free survival than standard-timing induction therapy (4-day treatment courses separated by two weeks or longer).[3] The MRC Group has intensified induction therapy by prolonging the duration of cytarabine treatment to 10 days.[1] Another way of intensifying induction therapy is by the use of high-dose cytarabine. While studies in non-elderly adults suggest an advantage for intensifying induction therapy with high-dose cytarabine (2-3 gm/m^2/dose) compared to standard-dose cytarabine,[7,8] a benefit for the use of high-dose cytarabine compared to standard-dose cytarabine in children was not observed using a cytarabine dose of 1 gm/m^2 given twice daily for 7 days with daunorubicin and thioguanine.[9]

Randomized trials evaluating hematopoietic growth factors during induction therapy for patients with AML have not been performed in children, and so the potential benefit of these agents for children with AML must be extrapolated from the adult experience. Hematopoietic growth factors such as granulocyte-macrophage colony-stimulating factor (GM-CSF) or granulocyte colony-stimulating factor (G-CSF) during AML induction therapy have been evaluated in multiple placebo-controlled studies in attempts to reduce the toxicity associated with prolonged myelosuppression.[10] Treatment with hematopoietic growth factor generally begins within a day or two following the completion of cytotoxic therapy and continues until granulocyte recovery. A reduction of several days in the duration of neutropenia with the use of either G-CSF or GM-CSF has been observed.[10] Most, but not all, randomized studies showed statistically significant reductions in the duration of hospitalization and antibiotic use in patients receiving hematopoietic growth factors.[10] However, significant effects on treatment-related mortality or overall survival were rarely observed.[10]

Central Nervous System Prophylaxis

Although the presence of central nervous system (CNS) leukemia at diagnosis (i.e., clinical neurologic features and/or leukemic cells in cerebral spinal fluid on cytocentrifuge preparation) is more common in childhood AML than in childhood acute lymphocytic leukemia (ALL), reduction in overall survival directly attributable to CNS involvement is presently less common in childhood AML. This finding is perhaps related to both the higher doses of chemotherapy used in AML (with potential cross-over to the CNS) and the fact that marrow disease has not yet been as effectively brought under long-term control in AML as in ALL. Children with M4 and M5 AML have the highest incidence of CNS leukemia (especially those with inv 16 or 11q23 chromosomal abnormalities). The use of some form of CNS treatment (intrathecal chemotherapy with or without cranial irradiation) is now incorporated into most protocols for the treatment of childhood AML and is considered a standard part of the treatment for this disease.[11]

Acute Promyelocytic Leukemia

Acute promyelocytic leukemia (APL) is a distinct subtype of AML and is treated differently than other types of AML. The characteristic chromosomal abnormality associated with APL is t(15;17). This translocation involves a breakpoint that includes the retinoid acid receptor and that leads to production of the PML-RARalpha fusion protein.[12] Clinically, APL is characterized by a severe coagulopathy often present at the time of diagnosis.[13] Mortality during induction due to bleeding complications is more common in this subtype than other FAB classifications. Due to the extremely low incidence of CNS disease in patients with APL, a lumbar puncture is not required at the time of diagnosis and prophylactic intrathecal chemotherapy is not administered. Studies have demonstrated that the absence of PML-RARalpha breakpoint at the end of therapy, as detected by RT-PCR monitoring, predicts a low risk of relapse.[14-16]

The leukemia cells from patients with APL are especially sensitive to the differentiation-inducing effects of all-trans retinoic acid (ATRA). The basis for the dramatic efficacy of ATRA against APL is the ability of pharmacologic doses of ATRA to overcome the repression of signaling caused by the PML RARalpha fusion protein at physiologic ATRA concentrations. Restoration of signaling leads to differentiation of APL cells and then to postmaturation apoptosis.[17] Most patients with APL achieve a complete remission when treated with ATRA, although single agent ATRA is generally not curative.[18,19] A series of randomized clinical trials have defined the benefit for combining ATRA with chemotherapy during induction therapy and also the utility of employing ATRA as maintenance therapy.[20-22] With the use of ATRA and chemotherapy, the 2-year survival rates for patients with APL have improved from approximately 40% to 50-80%.[20,22] Induction therapy for the current nationwide trial for children and adults with APL utilizes ATRA with standard-dose cytarabine and daunorubicin, and consolidation therapy employs ATRA with daunorubicin.[23]

There is an uncommon variant of APL associated with t(11;17) resulting in a PLZR-RARalpha fusion protein. This variant does not respond well to ATRA and has a worse prognosis than APL with t(15;17).[24-26]

Arsenic trioxide has also been identified as an active agent in patients with APL, with 70% to 90% of patients achieving remission following treatment with this agent.[27,28] There are limited data on the use of arsenic trioxide in children, though published reports suggest that children with APL have a response to arsenic trioxide similar to that of adults.[27,29] Because arsenic trioxide causes Q-T interval prolongation that can lead to life-threatening arrhythmias (e.g., torsades de pointes),[30] it is essential to monitor electrolytes closely in patients receiving arsenic trioxide and to maintain potassium and magnesium values at midnormal ranges.[31]

Children with Down Syndrome

Children with Down syndrome have an increased risk of developing leukemia, particularly AML M7 myelodysplastic syndrome. The majority of children with AML and Down syndrome can be cured of their leukemia.[32] Appropriate therapy for these children is less intensive than current AML therapy and bone marrow transplantation (BMT) is not indicated in first remission.[33]

Transient myeloproliferative syndrome (TMD) is a disorder primarily found in Down syndrome patients during the newborn period. It is characterized by an uncontrolled proliferation of myeloblasts. These blasts are frequently of megakaryocytic origin with varying degrees of differentiation and are clonal in nature. Information regarding the presentation and natural course of this disease is lacking. TMD can be distinguished from congenital AML primarily by its spontaneous resolution. Thus, TMD is managed with supportive care only during the first few months of life.

Juvenile Myelomonocytic Leukemia

Historically, more than 90% of juvenile myelomonocytic leukemia patients died despite the use of chemotherapy.[38] Patients appeared to follow three distinct clinical courses: 1) rapidly progressive disease and early demise; 2) transiently stable disease followed by progression and death; and 3) clinical improvement which lasted up to 9 years before progression or, rarely, long-term survival. A more recent retrospective review from the United Kingdom described 31 children (19 JMML; 12 Mo 7) in which chemotherapy (nonintensive and intensive) and marrow ablative therapy with marrow reconstitution from a sibling or unrelated, HLA-matched donor was used. The projected 5-year survival rate was 5% in patients with JMML and 40% in those with Mo 7.[34]

Based upon these laboratory observations, 12 patients with JMML were evaluated in a pilot study using cis-retinoic acid (C-RA).[39] Of ten patients who could be evaluated, responses were as follows: 2 CR, 3 partial responses (PR), 1 minimal response (MR), 4 progressive disease (PD). Toxicity was minimal. Responses were relatively slow and most children who experienced progressive disease did so within a few weeks of C-RA treatment. Transplantation seems to offer the best chance of cure for JMML.[40,41] A summary of the outcome of 91 patients with JMML treated with transplantation in 16 different reports is as follows: 38 patients (41%) were still alive at time of reporting, including 30 of the 60 (50%) patients who received grafts from HLA-matched or one-antigen mismatched familial donors, 2 of 12 (17%) with mismatched donors, and 6 of 19 (32%) with matched unrelated donors.[42]

References

1. Stevens RF, Hann IM, Wheatley K, et al.: Marked improvements in outcome with chemotherapy alone in paediatric acute myeloid leukemia: results of the United Kingdom Medical Research Council's 10th AML trial. MRC Childhood Leukaemia Working Party. *Br J Haematol* 101 (1): 130-40, 1998.

2. Creutzig U, Ritter J, Zimmermann M, et al.: Improved treatment results in high-risk pediatric acute myeloid leukemia patients after intensification with high-dose cytarabine and mitoxantrone: results of Study Acute Myeloid Leukemia-Berlin-Frankfurt-Münster 93. *J Clin Oncol* 19 (10): 2705-13, 2001.

3. Woods WG, Kobrinsky N, Buckley JD, et al.: Timed-sequential induction therapy improves postremission outcome in acute myeloid leukemia: a report from the Children's Cancer Group. *Blood* 87 (12): 4979-89, 1996.

4. Hann IM, Stevens RF, Goldstone AH, et al.: Randomized comparison of DAT versus ADE as induction chemotherapy in children and younger adults with acute myeloid leukemia. Results of the Medical Research Council's 10th AML trial (MRC AML10). Adult and Childhood Leukaemia Working Parties of the Medical Research Council. *Blood* 89 (7): 2311-8, 1997.

5. Creutzig U, Ritter J, Zimmermann M, et al.: Idarubicin improves blast cell clearance during induction therapy in children with AML: results of study AML-BFM 93. AML-BFM Study Group. *Leukemia* 15 (3): 348-54, 2001.

6. Berman E, Wiernik P, Vogler R, et al.: Long-term follow-up of three randomized trials comparing idarubicin and daunorubicin as induction therapies for patients with untreated acute myeloid leukemia. *Cancer* 80 (11 Suppl): 2181-5, 1997.

7. Weick JK, Kopecky KJ, Appelbaum FR, et al.: A randomized investigation of high-dose versus standard-dose cytosine

arabinoside with daunorubicin in patients with previously untreated acute myeloid leukemia: a Southwest Oncology Group study. *Blood* 88 (8): 2841-51, 1996.

8. Bishop JF, Matthews JP, Young GA, et al.: A randomized study of high-dose cytarabine in induction in acute myeloid leukemia. *Blood* 87 (5): 1710-7, 1996.

9. Becton D, Ravindranath Y, Dahl GV, et al.: A phase III study of intensive cytarabine (Ara-C) induction followed by cyclosporine (CSA) modulation of drug resistance in de novo pediatric AML; POG 9421. *Blood* 98: A-1929, 461a, 2001.

10. Ozer H, Armitage JO, Bennett CL, et al.: American Society of Clinical Oncology: 2000 update of recommendations for the use of hematopoietic colony-stimulating factors: evidence-based, clinical practice guidelines. American Society of Clinical Oncology Growth Factors Expert Panel. *J Clin Oncol* 18 (20): 3558-85, 2000.

11. Pui CH, Dahl GV, Kalwinsky DK, et al.: Central nervous system leukemia in children with acute nonlymphoblastic leukemia. *Blood* 66 (5): 1062-7, 1985.

12. Melnick A, Licht JD: Deconstructing a disease: RARalpha, its fusion partners, and their roles in the pathogenesis of acute promyelocytic leukemia. *Blood* 93 (10): 3167-215, 1999.

13. Tallman MS, Hakimian D, Kwaan HC, et al.: New insights into the pathogenesis of coagulation dysfunction in acute promyelocytic leukemia. *Leuk Lymphoma* 11 (1-2): 27-36, 1993.

14. Gameiro P, Vieira S, Carrara P, et al.: The PML-RAR alpha transcript in long-term follow-up of acute promyelocytic leukemia patients. *Haematologica* 86 (6): 577-85, 2001.

15. Jurcic JG, Nimer SD, Scheinberg DA, et al.: Prognostic significance of minimal residual disease detection and PML/RAR-alpha isoform type: long-term follow-up in acute promyelocytic leukemia. *Blood* 98 (9): 2651-6, 2001.

16. Hu J, Yu T, Zhao W, et al.: Impact of RT-PCR monitoring on the long-term survival in acute promyelocytic leukemia. *Chin Med J (Engl)* 113 (10): 899-902, 2000.

17. Altucci L, Rossin A, Raffelsberger W, et al.: Retinoic acid-induced apoptosis in leukemia cells is mediated by paracrine action of tumor-selective death ligand TRAIL. *Nat Med* 7 (6): 680-6, 2001.

18. Huang ME, Ye YC, Chen SR, et al.: Use of all-trans retinoic acid in the treatment of acute promyelocytic leukemia. *Blood* 72 (2): 567-72, 1988.

19. Castaigne S, Chomienne C, Daniel MT, et al.: All-trans retinoic acid as a differentiation therapy for acute promyelocytic leukemia. I. Clinical results. *Blood* 76 (9): 1704-9, 1990.

20. Fenaux P, Chastang C, Chevret S, et al.: A randomized comparison of all transretinoic acid (ATRA) followed by chemotherapy and ATRA plus chemotherapy and the role of maintenance therapy in newly diagnosed acute promyelocytic leukemia. The European APL Group. *Blood* 94 (4): 1192-200, 1999.

21. Fenaux P, Chevret S, Guerci A, et al.: Long-term follow-up confirms the benefit of all-trans retinoic acid in acute promyelocytic leukemia. European APL group. *Leukemia* 14 (8): 1371-7, 2000.

22. Tallman MS, Andersen JW, Schiffer CA, et al.: All-trans-retinoic acid in acute promyelocytic leukemia. *N Engl J Med* 337 (15): 1021-8, 1997.

23. Powell B, Cancer and Leukemia Group B: Phase III Randomized Study of Tretinoin, Cytarabine, and Daunorubicin With or Without Arsenic Trioxide as Induction/Consolidation Therapy Followed by Intermittent Tretinoin With or Without Mercaptopurine and Methotrexate as Maintenance Therapy in Patients With Previously Untreated Acute Promyelocytic Leukemia, CLB-C9710, Clinical trial, Active.

24. Licht JD, Chomienne C, Goy A, et al.: Clinical and molecular characterization of a rare syndrome of acute promyelocytic leukemia associated with translocation (11;17). *Blood* 85 (4): 1083-94, 1995.

25. Guidez F, Ivins S, Zhu J, et al.: Reduced retinoic acid-sensitivities of nuclear receptor corepressor binding to PML- and PLZF-RARalpha underlie molecular pathogenesis and treatment of acute promyelocytic leukemia. *Blood* 91 (8): 2634-42, 1998.

26. Grimwade D, Biondi A, Mozziconacci MJ, et al.: Characterization of acute promyelocytic leukemia cases lacking the classic t(15;17): results of the European Working Party. Groupe Français de Cytogénétique Hématologique, Groupe de Français d'Hematologie Cellulaire, UK Cancer Cytogenetics Group and BIOMED 1 European Community-Concerted Action "Molecular Cytogenetic Diagnosis in Haematological Malignancies." *Blood* 96 (4): 1297-308, 2000.

27. Soignet SL, Maslak P, Wang ZG, et al.: Complete remission after treatment of acute promyelocytic leukemia with arsenic trioxide. *N Engl J Med* 339 (19): 1341-8, 1998.

28. Niu C, Yan H, Yu T, et al.: Studies on treatment of acute promyelocytic leukemia with arsenic trioxide: remission induction, follow-up, and molecular monitoring in 11 newly diagnosed and 47 relapsed acute promyelocytic leukemia patients. *Blood* 94 (10): 3315-24, 1999.

29. Zhang P: The use of arsenic trioxide (As2O3) in the treatment of acute promyelocytic leukemia. *J Biol Regul Homeost Agents* 13 (4): 195-200, 1999 Oct-Dec.

30. Unnikrishnan D, Dutcher JP, Varshneya N, et al.: Torsades de pointes in 3 patients with leukemia treated with arsenic trioxide. *Blood* 97 (5): 1514-6, 2001.

31. Barbey JT: Cardiac toxicity of arsenic trioxide. *Blood* 98 (5): 1632; discussion 1633-4, 2001.

32. Lange BJ, Kobrinsky N, Barnard DR, et al.: Distinctive demography, biology, and outcome of acute myeloid leukemia and myelodysplastic syndrome in children with Down syndrome: Children's Cancer Group Studies 2861 and 2891. *Blood* 91 (2): 608-15, 1998.

33. Ravindranath Y, Abella E, Krischer JP, et al.: Acute myeloid leukemia (AML) in Down's syndrome is highly responsive to chemotherapy: experience on Pediatric Oncology Group AML Study 8498. *Blood* 80 (9): 2210-4, 1992.

34. Passmore SJ, Hann IM, Stiller CA, et al.: Pediatric myelodysplasia: a study of 68 children and a new prognostic scoring system. *Blood* 85 (7): 1742-50, 1995.

35. Luna-Fineman S, Shannon KM, Atwater SK, et al.: Myelodys-plastic and myeloproliferative disorders of childhood: a study of 167 patients. *Blood* 93 (2): 459-66, 1999.

36. Woods WG, Barnard DR, Alonzo TA, et al.: Prospective study of 90 children requiring treatment for juvenile myelomono-cytic leukemia or myelodysplastic syndrome: a report from the Children's Cancer Group. *J Clin Oncol* 20 (2): 434-40, 2002.

37. Creutzig U, Bender-Götze C, Ritter J, et al.: The role of inten-sive AML-specific therapy in treatment of children with RAEB and RAEB-t. *Leukemia* 12 (5): 652-9, 1998.

38. Freedman MH, Estrov Z, Chan HS: Juvenile chronic myelog-enous leukemia. *Am J Pediatr Hematol Oncol* 10 (3): 261-7, 1988 Fall.

39. Castleberry RP, Emanuel PD, Zuckerman KS, et al.: A pilot study of isotretinoin in the treatment of juvenile chronic myel-ogenous leukemia. *N Engl J Med* 331 (25): 1680-4, 1994.

40. Sanders JE, Buckner CD, Thomas ED, et al.: Allogeneic mar-row transplantation for children with juvenile chronic myelog-enous leukemia. *Blood* 71 (4): 1144-6, 1988.

41. Smith FO, King R, Nelson G, et al.: The National Marrow Do-nor Program: Unrelated donor bone marrow transplantation for children with juvenile myelomonocytic leukaemia. *Br J Haematol* 116 (3): 716-24, 2002.

42. Aricò M, Biondi A, Pui CH: Juvenile myelomonocytic leuke-mia. *Blood* 90 (2): 479-88, 1997.

Childhood Acute Myeloid Leukemia in Remission

Post-Remission Therapy

A major challenge in the treatment of children with acute myeloid leukemia (AML) is to prolong the duration of the initial remission with additional chemotherapy or bone marrow transplantation (BMT). In practice, most patients are treated with intensive chemotherapy after remission is achieved, as only a small subset have a matched-family donor. Such therapy includes the drugs used in induction and often includes high-dose cytarabine. Studies in adults with AML have demonstrated that consolidation with a high-dose cytarabine regimen improves outcome compared to consolidation with a standard-dose cytarabine regimen.[1,2] Randomized studies evaluating the contribution of high-dose cytarabine to post-remission therapy have not been conducted in children, but studies employing historical controls suggest that consolidation with a high-dose cytarabine regimen improves outcome compared to less intensive consolidation therapies.[3-5]

The use of BMT in first remission has been under evaluation since the late 1970s. Recent prospective trials of transplantation in children with AML suggest that greater than 60% to 70% of children with matched donors available who undergo allogeneic bone marrow transplantation during their first remission experience long-term remissions.[6,7] Prospective trials of allogeneic transplantation compared to chemotherapy and/or autologous transplantation have demonstrated a superior outcome for patients who were assigned to allogeneic transplantation based on availability of a family 6/6 or 5/6 donor.[6-10] In the MRC trial the difference (70% vs. 60%) did not reach statistical significance but the numbers of patients enrolled did not give the study the power to demonstrate this difference.[7] Several large cooperative group clinical trials for children with AML have found no benefit for BMT over intensive chemotherapy. [6-8, 10]

Two approaches have emerged for the use of allogeneic BMT in first remission. In the first approach, patients with favorable prognostic features at diagnosis are transplanted only after relapse. The Berlin-Frankfurt-Munster (BFM) group uses a combination of day 15 marrow response (<5% blasts), FAB subtype (M1 and M2 with Auer Rods, M3, or M4Eo) to define a good risk group.[11] Similarly, the United Kingdom Medical Research Council (MRC) has identified a group of good risk patients with a 7-year survival of 78%. The patients in this group include those with t(8;21), t(15;17), FAB M3, inv 16.[7] This most likely identifies an equivalent group of patients included in BFM standard risk group. The second approach is to offer allogeneic BMT to all patients who have a suitable donor. The current Children's Oncology Group (COG) studies assign all patients with suitable matched family donors to bone marrow transplantation. Of note, patients with Down syndrome, APL and FAB M3 or t(15;17), are treated on a separate protocol. The role of alternative donor transplants (unrelated marrow or cord blood) in first remission of AML has not been established. Although maintenance chemotherapy has been incorporated into pediatric AML therapy and continues to be used in BFM trials, no data demonstrate that maintenance therapy given after intensive post-remission therapy significantly prolongs remission duration.

References

1. Mayer RJ, Davis RB, Schiffer CA, et al.: Intensive post-remission chemotherapy in adults with acute myeloid leukemia. Cancer and Leukemia Group B. *N Engl J Med* 331 (14): 896-903, 1994.

2. Cassileth PA, Lynch E, Hines JD, et al.: Varying intensity of postremission therapy in acute myeloid leukemia. *Blood* 79 (8): 1924-30, 1992.

3. Wells RJ, Woods WG, Buckley JD, et al.: Treatment of newly diagnosed children and adolescents with acute myeloid leukemia: a Childrens Cancer Group study. *J Clin Oncol* 12 (11): 2367-77, 1994.

4. Wells RJ, Woods WG, Lampkin BC, et al.: Impact of high-dose cytarabine and asparaginase intensification on childhood acute myeloid leukemia: a report from the Childrens Cancer Group. *J Clin Oncol* 11 (3): 538-45, 1993.

5. Creutzig U, Ritter J, Zimmermann M, et al.: Improved treatment results in high-risk pediatric acute myeloid leukemia patients after intensification with high-dose cytarabine and mitoxantrone: results of Study Acute Myeloid Leukemia-Berlin-Frankfurt-Münster 93. *J Clin Oncol* 19 (10): 2705-13, 2001.

6. Woods WG, Neudorf S, Gold S, et al.: Children's Cancer Group: A comparison of allogeneic bone marrow transplantation, autologous bone marrow transplantation, and aggressive chemotherapy in children with acute myeloid leukemia in remission. *Blood* 97 (1): 56-62, 2001.

7. Stevens RF, Hann IM, Wheatley K, et al.: Marked improvements in outcome with chemotherapy alone in paediatric acute myeloid leukemia: results of the United Kingdom Medical Research Council's 10th AML trial. MRC Childhood Leukaemia Working Party. *Br J Haematol* 101 (1): 130-40, 1998.

8. Ravindranath Y, Yeager AM, Chang MN, et al.: Autologous bone marrow transplantation versus intensive consolidation chemotherapy for acute myeloid leukemia in childhood. Pediatric Oncology Group. *N Engl J Med* 334 (22): 1428-34, 1996.

9. Feig SA, Lampkin B, Nesbit ME, et al.: Outcome of BMT during first complete remission of AML: a comparison of two sequential studies by the Children's Cancer Group. *Bone Marrow Transplant* 12 (1): 65-71, 1993.

10. Amadori S, Testi AM, Aricò M, et al.: Prospective comparative study of bone marrow transplantation and postremission chemotherapy for childhood acute myelogenous leukemia. The Associazione Italiana Ematologia ed Oncologia Pediatrica Cooperative Group. *J Clin Oncol* 11 (6): 1046-54, 1993.

11. Creutzig U, Ritter J, Zimmermann M, et al.: Idarubicin improves blast cell clearance during induction therapy in children with AML: results of study AML-BFM 93. AML-BFM Study Group. *Leukemia* 15 (3): 348-54, 2001.

12. Lange BJ, Children's Oncology Group: Phase III Randomized Study of Intensively Timed Induction Chemotherapy Followed By Consolidation With the Same Chemotherapy Versus Fludarabine, Cytarabine, and Idarubicin, Followed By Intensification With Either High-Dose Cytarabine and Asparaginase With or Without Subsequent Interleukin-2 or Allogeneic Bone Marrow Transplantation in Children With Previously Untreated Acute Myelogenous Leukemia or Myelodysplastic Syndromes, COG-2961, Clinical trial, Closed.

13. Sievers EL, Lange BJ, Sondel PM, et al.: Children's cancer group trials of interleukin-2 therapy to prevent relapse of acute myelogenous leukemia. *Cancer J Sci Am* 6 Suppl 1:S39-44, 2000.

14. Sievers EL, Lange BJ, Sondel PM, et al.: Feasibility, toxicity, and biologic response of interleukin-2 after consolidation chemotherapy for acute myelogenous leukemia: a report from the Children's Cancer Group. *J Clin Oncol* 16 (3): 914-9, 1998.

Recurrent Childhood Acute Myeloid Leukemia

Despite second remission induction in about one-half of children with acute myeloid leukemia (AML) treated with drugs similar to drugs used in initial induction therapy, the prognosis for a child with recurrent or progressive AML is generally poor.[1] Approximately 50% to 60% of relapses occur within the first year following diagnosis with most relapses occurring by 4 years from diagnosis.[1] The vast majority of relapses occur in the bone marrow, with CNS relapse being very uncommon.[1] Length of first remission is an important factor affecting the ability to attain a second remission—children with a first remission of less than 1 year have substantially lower rates of remission than children whose first remission is greater than 1 year (<50% versus 70%-80%, respectively).[2,3] Survival for children with shorter first remissions is also substantially lower (approximately 10%) than that for children with first remissions exceeding one year (approximately 40%).[2,3]

Regimens that have been successfully used to induce remission in children with recurrent AML have commonly included high-dose cytarabine given in combination with other agents, including mitoxantrone,[4] fludarabine plus idarubicin,[5,6] and L-asparaginase.[7] The standard-dose cytarabine regimens used in the MRC AML 10 study for newly diagnosed children with AML (cytarabine plus daunorubicin plus either etoposide or thioguanine) have produced remission rates similar to those achieved with high-dose cytarabine regimens.[3]

For children with recurrent acute promyelocytic leukemia (APL), the use of arsenic trioxide or regimens including all-trans retinoic acid should be considered, depending on the therapy given during first remission. Arsenic trioxide is an active agent in patients with recurrent APL, with 70% to 90% of patients achieving remission following treatment with this agent.[8,9] There are limited data on the use of arsenic trioxide in children, though published reports suggest that children with APL have a response to arsenic trioxide similar to that of adults.[8,10] Because arsenic trioxide causes Q-T interval prolongation that can lead to life-threatening arrhythmias (e.g., torsades de pointes),[11] it is essential to monitor electrolytes closely in patients receiving arsenic trioxide and to maintain potassium and magnesium values at mid-normal ranges.[12]

The selection of further treatment following the achievement of a second remission depends on prior treatment as well as individual considerations. Consolidation chemotherapy followed by stem cell transplantation is often employed, though there is no definitive data as to the contribution of these modalities to the long-term cure of children with recurrent AML.[1] Clinical trials, including new chemotherapy and/or biologic agents and/or novel bone marrow transplant (autologous, matched or mismatched unrelated donor, cord blood) programs, should be considered.

References

1. Webb DK: Management of relapsed acute myeloid leukaemia. *Br J Haematol* 106 (4): 851-9, 1999.

2. Stahnke K, Boos J, Bender-Götze C, et al.: Duration of first remission predicts remission rates and long-term survival in children with relapsed acute myelogenous leukemia. *Leukemia* 12 (10): 1534-8, 1998.

3. Webb DK, Wheatley K, Harrison G, et al.: Outcome for children with relapsed acute myeloid leukaemia following initial therapy in the Medical Research Council (MRC) AML 10 trial. MRC Childhood Leukaemia Working Party. *Leukemia* 13 (1): 25-31, 1999.

4. Wells RJ, Odom LF, Gold SH, et al.: Cytosine arabinoside and mitoxantrone treatment of relapsed or refractory childhood leukemia: initial response and relationship to multidrug resistance gene 1. *Med Pediatr Oncol* 22 (4): 244-9, 1994.

5. Dinndorf PA, Avramis VI, Wiersma S, et al.: Phase I/II study of idarubicin given with continuous infusion fludarabine followed by continuous infusion cytarabine in children with acute leukemia: a report from the Children's Cancer Group. *J Clin Oncol* 15 (8): 2780-5, 1997.

6. Fleischhack G, Hasan C, Graf N, et al.: IDA-FLAG (idarubicin, fludarabine, cytarabine, G-CSF), an effective remission-induction therapy for poor-prognosis AML of childhood prior to allogeneic or autologous bone marrow transplantation: experiences of a phase II trial. *Br J Haematol* 102 (3): 647-55, 1998.

7. Capizzi RL, Davis R, Powell B, et al.: Synergy between high-dose cytarabine and asparaginase in the treatment of adults with refractory and relapsed acute myelogenous leukemia—a Cancer and Leukemia Group B Study. *J Clin Oncol* 6 (3): 499-508, 1988.

8. Soignet SL, Maslak P, Wang ZG, et al.: Complete remission after treatment of acute promyelocytic leukemia with arsenic trioxide. *N Engl J Med* 339 (19): 1341-8, 1998.

9. Niu C, Yan H, Yu T, et al.: Studies on treatment of acute promyelocytic leukemia with arsenic trioxide: remission induction, follow-up, and molecular monitoring in 11 newly diagnosed and 47 relapsed acute promyelocytic leukemia patients. *Blood* 94 (10): 3315-24, 1999.

10. Zhang P: The use of arsenic trioxide (As2O3) in the treatment of acute promyelocytic leukemia. *J Biol Regul Homeost Agents* 13 (4): 195-200, 1999 Oct-Dec.

11. Unnikrishnan D, Dutcher JP, Varshneya N, et al.: Torsades de pointes in 3 patients with leukemia treated with arsenic trioxide. *Blood* 97 (5): 1514-6, 2001.

12. Barbey JT: Cardiac toxicity of arsenic trioxide. *Blood* 98 (5): 1632; discussion 1633-4, 2001.

Additional Information

St. Jude Children's Research Hospital
332 N. Lauderdale Street
Memphis, TN 38101
Tel: 901-495-3306
Website: www.stjude.org

National Cancer Institute
6166 Executive Blvd., MSC 8322
Suite 3036A
Bethesda, MD 20892-8322
Toll-Free: 800-422-6237
Toll-Free TTY: 800-332-8615
Website: www.cancer.gov

Chapter 14

Statistics of Childhood Leukemia

In the United States, approximately 8,600 children were diagnosed with cancer and about 1,500 children died from the disease in 2001. While this makes cancer the leading cause of death by disease among U.S. children under age 15, cancer is still relatively rare in this age group, with, on average, 1 to 2 children developing the disease each year for every 10,000 children in the United States.

Among the 12 major types of childhood cancers, leukemias (blood cell cancers) and brain and other central nervous system tumors account for over one-half of the new cases. About one-third of childhood cancers are leukemias; approximately 2,700 children (younger than 15 years) were diagnosed with leukemia in 2001. The most common type of leukemia in children is acute lymphocytic leukemia. The most common solid tumors are brain tumors (e.g., gliomas and medulloblastomas), with other solid tumors (e.g., neuroblastomas, Wilms' tumors, and rhabdomyosarcomas) being less common.

Over the past 20 years, there has been some increase in the incidence of children diagnosed with all forms of invasive cancer; from 11.4 cases per 100,000 children in 1975 to 15.2 per 100,000 children in 1998. During this same time, however, death rates declined dramatically and survival increased for most childhood cancers. For example, the five-year survival rates for all childhood cancers combined increased from 55.7 percent in 1974–76 to 77.1 percent in 1992–97.

"National Cancer Institute Research on Childhood Cancers," Fact Sheet 6.40, National Cancer Institute (NCI), reviewed 2/12/2002.

This improvement in survival rates is due to significant advances in treatment, resulting in cure or long-term remission for a substantial proportion of children with cancer.

Long-term trends in incidence for leukemias and brain tumors, the most common childhood cancers, show a somewhat different pattern than the others. Childhood leukemias appeared to increase in incidence in the early 1980s, with rates in the preceding years at fewer than 4 cases per 100,000. Rates in the succeeding years have shown no consistent upward or downward trend and have ranged from 3.8 to 4.8 cases per 100,000.

For childhood brain tumors, the overall incidence rose from 1975 through 1998 (from 2.3 to 3.0 per 100,000), with the greatest increase occurring from 1983 through 1986. An article in the September 2, 1998, issue of the *Journal of the National Cancer Institute* suggests that the rise in incidence from 1983 through 1986 may not have represented a true increase in the number of cases, but may have reflected new forms of imaging equipment (magnetic resonance imaging or MRI) that enabled visualization of brain tumors that could not be easily visualized with older equipment. Other important developments during the 1983–86 period included the changing classification of brain tumors that resulted in tumors previously designated as benign being reclassified as malignant, and improvements in neurosurgical techniques in biopsy of brain tumors.

The causes of childhood cancers are largely unknown. A few conditions, such as Down syndrome, other specific chromosomal and genetic abnormalities, and ionizing radiation exposures, explain a small percentage of cases.

Environmental causes of childhood cancer have long been suspected by many scientists but have been difficult to pin down, partly because cancer in children is rare, and partly because it is so difficult to identify past exposure levels in children, particularly during potentially important periods such as pregnancy or even prior to conception. In addition, each of the distinctive types of childhood cancers develops differently—with a potentially wide variety of causes and a unique clinical course in terms of age, race, gender, and many other factors.

Results from Recent Studies Supported by the NCI

For several decades, the NCI has supported national and international collaborations devoted to studying causes of cancer in children. Some of the key findings from recent studies include:

- High levels of ionizing radiation from accidents or from radio-therapy have been linked with increased risk of some childhood cancers;

- Children treated with chemotherapy and radiation therapy for certain forms of childhood and adolescent cancers, such as Hodgkin's disease, brain tumors, sarcomas, and others, may develop a second primary malignancy;

- Low levels of radiation exposure from radon were not significantly associated with childhood leukemias;

- Ultrasound use during pregnancy has not been linked with childhood cancer in numerous large studies;

- Residential magnetic field exposure from power lines was not significantly associated with childhood leukemias;

- Certain types of chemotherapy drugs, including drugs that are alkylating agents or topoisomerase II inhibitors (e.g., epipodophyllotoxins), may cause increased risk of leukemia;

- Pesticides have been suspected to be involved in the development of certain forms of childhood cancer based on interview data. However, interview results have been somewhat inconsistent, and have not yet been validated by physical evidence of pesticides in the child's body or environment;

- No consistent findings have been observed linking specific occupational exposures of parents to the development of childhood cancers;

- Several studies have found no link between maternal cigarette smoking before pregnancy and childhood cancers, but increased risks were related to the father's prenatal smoking habits in studies in the United Kingdom and China;

- Little evidence has been found to link specific viruses or other infectious agents to the development of most types of childhood cancers, though investigators worldwide are exploring the role of exposure of very young children to some common infectious agents that may protect children from, or put them at risk for, developing certain leukemias;

- Recent research has shown that children with AIDS, like AIDS-stricken adults, have an increased risk of developing certain

159

cancers, predominantly non-Hodgkin's lymphoma and Kaposi's sarcoma. These children also have an additional risk of developing leiomyosarcoma (a type of muscle cancer);

- Specific genetic syndromes, such as the Li-Fraumeni syndrome, neurofibromatosis, and several others, have been linked to an increased risk of specific childhood cancers.

NCI's Current Research on Childhood Cancer

NCI is currently funding a large portfolio of studies (http://research portfolio.cancer.gov/) looking at the causes and most effective treatments for childhood cancers at an estimated cost of $128 million for the Fiscal Year 2001. Ongoing investigations include:

Studies to Identify Causes of the Cancers That Develop in Children

The Children's Oncology Group (www.childrensoncologygroup.org) is evaluating potential risk factors for a variety of childhood cancers. Very large studies of childhood acute lymphoblastic leukemia, acute myeloid leukemia, non-Hodgkin's lymphoma, primitive neuroectodermal tumors of the brain, astrocytoma, and neuroblastoma have recently been completed, while investigations of germ cell tumors are ongoing. These studies have included evaluation of diverse categories of suspected and possible risk factors including exposures linked to infectious agents (e.g., enrollment in daycare, spacing of siblings, and infectious diseases contracted during the first 12 months of life); parental occupational exposures to radiation or chemicals; parental medical conditions during pregnancy or before conception; parental, fetal, or childhood exposures to environmental toxins such as pesticides, solvents, or other household chemicals; maternal diet during pregnancy; early postnatal feeding patterns and dietary factors; reproductive history and other reproductive factors; and familial and genetic factors. The role of maternal exposures to oral contraceptives, fertility drugs, and diethylstilbestrol (DES) is being investigated in several ongoing studies. Researchers are looking at the role of familial and genetic disorders. The cancer risk of HIV-infected children is under investigation. The Childhood Cancer Survivor Study is evaluating the risks of second cancer related to ionizing radiation and chemotherapy received by survivors of childhood cancer as part of treatment for their primary cancer.

Monitoring of U.S. and International Trends in Incidence and Mortality Rates for Childhood Cancers

By identifying places where high or low cancer rates occur, researchers can uncover patterns of cancer that provide important clues for further in-depth studies into the causes and control of cancer.

Studies to Better Understand the Biology of Childhood Cancer

The hope is that this understanding will lead to new treatment approaches that target critical cellular processes required for cancer cell growth and survival. Researchers are investigating fundamental cellular processes, such as signal transduction, cell cycle control, transcriptional regulation, and tumor suppressor gene inactivation, to develop new prevention and treatment strategies.

Projects Designed to Improve the Health Status of Survivors of Childhood Cancers

A major component of NCI's survivorship research efforts is the Childhood Cancer Survivor Study (CCSS), which was created to learn about the long-term effects of cancer and its therapy on childhood cancer survivors (http://www.cancer.umn.edu/ltfu#CCSS). This knowledge may be useful in designing future treatment protocols and intervention strategies that increase survival and minimize harmful health effects. In addition, CCSS serves to educate survivors about the potential impacts of cancer diagnosis and treatment on their health. CCSS includes 14,000 childhood cancer survivors diagnosed with cancer before the age of 20 between 1970 and 1986 and approximately 3,500 siblings of survivors who serve as control subjects for the study. The CCSS cohort has been assembled through the efforts of 27 participating centers in the United States and Canada and is coordinated by investigators at the University of Minnesota. Initiated in 1993, the study has been funded by the NCI for continuation through 2004.

Clinical Trials

Clinical trials hope to identify superior treatments for childhood cancers, thereby leading to improved survival rates for children with cancer. Each year about 4,000 children enter 1 of approximately 100 ongoing clinical trials sponsored by NCI. The following groups are conducting these trials:

- Children's Oncology Group (COG) (www.childrensoncology group.org). COG is supported by NCI to conduct clinical trials devoted exclusively to children and adolescents with cancer at more than 200 member institutions, including cancer centers of all major universities, teaching hospitals throughout the United States and Canada, and sites in Europe and Australia. COG was formed in 2000 by the merger of four children's cancer cooperative groups in order to accelerate the search for a cure for the cancers of children and to make it possible for children with cancer, regardless of where they live, to have access to state-of-the art therapies and the collective expertise of world-renowned pediatric specialists.

- Pediatric Brain Tumor Consortium (PBTC) (http://www.pbtc. org). The primary objective of the PBTC is to rapidly conduct phase I and II clinical evaluations of new therapeutic drugs, intrathecal agents (agents injected into the cerebrospinal fluid), delivery technologies, biological therapies, and radiation treatment strategies in children up to 21 years of age with primary central nervous system (CNS) tumors. The PBTC includes nine leading academic institutions with extensive experience in the design and conduct of clinical trials for children with brain tumors. Another objective of the PBTC is to develop and coordinate innovative neuro-imaging techniques. Results from PBTC studies are made available to large international collaborative groups for confirmatory phase II and multi-agent phase III clinical trials.

- New Approaches to Neuroblastoma Therapy Consortium (NANT) (www.nant.org). NANT is a consortium of university and children's hospitals funded by the NCI to test promising new therapies for neuroblastoma. NANT members constitute a group of closely collaborating investigators linked with laboratory programs where novel therapies for high-risk neuroblastoma are being developed. The group conducts early trials to test new drugs and new combinations of drugs so that promising therapies can be tested nationally.

Evaluations of New Drugs

Evaluations are made of new drugs that may be more effective against childhood cancers and that may have less toxicity for children.

The Children's Oncology Group Phase I/Pilot Consortium is a major component of the NCI's pediatric drug development program (www.childrensoncologygroup.org). The primary objective of the consortium is to develop and implement pediatric phase I and pilot studies in order to promote the integration of advances in cancer biology and therapy into the treatment of childhood cancer. The consortium includes approximately 20 institutions that carefully monitor the drugs for toxicity and safety. After their initial evaluation for safety in children by the consortium, the agents and regimens can then be studied within the larger group of COG institutions to determine their role in the treatment of specific childhood cancers.

NCI's Future Investments

NCI is supporting a pilot study by the COG to evaluate the feasibility of establishing a Childhood Cancer Research Network that would create a national registry of children with cancer, including a tissue bank for tumor and blood specimens, to be used for identifying environmental and other causes of childhood cancer. This initiative seeks to build on the unique national clinical trials system for treating children with cancer.

Additional Information

National Cancer Institute
6166 Executive Blvd., MSC 8322
Suite 3036A
Bethesda, MD 20892-8322
Toll-Free: 800-422-6237
Toll-Free TTY: 800-332-8615
Website: www.cancer.gov

Chapter 15

Procedures That Diagnose and Treat Children with Leukemia

Understanding what will occur during a procedure and what other parents do to prepare their children will arm you with essential information. Knowing what to expect will lower the anxiety level of both you and your child and lay the foundation for years of tolerable tests. The descriptions of procedures in this chapter may not exactly mirror your experience. Practices vary by hospital and practitioner and this variability should be expected. What should be the same, however, is your comfort in asking questions and getting the support and help you need to prepare for and cope with your child's procedures.

Questions to Ask before Procedures

You need information prior to procedures in order to prepare yourself and your child. Some suggested questions to ask the physician are:

- Why is this procedure necessary and how will it affect my child's treatment?
- What information will it provide?
- Who will perform the procedure?
- Will it be an inpatient or outpatient procedure?

- Please explain the procedure in detail.
- Is there any literature available that describes it?
- Is there a child life specialist on staff who will help prepare my child for the procedure?
- Is the procedure painful?
- What type of anesthetic or sedation is used?
- What are the risks, if any?
- What are the common and rare side effects?
- When will we get the results?

Bone Marrow Aspiration

Protocols for children with leukemia require bone marrow aspirations, a process by which bone marrow is sucked out with a needle. The purpose of the first, or diagnostic, bone marrow aspiration is to see what percentage of the cells in the marrow are abnormal blasts. Then these cells are analyzed microscopically to determine which type of leukemia is present. The next bone marrow aspiration occurs on day seven or fourteen of treatment. At this time it is important to determine how many blasts are still present. This information helps the oncologists decide how intensive treatment should be. For instance, if the marrow shows less than 25 percent blasts, the child might continue on the intermediate-risk protocol. But if the marrow is still crowded with blasts, the child might be described as a "slow responder," who would require a more intensive course of treatment.

> Since the doctors knew that my daughter had leukemia from the blood work, they did her first bone marrow while she was under anesthesia to implant her Port-a-cath. This was a blessing as her marrow was packed tight with blasts.

Most centers require additional bone marrow aspirations at the end of each phase of treatment and at the end of maintenance (or post-remission treatment, if your child does not require the maintenance phase).

To obtain a sample of the bone marrow, doctors usually use the iliac crest of the hip (the top of the hip bone in back or front). This bone is right under the skin and contains a large amount of marrow.

The child is placed face down on a table, sometimes on a pillow to elevate the hip. The doctor will feel the site, then wipe it several times with an antiseptic to eliminate any germs. Sterile paper may be placed around the site, and the doctor will wear sterile gloves. Then an anesthetic (usually Xylocaine) may be injected into the skin and a small area of bone. This causes a burning and stinging sensation that passes quickly. The physician usually rubs the area to allow the drug to fully anesthetize the area. The physician then pushes a hollow needle (with a plug inside) through the skin into the bone, withdraws the plug, and attaches a syringe. The liquid marrow is then aspirated (sucked out) through the syringe. After a sample is obtained, the needle is removed and a bandage is put on.

If the child or teen is not sedated, removing the marrow can be very painful. Here are some descriptions from children and adult survivors who have experienced it:

> *It was the worst thing of all. It felt really, really bad.*

> *It hurts a lot. It feels like they are pulling something out and then it aches. You know, it hurts so much that now they put the kids to sleep. Boy, am I glad about that.*

> *It feels like they are trying to suck thick Jell-O from inside the bone. Brief but incredible pain.*

> *I would become very anxious when they were cleaning my skin and laying the towels down. Putting the needle in was a sharp, pressure kind of pain. Drawing the marrow feels tingly, like they hit a nerve. I always asked a nurse to hold my legs because I felt like my legs were going to jump up off the table.*

Spinal Tap (Lumbar Puncture or LP)

Due to the blood-brain barrier, systemic chemotherapy usually cannot destroy any blasts in the central nervous system (brain and spinal cord). Chemotherapy drugs must be directly injected into the cerebrospinal fluid in order to kill any blasts present and prevent a possible central nervous system relapse. The drugs most commonly used intrathecally are methotrexate, ARA-C, and hydrocortisone. The number of spinal taps required varies depending on the child's risk level, the clinical study involved, and whether radiation is used.

Some hospitals routinely sedate children for spinal taps, and others do not. If the child is not sedated, EMLA cream is usually prescribed.

EMLA is an anesthetic cream put on the spinal tap site one to two hours prior to the procedure. It anesthetizes deep into the tissue, preventing some or all of the pain associated with the procedure.

To perform a spinal tap, the physician or nurse practitioner will ask the child to lie on her side with her head tucked close to the chest and knees drawn up. A nurse or parent usually helps hold the child in this position. The doctor will feel the designated spot in the lower back, and will swab it with antiseptic several times. The antiseptic feels very cold on the skin. A sterile sheet may drape the area, and the doctor will wear sterile gloves. One or two shots of an anesthetic (usually Xylocaine) may be injected into the skin and deeper tissues. This causes a painful stinging or burning sensation that lasts about a minute. If EMLA was used, the doctor may still inject anesthetic into the deep tissues. A few minutes wait is necessary to ensure that the area is fully anesthetized.

My four-year-old daughter had finished eighteen months of her treatment for ALL when EMLA was first prescribed. She had been terrified of going to the clinic. After using EMLA for her next LP, a dramatic change occurred. She was no longer frightened to go for treatment, and her behavior at home improved unbelievably. We use it for everything now: finger pokes, accessing port, bone marrows, even flu shots.

It is essential that the child hold very still for the rest of the procedure. The doctor will push a needle between two vertebrae into the space where cerebrospinal fluid (CSF) is found. The CSF will begin to drip out of the hollow needle into a container. After a small amount is collected, a syringe is attached to the needle in the back and the medicine is slowly injected, causing a sensation of coldness or pressure down the leg. The needle is then removed and the spot bandaged. The CSF is sent to the laboratory to see if any cancer cells are present and to measure glucose and protein. Occasionally, older children and teenagers get severe headaches from spinal taps. These can sometimes be prevented by lying still for up to an hour after the procedure.

During spinals, Brent listens to rock and roll on his Walkman, but he keeps the volume low enough so that he can still hear what is going on. He likes me to lift up the earpiece and tell him when each part of the procedure is finished and what's coming next.

Starting an IV

Most children with leukemia have a permanent right atrial catheter implanted in their chest within a week after diagnosis to avoid the pain of years of IV sticks. However, some physicians do not recommend catheters, and there are many medical reasons why surgery for a catheter may be postponed. Even if your child has a catheter, there may be times when your child will need an intravenous line started, as well.

Most pediatric hospitals have teams of technicians who specialize in starting IVs and drawing blood. The IV technician will generally use a vein in the lower arm or hand. First, a constricting band is put above the site to make the veins larger and easier to see and feel. The vein is felt by the technician, the area is cleaned, and the needle is inserted. Sometimes a needle is left in place and sometimes it is withdrawn, leaving only a thin plastic tube in the vein. The technician will make sure that the needle (or tube) is in the proper place, then cover the site with a clear dressing and secure it with tape.

Some methods that help when having an IV started are:

- **Stay calm.** The body reacts to fear by constricting the blood vessels near the skin surface. Small children are usually more calm with a parent present; teenagers may or may not desire privacy. Listening to music, visualizing a tranquil scene (mountains covered with snow, floating in a pool), or using the same technician each time can help.

- **Use EMLA cream.** EMLA—a cream anesthetic—is applied to the skin one hour prior to the procedure to prevent pain. In some cases, it can constrict the veins, so experiment to see if it works for your child.

- **Keep warm.** Cold temperatures also cause the surface blood vessels to constrict. Wrapping the child in a blanket and putting a hot water bottle on the arm can enlarge the veins.

- **Drink lots of fluids.** Dehydration decreases the fluid in the veins, so encourage lots of drinking.

- **Let gravity help.** If the child is lying in bed, have her hang her arm down over the side to increase the size of the vessels in the arm and hand.

- **Let the child be in control.** If the child has a preference, let him pick the arm to be stuck. If the child is a veteran of many IVs, let him point out the best vein.

- **Stop if problems develop.** The art of treating children is lots of time on preparation and not much time on procedures. If a conflict arises, take a time-out and regroup. Children can be remarkably cooperative if their needs are respected and they are given some control over the situation.

You'll think I'm crazy, but I'll tell you this story anyway. After getting stuck constantly for a year, my daughter (five years old) just lost it one day when she needed an IV. She started screaming and crying, just flew into a rage. I told the tech, "Let's just let her calm down. Why don't you stick me for a change?" She was a sport and started a line in my arm. I told my daughter that I had forgotten how much it hurt and I could understand why she was upset. I told her to let us know when she was ready. She just walked over and held out her arm.

Subcutaneous Injections

Some children require medications given by subcutaneous injection during their treatment. For example, Neupogen (G-CSF), a colony-stimulating factor that is often used to boost the white blood cell count, and methotrexate are usually given by injection.

To minimize pain caused by subcutaneous injections, apply EMLA cream one to two hours before administration. Parents can also reduce pain by rubbing ice over the site to numb the area prior to injection.

We always used EMLA cream before our son needed a subcutaneous injection. I think part of the benefit to him was pharmacological, and part of it was psychological. He just seemed to be more at ease with the injections when he knew the EMLA was applied a few hours before the needle was given.

My two boys have ALL. Brian and Kevin both receive[d] IM methotrexate as part of their protocols. Brian, because of his age (twelve), was very macho about it, used "freezy" spray to numb the thigh, then giggled or made funny faces while the methotrexate was pushed. He had no aftereffects. Kevin, only four when they began, still doesn't like them. There were three or four months of overlap, when both boys got shots at the same time every week. This made it easier for Kevin, but he still insisted on an ice pack and "freezy" spray. Now, he's graduated to doing it alone and uses the spray only.

Blood Draws

Frequent blood samples are a part of life during leukemia treatment. A complete blood count (CBC) tells the physician how effective the drugs are and helps determine the child's susceptibility to infection. It is important to measure blood chemistries to make sure that the liver and kidneys are not being damaged by treatment. During induction and consolidation, transfusions are necessary when the red cell count or platelet count gets too low.

Blood specimens are primarily used for three purposes: to obtain a CBC, evaluate blood chemistries, or culture the blood to check for infection. A CBC measures the types and numbers of cells in the blood. Blood chemistries measure substances contained in the blood plasma to determine if the liver and kidneys are functioning properly. Blood cultures help evaluate whether the child is developing a bacterial or fungal infection. If only a CBC is needed, a finger poke will provide enough blood. Blood chemistries or cultures require one or more vials of blood obtained from a vein in the arm or the right atrial catheter.

Blood is usually drawn from the large vein on the inside of the elbow using a procedure similar to starting an IV, except that the needle is removed rather than left in the arm. The advice for starting an IV also applies to drawing blood from the arm.

Catheters

Children with catheters usually have blood drawn from the catheter rather than the arm or finger.

Finger Pokes

Finger pokes are different from blood draws in several ways. First, EMLA can be used successfully. Put a blob of EMLA on the tip of the middle finger. Cover the fingertip with plastic wrap, and tape it on the finger. Another method is to buy long, thin balloons with a diameter a bit wider than the child's finger. Cut off the open end, leaving only enough balloon to cover the finger up to the first knuckle. Fill the tip of the balloon with EMLA and slide it on the fingertip. EMLA needs to be applied an hour before a finger poke to be effective. At the laboratory, remove the plastic wrap or balloon, wipe off the EMLA, and ask for a warm pack. Wrapping this heated pack around the finger for a few minutes opens the capillaries to allow the blood to flow out more readily. Now the child is ready for a pain-free finger poke.

The technician will hold the finger and quickly stick it with a small sharp instrument. Blood will be collected in narrow tubes or a small container. It is usually necessary for the technician to squeeze the fingertip to get enough blood. If EMLA is not used, the squeezing part is uncomfortable and the finger can ache for quite a while.

> *Even though we use EMLA, Katy (five years old) still becomes angry when she has to have a finger poke. I asked her why it was upsetting if there was no pain, and she replied, "It doesn't hurt my body anymore, but it still hurts my feelings."*

Blood Transfusions

Treatment for leukemia can cause severe anemia (a low number of oxygen-carrying red cells). The normal life of a red cell is three to four months and, as old cells die, the diseased (or suppressed by treatment) marrow cannot replace them. Many children require transfusions of red cells when first admitted, and periodically throughout treatment.

> *Whenever my son needed a transfusion, I brought along bags of coloring books, food, and toys. The number of VCRs at the clinic was limited, so I tried to make arrangements for one ahead of time. When anemic (hematocrit below 20 percent), he didn't have much energy, but by the end of the transfusion, his cheeks were rosy and he had tremendous vitality. It was hard to keep him still. After one unit (bag) of red cells, his hematocrit usually jumped up to around 30.*

One bag (called a unit) of red cells takes approximately two to four hours to administer and is given through an IV or catheter. If your child develops chills and/or fever during a transfusion, the nurse should be notified so that the transfusion can be stopped immediately.

There are some risks of infection from red cell transfusions. Since new tests have been devised to detect the AIDS virus, the risk of exposure is minuscule, less than 1 in 450,000. Although there are excellent tests for the various types of hepatitis, exposure to this disease is still possible (the risk is less than 1 in 4,000). Exposure to cytomegalovirus is also a concern. These risks are the reason transfusions are given only when absolutely necessary.

Platelet Transfusions

Platelets are an important component of the blood. They help form clots and stop bleeding by repairing breaks in the walls of blood vessels. A normal platelet count for a healthy child is 150,000/mm to 420,000/ mm. Chemotherapy can severely depress the platelet count for some children. If a transfusion is not given when counts are very low, uncontrollable bleeding can result. Many centers require a transfusion when the child's platelet count goes below 10,000 to 20,000/mm, and sometimes repeat transfusions are required every two or three days until the marrow recovers.

> *Brent (six years old) had several platelet transfusions during induction and consolidation. He had no problems and his counts would immediately jump up to around 40,000/mm.*

> *Three-year-old Matthew had countless platelet transfusions, and only once did he have a reaction. It was an awful thing to watch, but the nurse who was monitoring him was very calm and professional, which helped both of us. Matthew was always premedicated for his platelet transfusions with Benadryl, which made him very drowsy. Most often he would sleep through the entire transfusion.*

Infections transmitted by platelets are identical to those of other blood products: hepatitis, cytomegalovirus, and HIV (the virus that causes AIDS). The chance of contracting these infections, although small, is the reason that platelet transfusions are also given only when absolutely necessary. Because uncontrollable bleeding can be life threatening, prevention is paramount.

Taking Pills

When giving oral medications, it is essential to get off to a good start and establish cooperation early. In the following suggestions from veteran parents, you may find a technique that works well for your child.

> *To teach Brent (six years old) to swallow pills, when we were eating corn for dinner I encouraged him to swallow one kernel whole. Luckily, it went right down and he got over his fear of pills.*

> *I wanted Katy (three years old) to feel like we were a team right from the first night. So I made a big deal out of tasting each of*

her medications and pronouncing it good. Thank goodness I tasted the prednisone first. It was nauseating—bitter, metallic, with a lingering aftertaste. I asked the nurse for some small gel caps, and packed them with the pills which I had broken in half. I gave Katy her choice of drinks to take her pills with and taught her to swallow gel caps with a large sip of liquid. Since I gave her over 3,000 pills and 1,100 teaspoons of liquid medication during treatment, I'm very glad we got off to such a good start.

Gel caps come in many sizes. Number 4s are small enough for a three- or four-year-old to swallow, but big enough to hold half a 10 mg. prednisone tablet. Dexamethasone also tastes awful to many kids. Most of the other pills can be chewed or swallowed whole without taste problems. Just remember that children develop different taste preferences and aversions to medications, and gel caps are useful for any medication that bothers them.

After much trial and error with medications, Meagan's method became chewing up pills with chocolate chips. She's kept this up for the long haul.

I always give choices such as, "Do you want the white pill or the six yellow pills first?" It gives them a little control in their chaotic world.

For younger children, many parents crush the pills in a small amount of pudding, applesauce, jam, frozen juice concentrate, or other favorite food.

Jeremy was four when he was diagnosed, and we used to crush up the pills and mix them with ice cream. This worked well for us.

We used the liquid form of prednisone for my son, mixed it with a chocolate drink, and followed this with M&Ms. The chocolate seemed to mask the taste.

Most children on maintenance take SMZ-TMP (sulfamethoxazole and trimethoprim) three times a week to prevent pneumonia. The brand names are Bactrim or Septra. They come in liquid or pill form, and are produced by several different manufacturers. Ask your pharmacist (you'll know her quite well after a few years) for a kid taste test. Letting your child choose a medicine that appeals to him encourages compliance.

Whenever my son had to take a liquid medicine, such as antibiotics, he enjoyed taking it from a syringe. I would draw up the proper amount, then he would put it in his mouth and push the plunger.

Since children associate taking medicine with being sick, it is helpful to explain why they must continue taking pills for years after they feel well. Some parents use the Pac-man analogy, "The pills are needed to gobble up the last few bad cells." Others explain that the leukemia can return, so medicine is needed to prevent it from growing again. It is important that parents give children all the required medications; there are many studies showing low compliance results in lower survival rates.

Issues for teenagers about taking pills are completely different from those for young children. The problems with teens revolve around autonomy, control, and feelings of invulnerability. It is normal for teenagers to be noncompliant, and they cannot be forced to take pills if they choose not to cooperate. Trying to coerce teens fuels conflict and tends to frustrate everyone. If you need help, ask for an assessment by the psychosocial team at the hospital to work out a plan for adherence to treatment. Everyone will need to be flexible to reach a favorable outcome.

I think the main problem with teens is making sure that they take the meds. Joel (fifteen years old) has been very responsible about taking his nightly pills. I've tried to make it easy for him by having an index card for the week and he marks off the med as he takes it. I also put the meds on a dry erase board on the fridge as a reminder. As he takes the med, he erases it. That way it's easy for him (and me) to see at a glance if he's taken his stuff. The index card alone wasn't working because he couldn't find a pen or forgot to mark it off.

One of the biggest concerns with teens and maintenance is non-compliance. I think it's a delicate balancing act to allow the teen to be responsible for taking his own meds and yet have some supervision of the process. Our meds are kept in a small plastic basket on the kitchen counter. All meds are taken there. I'd never want him to keep his meds in his room where I would have no idea if he had taken them or not.

On Friday nights when he is to take his weekly methotrexate—a sixteen-pill dose—I will count it out and put it in a medicine cup

*on the counter. I am not always an awake and alert person when
he comes home at midnight on Friday night. When I get up Saturday morning, I know immediately if he's taken his meds.*

*If he had shown any resistance to taking the meds, or any sign of
telling me that he had taken them when he had not, I'd be doing
this differently. But he's aware of the importance of each dose
and the importance of his participation in the team beating the
leukemia.*

*My only other advice is to be sure and ask the doctors what to do
about a missed dose for each med. In three-plus years of treatment, you are going to have a missed dose and it helps to know
how to handle it.*

Taking a Temperature

In the years a child is treated for childhood leukemia, fever becomes
an enemy because it may signal the start of an infection. Parents take
hundreds of temperatures, often when their child is not feeling well.
Temperatures can be taken under the tongue, under the arm, or in
the ear using a special type of thermometer. Rectal temperatures are
not recommended due to the risk of tears and infection, especially
when the blood counts are depressed. Here are a few suggestions that
might help:

- Use a glass thermometer under the tongue.

- Digital thermometers can be purchased at any drug store. Some
  have an alarm that beeps when it is time to remove the thermometer.

  *We bought a digital thermometer that we only use under his
  arm. It has worked well for us.*

- Tympanic thermometers measure infrared waves and are very
  easy to use.

  *When my in-laws asked at diagnosis if there was anything that
  we needed, I asked them to try to buy a tympanic (ear) thermometer. The device cost over a hundred dollars then, but it worked
  beautifully. It takes only one second to obtain a temperature. You
  can even use it when she is asleep without waking her. They are
  now sold at pharmacies and drug stores, and cost much less.*

Before you leave the hospital, you should know when to call the clinic because of fever. Usually, parents are told not to give any medication for fever and to call if the fever goes above 101°F (38.5°C). It is especially important for parents of children with implanted catheters to know when to call the clinic, as an untreated infection can be life threatening.

Providing a Urine Specimen

Chemotherapy requires frequent urine specimens. One way to help obtain a sample is to encourage lots of drinking the hour before or ask the nurse to increase the drip rate on the IV. Explain to the child why the test is necessary. Ask the nurse to show how the dip sticks work (they change color, so they are quite popular with the preschoolers). Use a "hat" under the toilet seat. This is a shallow plastic bucket that fits under the seat and catches the urine.

Turn on the water while the child sits on the toilet. I don't know why it works, but it does.

As all parents learn, eating and elimination are areas that the child controls. If she just can't or won't urinate in the hat, go out, buy her the largest drink you can find, and wait.

Echocardiogram

Several drugs used to fight leukemia can damage the muscle of the heart, decreasing its ability to contract effectively. Many protocols require a baseline echocardiogram to measure the heart's ability to pump before any chemotherapy drugs are given. Echocardiograms are then given periodically during treatment and after treatment ends to see if any heart muscle damage has occurred.

An echocardiogram uses ultrasound waves to measure the amount of blood that leaves the heart each time it contracts. This percentage (blood ejected during a contraction compared to blood in the heart when it is relaxed) is called the ejection fraction.

The echocardiogram is performed by a technician, nurse, or doctor. The child or teen lies on a table and has conductive jelly applied to the chest. Then the technician puts a transducer (which emits the ultrasound waves) on the jelly and moves the device around on the chest to obtain different views of the heart. Pressure is applied on the transducer, and can sometimes cause mild discomfort. The test results are displayed on a videotape and photographed for later interpretation.

Meagan used to watch a video during the echocardiogram. Sometimes she would eat a sucker or a popsicle. She found it to be boring, not painful.

MUGA Scan

MUGA stands for multiple-gated acquisition scan; a MUGA scan is another way to test cardiac function. Prior to having a MUGA scan, children are sometimes given a sedative to relax and help them stay perfectly still for the fifteen- to twenty-minute test. An injection of red cells or proteins tagged with a mildly radioactive substance (called technetium) is also given. The child lies on a table with a large movable camera above. This special camera records sequential images of the technetium as it moves through the heart. These pictures of the heart's function allow doctors to determine how efficiently the heart muscle is pumping and if any damage to the heart has occurred.

My three-year-old daughter had a MUGA scan before she received any chemotherapy. They gave her an injection, and she fell asleep. They laid her on her back on a big table and moved a huge contraption around her to take pictures of her heart beating. We watched on a screen, and they printed out a copy on paper for the doctors.

If either the echocardiogram or MUGA scan shows heart damage, the oncologist may reduce the dosage or remove the drug causing the damage from the child's protocol.

Chapter 16

Guidelines for Parents of Children with Leukemia

When Your Child Is Diagnosed

After your child's leukemia has been diagnosed, a series of tests will be done to help identify your child's specific type of leukemia. Called staging, this series of tests is sometimes done during diagnosis. Staging determines how much cancer is in the body and where it is located. To stage leukemia, the doctor checks the bone marrow, liver, spleen, and lymph nodes around the sites where the leukemia can hide. Staging must be done to determine the best treatment. Many different tests can be used in staging, such as x-rays, MRIs, CT (or CAT) scans, and others. See Chapter 15, *Procedures That Diagnose and Treat Children with Leukemia* for a description of the various tests.

As soon as your child is suspected to have or is diagnosed with leukemia, you will face decisions about who will treat your child, whom to ask for a second opinion (if desired or if the diagnosis is not clear), and what the best treatment is. After your child's staging is complete, the treatment team develops a plan that outlines the exact type of treatment, how often your child will receive treatment, and how long it will last.

Talking with Your Child's Doctor

Your child's doctor and the treatment team will give you a lot of details about the type of leukemia and possible treatments. Ask your

Excerpts from "Young People with Cancer: A Handbook for Parents," National Cancer Institute (NCI), NIH Publication No. 01-2378, revised January 2001.

doctor to explain the treatment choices to you. It is important for you to become a partner with your treatment team in fighting your child's leukemia. One way for you to be actively involved is by asking questions. You may find it hard to concentrate on what the doctor says, remember everything you want to ask, or remember the answers to your questions. Here are some tips for talking with those who treat your child:

- Write your questions in a notebook and take it to the appointment with you. Record the answers to your questions and other important information.

- Tape record your conversations with your child's health care providers.

- Ask a friend or relative to come with you to the appointment. The friend or relative can help you ask questions and remember the answers.

Questions to Ask the Doctor and Treatment Team

When your child's treatment team gives you information about your child's leukemia, you may not remember everything. That is natural. It is a lot of information, and your emotions will get in the way as you try to take it all in. Use the three techniques listed—write, tape record, and ask a friend for help—to help you retain the information you need to be an effective partner with your child's treatment team. Make sure you know the answers to these questions:

About the Diagnosis

- What kind of leukemia does my child have?

- What is the stage, or extent, of the disease?

- Will any more tests be needed? Will they be painful? How often will they be done?

About Treatment Choices

- What are the treatment choices? Which do you recommend for my child? Why?

- Would a clinical trial be right for my child? Why?

- Have you treated other children with this type of leukemia? How many?

- What are the chances that the treatment will work?

- Where is the best place for my child to receive treatment? Are there specialists—such as surgeons, radiologists, nurses, anesthesiologists, and others—trained in pediatrics? Can my child have some or all of the treatment in our hometown?

About the Treatment

- How long will the treatment last?

- What will be the treatment schedule?

- Whom should we ask about the details of financial matters?

- Will the treatment disrupt my child's school schedule?

About Side Effects

- What possible side effects of the treatment can occur, both right away and later?

- What can be done to help if side effects occur?

About the Treatment Location

- How long will my child be in the hospital?

- Can any treatment be done at home? Will we need any special equipment?

- Does the hospital have a place where I can stay overnight during my child's treatment?

About School and Other Activities

- Is there a child-life worker specialist (a professional who is responsible for making the hospital and treatment experience less scary for the child) to plan play therapy, schoolwork, and other activities?

- When can my child go back to school?

- Are there certain diseases my child cannot be around? Should I have my child and his or her siblings immunized against any diseases?

- Will my child need tutoring?

- Is information available to give to the school system about my child's needs as he or she receives treatment?

Talking with Your Child

Your first question may be, "Should I tell my child about the leukemia?" You may want to protect your child, but children usually know when something is wrong. Your child may not be feeling well, may be seeing the doctor often, and may have already had some tests. Your child may notice that you are afraid. No matter how hard you try to keep information about the illness and treatment from your child, others—such as family, friends, and clinic or hospital staff—may inadvertently say things that let your child know about the leukemia. In addition, it will upset your child to find out that you were not telling the truth; your child depends on you for honest answers.

Why Should I Tell My Child?

Telling your child about his or her leukemia is a personal matter, and family, cultural, or religious beliefs will come into play. It is important to be open and honest with your child because children who are not told about their illness often imagine things that are not true. For example, a child may think he or she has leukemia as punishment for doing something wrong. Health professionals generally agree that telling children the truth about their illness leads to less stress and guilt. Children who know the truth are also more likely to cooperate with treatment. Finally, talking about leukemia often helps to bring the family closer together and makes dealing with the leukemia a little easier for everyone.

Parent's Questions

Parents have many questions about talking with their children about the diagnosis. Perhaps you have asked some of these yourself.

When Should My Child Be Told?

Because you are probably the best judge of your child's personality and moods, you are the best person to decide when your child should be told. Keep in mind, though, that your child is likely to know early on that something is wrong, so you may want to tell your child soon after the diagnosis. In fact, most parents say it is easiest to tell them then. Waiting days or weeks may give your child time to imagine worse things than the truth and develop fears that may be hard to dispel later. Certainly, it would be easier for your child if he or she is told before treatment starts.

Who Should Tell My Child?

The answer to this question is personal. As a parent, you may feel that it is best for you to tell your child. Some parents, however, find it too painful to do so. Other family members or the treatment team—doctor, nurse, or social worker—may be able to help you. They may either tell your child for you or help you explain the illness.

Thinking about what you are going to say and how to say it will help you feel more relaxed. But how do you decide just what to say? Family and close friends, members of the treatment team, parents of other children who have leukemia, members of support groups, and clergy members can offer ideas.

Who Should Be There?

Your child needs love and support when hearing the diagnosis. Even if the doctor explains the illness, someone your child trusts and depends upon should be present. Having the support of other family members at this time can be very helpful.

What Should My Child Be Told?

How much information and the best way to relate this information depends on your child's age and what your child can understand. Being gentle, open, and honest is usually best. The following sections describe what most children in various age groups are likely to understand. These guidelines are general—each child is different. Your child may fit into more than one or none of these categories.

Up to 2 Years Old

Children this young do not understand leukemia. They understand what they can see and touch. Their biggest concern is what is happening to them right now. They worry most about being away from their parents.

After children are a year old, they think about how things feel and how to control things around them. Very young children are most afraid of medical tests. Many cry, run away, or squirm to try to control what is happening.

Because children begin to think about and understand what is going on around them at about 18 months, it is best to be honest. Be truthful about trips to the hospital and explain procedures that may hurt. You can tell your child that needle sticks will hurt a minute and that it is okay to cry. Being honest lets your child know that you understand and accept his or her feelings and helps your child trust you.

When you can, give your child choices. For example, if a medicine is taken by mouth, you might ask if your child would like it mixed in apple juice, grape juice, or applesauce.

2 to 7 Years Old

When children are between the ages of 2 and 7, they link events to one thing. For example, they usually tie illness to a specific event such as staying in bed or eating chicken soup. Children this age often think their illness is caused by a specific action. Therefore, getting better will "just happen" or will come if they follow a set of rules.

These approaches might help when talking with a child in this age group:

- Explain that treatment is needed so the hurting will go away or so the child can get better and play without getting so tired.

- Explain that the illness or treatment is not punishment for something the child has done, said, or thought.

- Be honest when you explain tests and treatments. Remind the child that all of these things are being done to get rid of the leukemia and to help him or her get well.

- Use simple ways to explain the illness. For example, try talking about the leukemia as a contest between good cells and bad cells. Having treatment will help the good cells to be stronger so that they can beat the bad cells.

7 to 12 Years Old

Children ages 7 to 12 are starting to understand links between things and events. For example, a child this age sees his or her illness as a set of symptoms, is less likely to believe that something he or she did caused the illness, understands that getting better comes from taking medicines and doing what the doctor says, and is able to cooperate with treatment.

You can give more details when explaining leukemia, but you should still use situations your child may be used to. You might say that the body is made of up different types of cells, and these cells have different jobs to do. Like people, these cells must work together to get the job done. You might describe the leukemia cells as troublemakers that get in the way of the work of the good cells. Treatment helps to get rid of the troublemakers so that other cells can work well together.

12 Years and Older

Children over 12 years old can often understand complicated relationships between events. They can think about things that have not happened to them. Teenagers tend to think of illness in terms of specific symptoms, such as tiredness, and in terms of limits or changes in their everyday activity. But because they also can understand the reason for their symptoms, you can explain leukemia as a disease in which a few cells in the body go haywire. These haywire cells grow more quickly than normal cells, invade other parts of the body, and get in the way of how the body usually works. The goal of treatment is to kill the haywire cells. The body can then work normally again, and the symptoms will go away.

Questions Children May Ask

Children are naturally curious about their disease and have many questions about leukemia and leukemia treatment. Your child will expect you to have answers to most questions. Children may begin to ask questions right after diagnosis or may wait until later. Here are some common questions and some ideas to help you answer them.

Why Me?

A child, like an adult, wonders "Why did I get leukemia?" A child may feel that it is his or her fault, that somehow he or she caused the illness. Make it clear that not even the doctors know exactly what caused the leukemia. Neither you, your child, nor his or her brothers or sisters did, said, or thought anything that caused the leukemia. Stress also that leukemia is not contagious, and your child did not catch it from someone else.

Will I Get Well

Children often know about family members or friends who died of leukemia. As a result, many children are afraid to ask if they will get well because they fear that the answer will be no. Thus, you might tell your child that leukemia is a serious disease, but that treatment—such as medicine, radiation, or an operation—has helped get rid of leukemia in other children, and the doctors and nurses are trying their best to cure your child's leukemia, too. Knowing that caring people—such as family, doctors, nurses, counselors, and others—surround your child and your family may also help him or her feel more secure.

What Will Happen to Me?

When your child is first diagnosed with leukemia, many new and scary things will happen. While at the doctor's office, hospital, or clinic, your child may see or play with other children with leukemia who may not be feeling well, have lost their hair, or have had limbs removed because of leukemia. Your child may wonder, "Will these things happen to me?" Yet, your child may be too afraid to ask questions. It is important to try to get your child to talk about these concerns. Explain ahead of time about the leukemia, treatment, and possible side effects. Discuss what the doctor will do to help if side effects occur. You can also explain that there are many different types of leukemia and that even when two children have the same leukemia, what happens to one child will not always happen to the other. Children should be told about any changes in their treatment schedule or in the type of treatment they receive. This information helps them prepare for visits to the doctor or hospital. You may want to help your child keep a calendar that shows the days for doctor visits, treatments, or tests. Do not tell younger children about upcoming treatments far ahead of time if it makes them nervous.

Why Do I Have to Take Medicine When I Feel Okay?

With leukemia, your child may feel fine much of the time but need to take medicine often. Children do not understand why they have to take medicine when they feel well. You may want to remind your child of the reason for taking the medicine in the first place. For example, a child could be told: "Although you are feeling well, the bad cells are hiding. You must take the medicine for a while longer to find the bad cells and stop them from coming back."

What about Treatment?

To plan the best treatment, the doctor and treatment team will look at your child's general health, type of leukemia, stage of the disease, age, and many other factors. Based on this information, the doctor will prepare a treatment plan that outlines the exact type of treatment, how often your child will receive treatment, and how long it will last. Each child with leukemia has a treatment plan that is chosen just for that child; even children with the same type of leukemia may receive different treatments. Depending on how your child responds to treatment, the doctor may decide to change the treatment plan or choose another plan.

Before treatment begins, your child's doctor will discuss the treatment plan with you, including the benefits, risks, and side effects. Then you and the treatment team will need to talk with your child about the treatment. After the doctor fully explains the treatment and answers your questions, you will be asked to give your written consent to go ahead with treatment. Depending on your child's age and hospital policy, your child may also be asked to give consent before treatment.

The treatment plan may seem complicated at first. But the doctor and treatment team will explain each step, and you and your child will soon become used to the routine. Many parents find it helpful to get a copy of the treatment plan to refer to as the treatment proceeds. It also helps them in arranging their own schedules. Do not be afraid to ask questions or speak up if you feel something is not going right. Your child's doctor is often the best person to answer your questions, but other members of the treatment team can give you information, too. If you feel as though you need extra time with the doctor, schedule a meeting or phone call. Remember, you are part of the treatment team and should be involved in your child's treatment.

What Are the Different Types of Cancer Treatment?

The types of treatment used most often to treat cancer are surgery, chemotherapy, radiation therapy, immunotherapy, and bone marrow or peripheral blood stem cell transplantation. Doctors use these treatments to destroy cancer cells. Depending on the type of cancer, children may have one kind of treatment or a combination of treatments. Most children receive a combination of treatments, called combination therapy. Treatments for cancer often cause unwanted or unpleasant side effects such as nausea, hair loss, and diarrhea. Side effects occur because cancer treatment that kills cancer cells can hurt some normal cells, too. As your child begins treatment, you may want to keep the following in mind.

The kinds of side effects and how bad they will be depend on the kind of drug, the dosage, and the way your child's body reacts. The doctor plans treatment so that your child has as few side effects as possible. The doctor and treatment team have ways to lessen your child's side effects. Talk with them about things that can be done before, during, and after treatment to make your child comfortable. Lowering the treatment dosage slightly to eliminate unpleasant side effects usually will not make the treatment less able to destroy cancer cells or hurt your child's chances of recovery. Most side effects go away soon after treatment ends. Remember that not every child gets every side effect, and some children get few, if any. Also, how serious the side effects are varies from child to child, even among children who are receiving the same treatment. The doctor or treatment team can tell you which, if any, side effects your child is likely to have and how to handle them. If you know what side effects can occur, you can recognize them early.

Chapter 17

Helping Children and Teens Understand Clinical Trial Participation

If you are considering enrolling your child in a clinical trial, this chapter should help you better understand the concept of assent (a child's agreement to participate) as well as some of the larger issues surrounding young people's participation in trials.

What happens if the prospective participant in a clinical trial is not an adult, but a child or teenager? What, if anything, should be done to educate the young person about the trial and ensure that he or she is given a say in whether or not to participate?

At one time, it was assumed that young people lacked the ability to consent to participation in clinical research. Instead, parents or guardians went through the informed consent process on their behalf and gave what was known as proxy consent.

Over the past couple of decades, medical and legal experts have given much thought to the special issues surrounding children's participation in clinical trials. In the eyes of the law, children under 18 are not adults; therefore, legal permission for their participation must be given by parents or guardians after going through the informed consent process on their behalf.

Health care providers want young people to know that they have a say in what happens to them and that their questions and input are valued. Encouraging their involvement in decision-making is done out of respect for their rights as individuals and the desire to give

"Children's Assent to Clinical Trial Participation," National Cancer Institute (NCI), updated: 1/11/2001.

them a sense of ownership in what happens during the trial. Even though children cannot consent, because true consent implies full understanding, they are now routinely asked whether they agree (assent) or do not agree (dissent) to participate. Their parents or guardians are no longer asked to give proxy consent but instead give informed permission.

Parents reviewing written information about a clinical trial for their child can interact with the research team and learn how the study will work, its objectives, the possible benefits and risks of participating, and the child's rights and responsibilities. In this way, they can make a fully informed decision about whether or not to give informed permission for their child's participation in the clinical trial.

Informed Consent

Federal regulations state that parents and guardians must participate in an informed consent process— just as they would do if they themselves were considering enrolling in a clinical trial—and give legal permission for their child to enroll. This process must follow the guidelines established for the general requirements of informed consent.

The Assent Process

Federal regulations entrust each research institution's Institutional Review Board (IRB) with determining what the assent process should involve and how the child's assent (or dissent) should be documented. IRBs are panels of medical specialists, nurses, social workers, medical ethicists, and patient advocates who review clinical trial protocols at institutions that conduct medical research.

The *Institutional Review Board Guidebook* published by the Department of Health and Human Services (DHHS) Office for Human Research Protections suggests that "the child should be given an explanation of the proposed research procedures in a language that is appropriate to the child's age, experience, maturity, and condition. This explanation should include a discussion of any discomforts and inconveniences the child may experience if he or she agrees to participate."

Tip for Parents and Guardians—Children's Expectations

Many parents feel the desire to protect their child from learning about the possible discomforts and inconveniences of the trial, and only tell them about the good that may come of it. However, it's essential they be given a complete picture of what the trial involves and have access to as much information as they want. This is likely to help them understand what is expected of them, and how they may feel, as they participate in research.

Like the informed consent process, the assent process is intended to be an ongoing, interactive conversation between the research team and the child or young adult. The research team may include doctors (who are often principal investigators and leading the study), nurses, social workers, and other health care professionals. The process is not about getting the young person to sign on the dotted line; rather, it is about making sure they understand the trial and what it means to participate. By engaging young people in understanding the research project, health care providers and young patients may become partners in the project. Children are likely to feel more in control and more involved in the trial as a result.

Although the assent process varies from institution to institution, certain elements remain constant. Before the process can begin, parents or guardians must give permission for their children to participate. Then, the child or teenager may be provided with a form that explains, in concrete and age-appropriate terms, the purpose of the research, what they will be asked to do, and what procedures they will undergo. For older adolescents (ages 16 or older), this might look very much like the adult informed consent document. For younger children, the terms and explanations will be greatly simplified into words they can understand.

Usually, the principal investigator in charge of the study, or a nurse or other health professional working with the investigator, explains the information and gives the child a chance to ask questions. The process typically takes place apart from parents or the key researchers on the study, so that the young person does not feel undue pressure. In some cases, though, especially when teenagers are involved, the assent process may turn into a discussion that includes parents, the potential participant, and researchers.

Whatever form it takes, the process should always make clear that the young person has the right to leave the trial, at any time and for any reason, without penalty or consequences, and that any information gathered will be kept confidential.

The research team may use other approaches in addition to written forms, conversations, and question and answer sessions. These might include videotapes, diagrams, pictures, or drawings. Researchers also may provide a chance for the young person to speak with other children or teens who have been in similar trials and are willing to talk about their experiences.

Tip for Parents and Guardians—Learning Styles

If your child seems to be struggling with the information the research team presents, ask about other strategies that might be tried. For instance, if your child learns better through seeing or hearing information, rather than just reading it, ask about videotapes or other visual aids.

It may take several sessions before the research team feels that the young person has developed a clear understanding of what the trial involves. At that point, he or she is asked to indicate assent or dissent either by signing the form or checking off a box that says yes or no (again, it will depend on age and capabilities). A no answer, or dissent to participation, should be considered binding. Occasionally, situations exist where a young person's assent is not required.

Tip for Parents and Guardians—Watch for Gaps

Although a child or adolescent may say that he or she understands that a choice exists, they may not be able to identify all the possible options and consequences. If there seem to be gaps in your child's understanding, it may help to go back over the information.

When Assent Is Not Required

An assent process for children or young adults is not required if one or the other of the following situations exists (but parent or guardian consent is still required):

1. The child is found incapable of participating, or

2. The clinical trial offers a treatment or procedure that "holds out a prospect of direct benefit that is important to the health or well-being of the child and is available only in the context of the research." In other words, researchers are not required to ask for children's assent to participation if the study offers a treatment that is thought to be a better option than those currently available, or if it offers the only alternative.

In life-threatening situations, such as that of a child with cancer, the second situation listed may be especially relevant. In the case of Phase III clinical trials, the trial will compare a standard treatment (with known risks and benefits) to an experimental new treatment. The experimental treatment is under study because it has not been proven and is not known whether the new treatment is better or worse than the standard treatment.

While the experimental treatment is always hoped to be better, researchers cannot make any firm conclusions about the benefits and risks of the new treatment until the clinical trial is completed and the results are carefully analyzed. Usually patients are randomized to either the standard or experimental arm of the clinical trial. In this situation, even though a child usually cannot receive the experimental treatment without participating in the clinical trial, the patient can always receive standard treatment without enrolling in a clinical trial.

There are occasionally medical diagnoses or circumstances, such as relapse of the cancer, for which the available treatment methods have an acknowledged poor outcome and enrollment in a clinical trial is the only means to receive a promising new treatment intervention. In such a situation, a child's assent is not required for a clinical trial, although permission from a parent or guardian is still required.

Tip for Parents and Guardians—You Have Final Say

> *Some of the newest approaches to treating children's cancers are available only through clinical trials, and your doctor may recommend one as essential to your child's treatment plan. In such critical cases, you have the final say over whether or not your child will participate. Nevertheless, the child should still be actively involved in the decision-making process.*

Although a legal requirement for assent is waived in these circumstances, the research team is still expected and encouraged to obtain a young person's assent, even if parents or guardians must give the final say. In all other cases, though, the young person's decision should be considered binding.

Other types of clinical trials may not be as critical to a young person's well-being. For example, some clinical trials may study the effects of support groups on children's or teens' recovery from cancer. While participating in such a study might help young people, it is not critical to their survival; therefore, they have the right to make the final decision about whether or not to take part.

Tip for Parents and Guardians—Participation Not Required

Keep in mind that your child always has the right to receive treatment off a clinical trial (that is, to not participate in any clinical trial).

What's Required by Law

The Department of Health and Human Services' (DHHS) *Regulations for the Protection of Human Subjects* (Title 45, Part 46 of the Code of Federal Regulations, Protection of Human Subjects; also referred to as 45 CFR 46) set standards for the informed consent process, the formation and function of Institutional Review Boards, and many other protective measures. Subpart D of 45 CFR 46 specifies "[A]dditional DHHS Protections for Children Involved as Subjects in Research." Established in 1983 and reviewed in 1991, these additional protections apply to all research involving children and is conducted or supported by DHHS, which includes National Cancer Institute-sponsored clinical trials.

The Subpart D regulations assign Institutional Review Boards with the responsibility for ensuring that any clinical trials involving children meet the following criteria:

- The research does not involve greater than minimal risk.

- If it does present more than minimal risk, it must offer an intervention or procedure that holds out the prospect of direct benefit for the individual child, or a monitoring procedure that is likely to contribute to [their] well-being. However, the IRB must ensure that the risk is justified by anticipated benefits, and that the risk-benefit ratio is at least as favorable as that of alternative approaches.

- If the research involves greater than minimal risk and no prospect of direct benefit to the child, it must be likely to yield general knowledge about their disease or condition. The IRB is charged with ensuring that the level of risk is reasonable, and that the research will most likely provide important general information that leads to better understanding of the condition.

- Any other research that does not appear to meet these criteria but presents an opportunity to understand, prevent, or alleviate a serious problem affecting the health or welfare of children must be considered by the IRB on a case-by-case basis, and must be approved by the Secretary of the Department of Health and Human Services.

These Federal regulations go on to state that adequate provisions must be made for soliciting the assent of children, when the IRB determines that they are capable of participating in such a process based on their age, maturity, and state of mind.

Tip for Parents and Guardians—Level of Risk

Institutional Review Boards (IRBs) are required to make sure that any clinical trial is likely to provide important information about how to better help young people, without posing an unacceptable level of risk. Whatever trial you are considering has already undergone intensive review by an IRB with this goal in mind.

Assent is Essential

Over the past few years, the National Institutes of Health, the U.S. Food and Drug Administration, and the American Academy of Pediatrics have emphasized the need to include more children and adolescents in clinical trials. You may be wondering why this is even necessary—wouldn't it just be simpler to require that all trial participants be over age 18? While it might be simpler, it would not be good medical practice. Many diseases only affect children, and advances in treating these diseases depends on research studies. For those diseases that do affect both adults and children, a treatment that helps adults may not help children in the same way.

Fortunately, there are many cancer clinical trials designed specifically for children because childhood forms of cancer are often very different from adult forms. Researchers studying new treatments for adults with cancer generally do not include children in their clinical trials, but instead are encouraged to work with pediatric cancer specialists to assure timely and appropriate evaluations of their new treatment approaches in children.

Additional Information

National Cancer Institute
6166 Executive Blvd., MSC 8322
Suite 3036A
Bethesda, MD 20892-8322
Toll-Free: 800-422-6237
Toll-Free TTY: 800-332-8615
Website: www.cancer.gov

Chapter 18

Blood Counts and Record Keeping

Keeping track of their child's blood counts becomes a way of life for parents of children with leukemia. Unfortunately, misunderstandings about the implications of certain changes in blood values can cause unnecessary worry and fear. To help prevent these concerns, and to better enable parents to help spot trends in the blood values of their child, this chapter explains the blood counts of healthy children, the blood counts of children being treated for leukemia, and what each blood value means.

Values for Healthy Children

Each laboratory and lab handbook has slightly different reference values for each blood cell, so your lab sheets may differ slightly from these charts. There is also variation in values for children of different ages. For instance, in children from newborn to four years old, granulocytes are lower and lymphocytes higher than the numbers listed. Geographic location affects reference ranges as well.

Values for Children on Chemotherapy

Blood counts of children being treated for leukemia fluctuate wildly. White blood cell counts can go down to zero, or be above normal. Red

"Blood Counts and Record Keeping," Excerpted from: *Childhood Leukemia: A Guide for Families, Friends, and Caregivers,* 3rd Edition by Nancy Keene, © 2002 by O'Reilly & Associates, Inc., reprinted with permission.

cell counts go down periodically during treatment, necessitating transfusions of packed red cells. Platelet levels also decrease, requiring platelet transfusions. Absolute neutrophil counts (ANC) are closely watched as they give the physician an idea of the child's ability to fight infection. ANCs vary from zero to in the thousands.

Oncologists consider all of the blood values to get the total picture of the child's reaction to illness, chemotherapy, radiation, or infection. Trends are more important than any single value. For instance, if the values were 5.0, 4.7, 4.9, then the second result was insignificant. If, on the other hand, the values were 5.0, 4.7, 4.6, then there is a decrease in the cell line.

The following explanations will describe each blood value. If you have any questions about your child's blood counts, ask your child's

Table 18.1. Values for Healthy Children

Hemoglobin (Hgb)	11.5-13.5 g/100ml.
Hematocrit	34-40%
Red Blood Count	3.9-5.3 m/cm or 3.9-5.3 x 10^{12}/L
Platelets	160,000-500,000 mm^3
White Blood Count	5,000-10,000 mm^3 or 5-10 K/ul
WBC Differential:	
• Segmented neutrophils	50-70%
• Band neutrophils	1-3%
• Basophils	0.5-1%
• Eosinophils	1-4%
• Lymphocytes	12-46%
• Monocytes	2-10%
Bilirubin (total)	0.3-1.3 mg./dl
Direct (conjugated)	0.1-0.4 mg./dl
Indirect (unconjugated)	0.2-0.18 mg./dl
AST (SGOT)	0-36 IU./l.
ALT (SGPT)	0-48 IU./l.

doctor for a clear explanation. Especially in the beginning, many parents agonize over whether the rapid changes in blood counts (often requiring transfusions, changes in chemo dosages, or whether the child can have visitors) are normal or expected. The only way to address your worries, and prevent them from escalating, is to ask what the changes mean.

What Do These Blood Values Mean?

The following sections explain each line of the blood values in Table 18.1.

Hemoglobin (Hgb)

Red cells contain hemoglobin, the molecules that carry oxygen and carbon dioxide in the blood. Measuring hemoglobin gives an exact picture of the ability of the blood to carry oxygen. Children will have low hemoglobin levels at diagnosis and during the intensive parts of treatment. This is because both cancer and chemotherapy decrease the bone marrow's ability to produce new red cells. During maintenance, your child's hemoglobin level will be higher than during induction and consolidation, but still lower than that of a healthy child. Usually, signs and symptoms of anemia—pallor, shortness of breath, fatigue—will start to show when the hemoglobin gets to or below 10g/dl.

Hematocrit (HCT), Also Called Packed Cell Volume (PCV)

The purpose of this test is to determine the ratio of plasma (clear liquid part of blood) to red cells in the blood. Blood is drawn from a vein, finger prick, or from a Hickman or Port-a-Cath and is spun in a centrifuge to separate the red cells from the plasma. The hematocrit is the percentage of cells in the blood; for instance, if the child has a hematocrit of 30 percent, it means that 30 percent of the amount of blood drawn was cells and the rest was plasma. When the child is on chemotherapy, the bone marrow does not make many red cells, and the hematocrit will go down. Usually the child will be given a transfusion of packed red cells when the hematocrit goes below 18 to 19 percent. Even during maintenance the bone marrow is partially suppressed, so the hematocrit is often in the low to mid-thirties. This results in less oxygen being carried in the blood, and your child may have less energy.

Red Blood Cell Count (RBC)

Red blood cells are produced by the bone marrow continuously in healthy children and adults. These cells contain hemoglobin which carries oxygen and carbon dioxide throughout the body. To determine the RBC, an automated electronic device is used to count the number of red cells in a liter of blood.

Red cell indices (MCV, MCH, MCHC) are mathematical relationships of hematocrit to red cell count, hemoglobin to red cell count, and hemoglobin to hematocrit. This gives a mathematical expression of the degree of change in shape found in red cells. The higher the number (low teens are fine) the more distorted the red cell population is.

White Blood Cell Count (WBC)

The total white blood cell count determines the body's ability to fight infection. Treatment for cancer kills healthy white cells as well as diseased ones. Parents need to expect prolonged periods of low white counts during treatment. To determine the WBC, an automated electronic device counts the number of white cells in a liter of blood. If your lab sheet uses K/ul instead of mm^3, multiply by 1000 to get the value in mm^3. For example, the total WBC is 0.7 K/ul. Therefore, 0.7 x 1000 = 700 mm^3.

White Blood Cell Differential

When a child has blood drawn for a complete blood count (CBC) one section of the lab report will state the total white blood cell count and a differential. This means that each type of white cell will be listed as a percentage of the total, as in Table 18.2.

Table 18.2. White Blood Cells (WBC)–1,500 mm^3

Segmented neutrophils	49% (also called polys or segs)
Band neutrophils	1% (also called bands)
Basophils	1% (also called basos)
Eosinophils	1% (also called eos)
Lymphocytes	38% (also called lymphs)
Monocytes	10% (also called monos)

You might also see cells called metamyelocytes, myelocytes, promyelocytes, and myeloblasts listed. These cells are nonfunctional and are seen in a variety of serious illnesses. The appearance or disappearance of these immature cells are early signals of change.

The differential is obtained by microscopic analysis of a blood sample on a slide.

Absolute Neutrophil Count (ANC)

The absolute neutrophil count (also called the absolute granulocyte count or AGC) is a measure of the body's ability to withstand infection. Generally, an ANC above 1,000 means that the child can go to school and participate in normal activities.

To calculate the ANC, add the percentages of neutrophils (both segmented and band) and multiply by the total WBC. Using the example in Table 18.2, the ANC is 49% + 1% = 50%. 50% of 1,500 (.50 X 1,500) = 750. The ANC is 750.

Platelet Count

Platelets are necessary to repair the body and to stop bleeding through the formation of clots. Because platelets are produced by the bone marrow, platelet counts decrease when a child is on chemotherapy. Signs of lowering platelet counts are small vessel bleeding such as bruises, gum bleeding, or nose bleeding. Platelet transfusions are usually given when the count is between 10,000-20,000 mm^3. Platelets are counted by passing a blood sample through an electronic device.

Approximately one-third of all platelets spend a great deal of time in the spleen. Any splenic dysfunction such as enlargement may cause the counts to drop precipitously. If the spleen is removed, platelet counts may skyrocket. This transient thrombocytosis (elevated platelet count) will abate within a month.

ALT (Alanine Aminotransferase), Also Called SGPT (Serum Glutamic Pyruvic Transaminase)

When doctors talk about liver functions, they are usually referring to tests on blood samples that measure liver damage. If the chemotherapy is proving to be toxic to your child's liver, the damaged liver cells release an enzyme called ALT into the blood serum. ALT levels can go up in the hundreds or even thousands in some children on chemotherapy. Each institution and protocol has different points at which they decrease dosages or stop chemotherapy to allow the child's liver to recover. If you notice a change in your child's ALT, ask for an explanation and plan of action (for example, "John's ALT is now 450, what is your plan to reduce or stop the chemotherapy to allow his liver to recover?")

> *I was very interested in my daughter's blood counts throughout her treatment. I also tried to get information without making people mad. If I asked a question and received an unsatisfactory answer, I would reply in a nice way, "I am worrying about this and would really appreciate a few minutes of your time to explain it to me." I found the attendants and clinic director to be the most willing to provide explanations. If you get a ridiculous reply (once a fellow patted me on the head and said, "It's our job to think about these things, not yours") go find someone else to ask.*

AST (Aspartate Aminotransferase), Also Called SGOT (Serum Glutamic Oxaloacetic Transaminase)

SGOT is an enzyme present in high concentrations in tissues with high metabolic activity, including the liver. Severely damaged or killed cells release SGOT into the blood. The amount of SGOT in the blood is directly related to the amount of tissue damage. Therefore, if your child's liver is being damaged by the chemotherapy, the SGOT can rise into the thousands. In addition, there are other causes for an elevated SGOT, such as viral infections, reaction to an anesthetic, and many others. If your child's level jumps unexpectedly, ask the physician for an explanation and a plan of action.

Bilirubin

The body converts hemoglobin released from damaged red cells into bilirubin. The liver removes the bilirubin from the blood, and excretes it into the bile, which is released into the small intestine to aid digestion.

Normally there is only a small amount of bilirubin in the bloodstream. Bilirubin rises if there is excessive red blood cell destruction or if the liver is unable to excrete the normal amount of bilirubin produced.

There are two types of bilirubin: indirect (also called unconjugated), and direct (also called conjugated) bilirubin. An increase in indirect (unconjugated) is seen when destruction of red cells has occurred, while an increase of direct (conjugated) is seen when there is a dysfunction or blockage of the liver.

If excessive amounts of bilirubin are present in the body, the bilirubin seeps into the tissues producing a yellow color called jaundice.

If your child's total bilirubin rises above normal levels, ask the physician for an explanation and plan of action.

Your Child's Pattern

Each child develops a unique pattern of blood counts during treatment, and observant parents can help track these changes. If there is a change in the pattern, show it to your child's doctor and ask for an explanation. Doctors consider all of the laboratory results to decide how to proceed, but they should be willing to explain their plan of action to you so that you better understand what is happening and worry less.

If your child is participating in a clinical trial and you have obtained the entire clinical trial protocol, it will contain a section that clearly outlines the actions that should be taken by the oncologist if certain changes in blood counts occur. For example, my daughter's protocol has an extensive section which lists each drug and when the dosage should be modified. For vincristine it states:

Vincristine

1.5 mg/m^2 (2 mg maximum) IV push weekly x 4 doses days 0,7,14,21.

Seizures: Hold one dose, then reinstitute.

Severe foot drop, paresis, or ileus: Hold dose(s); when symptoms abate, resume at 1.0 mg/m^2; escalate to full dose as tolerated.

Jaw pain: Treat with analgesics; do not modify vincristine dose.

Withhold if total bilirubin >1.9 mg/dl. Administer 1/2 dose if total bilirubin 1.5-1.9 mg/dl.

Chapter 19

Interactions with Friends When a Child Has Leukemia

Like family, friends can cushion the shock of diagnosis and ease the difficulties of treatment with their words and actions.

Notifying Friends

The easiest way to notify friends is to delegate one person to do the job. Calling one neighbor or close friend prevents numerous tearful conversations. Most parents are at their child's bedside and want to avoid more emotional upheaval, especially in front of their child. Parents need to recognize that friends' emotions will mirror their own: shock, fear, worry, helplessness. Since most friends want to help but don't know what to do or say, giving cues of what would be helpful are welcome.

Helpful Things for Friends to Do

Mother Theresa once said, "We can do no great things—only small things with great love." It is a given that the family of a newly diagnosed child is overwhelmed. The list of helpful things to do is endless, but here are some suggestions from veteran parents.

"Interactions with Friends," excerpted from *Childhood Leukemia: A Guide for Families, Friends, and Caregivers*, 3rd Edition by Nancy Keene, © 2002 by O'Reilly & Associates, Inc., reprinted with permission.

Household

- Provide meals.

  One of the nicest things that friends did was to bring us a huge picnic basket full of food to the hospital. We spread a blanket on the floor, Erica crawled out of bed, and the entire family sat down together and ate. Most people don't realize how expensive it is to have to eat every meal at the hospital cafeteria, so the picnic was not only fun, but helped us to save a few dollars.

- Take care of pets or livestock.

- Mow grass, shovel snow, rake leaves, weed gardens.

  We came home from the hospital one evening right before Christmas, and found a freshly cut, fragrant Christmas tree leaning next to our door. I'll never forget that kindness.

- Clean the house.

  My husband's cousin sent her cleaning lady over to our house. It was so neat and such a luxury to come home to find the stove and windows sparkling clean.

- Grocery shop (especially when the family is due home from the hospital).

- Do laundry. Drop off and pick up dry cleaning.

- Provide a place to stay near the hospital.

  One of the ladies from the school where I worked came up to the ICU waiting room where we were sleeping and pressed her house key into my hand. She lived five minutes from the hospital. She said, "My basement is made up, there's a futon, there's a TV, you are coming and staying at my house." I hardly knew her, but we accepted. Every day when we came in from the hospital there was some cute little treat waiting for us like a bowl of cookies, or two packages of hot chocolate and a thermos of hot milk.

Siblings

- Baby-sit whenever parents go to the clinic, emergency room, or for a prolonged hospital stay.

  The mother of a secretary from my office called me, introduced herself, and offered to care for my newborn daughter while I spent time at the hospital. I had never met this woman, but she turned out to be a real lifesaver and a jewel. She would come every day, bathe, dress, and feed my daughter, clean up the house, and stay from morning until evening. She did this for several months. I will never forget her for being so kind. I would not have been able to get through those first few difficult months without this type of support—and to find it in a complete stranger certainly renewed my faith in mankind!

- When parents are home with a sick child, take sibling(s) to the park, sports event, or a movie.

- Invite sibling(s) over for meals.

- If you bring a gift for the sick child, bring something for the sibling(s), too.

  Friends from home sent boxes of art supplies to us when the whole family spent those first ten weeks at a Ronald McDonald house far from our home. They sent scissors, paints, paper, colored pens. It was a great help for Carrie Beth and her two sisters. One friend even sent an Easter package with straw hats for each girl, and flowers, ribbons, and glue to decorate them with.

- Offer to help sibling(s) with homework.

- Drive sibling(s) to lessons, games, or school.

- Listen to how they are feeling and coping. Siblings' lives have been disrupted, they have limited time with their parents, and they need support and care.

Psychological Support

- Call frequently, and be open to listening if the parents want to talk about their feelings. Also, talk about non-cancer-related topics such as sharing the neighborhood and school news.

- Visit the hospital and bring fun stuff like bubbles, silly string, water pistols, joke books, funny videotapes, rub-on tattoos, and board games.

- Bring lots of prepaid phone cards to the hospital so the family can call distant friends and relatives.

- If one parent had to leave work to stay in the hospital with the sick child, coworkers can send messages by mail or tape.

  One very neat thing that was an emotional boost was that my friends and former coworkers from Kansas faxed us messages and pictures and things to Meagan while we were in the hospital. It was very nice to get such fresh messages—it really shortened the miles.

- If you think the family might be interested, call Candlelighters, the American Cancer Society, or the social worker at the local hospital to find out if there are support groups for parents and/ or kids in your area.

- Offer to take the children to the support groups or go with the parents. For most families, the parent support group becomes a second family with ties of shared experience as deep and strong as blood relations.

- Drive parent and child to clinic visits.

- Buy books (uplifting ones) for the family if they are readers.

- Send cards or letters.

  Word got around my parents' hometown, and I received cards from many high school acquaintances, who still cared enough to call or write and say we're praying for you, please let us know how things are going. It was so neat to get so many cards out of the blue that said, "I'm thinking about you."

- Baby-sit the sick child so that the parents can go out to eat, exercise, take a walk, or just get out of the hospital or house.

- Donate blood. Your blood will not be used specifically for the ill child, but will replenish the general supply, which is depleted by children with cancer.

- If the child has a type of leukemia that may require a bone marrow transplant, organize a drive to have lots of people typed and entered into the marrow registry. Contact information is at the end of the chapter.

- Give lots of hugs.

  Grandpa Fred is a seventy-one-year-old retiree who has been visiting pediatric oncology patients at Children's for almost twelve years. He begins his day at 9:30 every morning on the teens ward, then he moves on to visit the younger patients, the playroom, and the clinic. Grandpa Fred always takes pictures of his young friends, very good ones, and has filled twenty-three photo albums with them. Fred has two prints made of each picture he takes and gives one to the families. He also helps Santa on

Christmas and visits on Halloween. He has been the camp manager at Camp Good Times every summer for eight years. Fred feels that a hug is more important than anything he can say to someone. "Listening and giving a hug," he says, "That's the best I can do."

Financial Support

Helping families avoid financial disaster can be the next greatest gift after the life of the child and the strength of the family. It is estimated that even fully insured families spend 25 percent or more of their income on co-payments, travel, motels, meals, and other uncovered items. Uninsured or underinsured families may lose their savings or even their house. Most families need financial help. Here are some suggestions:

- Start a support fund.

  A friend of mine called and asked very tentatively if we would mind if she started a support fund. We felt awkward, but we needed help, so we said okay. She did everything herself, and the money she raised was very, very helpful. We did ask her to stop the fund when people started calling us to ask if they could use giving to the fund as an advertisement for their business.

- Help them apply for financial aid from the Leukemia & Lymphoma Society. Ask for the "Guidelines for Patient Aid Program Application and Reimbursement Process."

- Share leave. Governments and some companies have leave banks that permit persons who are ill or taking care of someone who is ill to use other coworkers' leave so they won't have their pay docked.

- Job share. Some families work out job-share arrangements in which a coworker donates time to perform part of one job to enable one parent to spend time at the hospital. Job sharing allows the job to get done, keeps peace at the job site, and prevents financial losses for the family. Another possibility would be for one or more friends with similar skills (e.g., word processing, filing, sales, etc.) to rotate through the job on a volunteer basis to cover for the parent of the ill child.

- Collect money at church or work to give informally.

  The day my daughter was diagnosed, my husband's coworkers passed the hat and gave us over $250. I was embarrassed, but it *paid for gas, meals, and the motel until there was an opening in the Ronald McDonald House.*

Finances were a main concern for us because I wanted to cut back on work to be at home with Meagan. Sometimes my coworkers would pool money and present it with a card saying, "Here's a couple of days work that you won't have to worry about.

My husband's coworkers didn't collect money, they did something even more valuable. They donated sick leave hours, so that he was able to be at the hospital frequently during those first few months without losing a paycheck.

- Collect money by organizing a bake sale, dance, or raffle.

Coworkers of my husband held a Halloween party and charged admission. We were very uncomfortable with the idea at first, but they were looking for an excuse to have a party, and it helped us out.

- Keeping track of medical bills is time-consuming, frustrating, and exhausting. If you are a close relative or friend, you could offer to review, organize, and file (or enter into a computer) the voluminous paperwork. Making the calls and writing the letters over contested claims or errors in billing are very helpful.

Help from Schoolmates

- Encourage visits (if appropriate), cards, and phone calls from classmates.
- Ask the teacher to send the school newspaper and other news along with assignments.
- Classmates can sign a brightly colored banner to send to the hospital.

Brent's kindergarten class sent a packet containing a picture drawn for him by each child in the class. They also made him a book. Another time they sent him a letter written on huge poster board. He couldn't wait to get back to school.

Religious Support

- If the family goes to church, contact a member of the clergy.
- Arrange for church members and clergy to visit the hospital, if that is what the family wants.

- Arrange prayer services for the sick child.

- Have the child's Sunday school class (or whatever class is appropriate for the family's denomination) send pictures, posters, letters, balloons, or tapes to the sick child.

The day our son was diagnosed, we raced next door to ask our wonderful neighbors to take care of our dog. The news of his diagnosis quickly spread, and we found out later that five neighborhood families gathered that very night to pray for Brent.

Accepting Help

One of the kindest things you can do for your friends is to let them help you. Let them channel their time and worry into things that make your life easier. Think of the many times you have visited a sick friend, made a meal for a new mom, baby-sat someone else's child in an emergency, or just pitched in to do what needed to be done. These actions probably made you feel great and provided a good example for your children. When your child is diagnosed with cancer, both you and your friends will immensely benefit if you let them help you and give them guidance on what you need.

One father's thoughts on accepting help:

Fathers have a deep-seated need to protect their family. Yet here I was with a child with leukemia, and there wasn't a single thing that I could do about it. The loss of control really bothered me. The very hardest thing that I had to learn was to let go enough to let people help us.

One mother's thoughts on accepting help:

The most important advice I received as the parent of a child newly diagnosed with cancer came from a hospital nurse whom I turned to when I was overwhelmed with all the advice being offered by family and friends. This wise nurse said, "Don't discount anything. You're going to need all the help you can get." I think it is very important for families to remain open and accept the help that is offered. It often comes when least expected and from unlikely sources. I was totally unprepared at diagnosis for how much help I would need, and I'm glad that I remained open to offers of kindness. This is not the time to show the world how strong you are.

What to Say

The following are some suggestions on what to say and how to offer help. Of course, much depends on the type of relationship that already exists, but a specific offer can always be accepted or graciously declined:

- I am so sorry.
- I didn't call earlier because I didn't know what to say.
- Our family would like do your yardwork. It will make us feel as if we are helping in a small way.
- We want to clean your house for you once a week. What day would be convenient?
- Would it help if we took care of your dog (or cat, or bird)? We would love to do it.
- I walk my dog three times a day. May I walk yours, too?
- The church is setting up a system to deliver meals to your house. When is the best time to drop them off?
- I will take care of Jimmy whenever you need to take John to the hospital. Call us anytime, day or night, and we will come pick him up.

Things That Do Not Help

Out of ignorance, people sometimes say hurtful things to parents of children with cancer. If you are a family member or friend of a parent in this situation, please do not say any of the following:

- "God only gives people what they can handle." (Some people cannot handle the stress of childhood leukemia.)
- "I know just how you feel." (Unless you have a child with cancer, you simply don't know.)
- "You are so brave," or "so strong," etc. (Parents are not heroes; they are normal people struggling with extraordinary stress.)
- "They are doing such wonderful things to save children with leukemia these days." (Yes, the prognosis is good, but what parents and children are going through is not wonderful.)
- "Well, we're all going to die one day." (True, but parents do not need to be reminded of this fact.)

- "It's God's will." (This is just not a helpful thing to hear.)

- "At least you have other kids," or

- "Thank goodness you are still young enough to have other children." (A child cannot be replaced.)

  A woman whom I worked with, but did not know well, came up to me one day and out of the blue said, "When Erica gets to heaven to be with Jesus, He will love her." All I could think to say was, "Well, I'm sorry, but Jesus can't have her right now."

Parents also make the following suggestions of things to avoid doing:

- Do not say, "Let us know if there is anything we can do." It is far better to make a specific suggestion.

  Many well-wishing friends always said, "Let me know what I can do." I wish they had just "done," instead of asking for direction. It took too much energy to decide, call them, make arrangements, etc. I wish someone would have said, "When is your clinic day? I'll bring dinner," or "I'll baby-sit Sunday afternoon so you two can go out to lunch."

- Do not make personal comments in front of the child: when will his hair grow back in, he's lost so much weight, she's so pale, etc.

- Do not do things that require the parent to support you (for example, repeatedly call up, crying).

- Do not talk continually about the cancer; some normal conversations are welcome.

- Do not ask "what if" questions: What if he can't go to school? What if your insurance won't cover it? What if she dies? The present is really all the parents can deal with.

- Stories of children you know who have survived leukemia and are doing fine are welcome. Stories of those who have died or who have long-term side effects should not be shared.

Losing Friends

It is an unfortunate reality that most parents of children with leukemia lose friends. For a variety of reasons, some friends just can't cope and either suddenly disappear or gradually fade away. Many times this can be prevented by calling them to keep them involved, but sometimes, they just can't handle the stress.

Except for one good friend, none of my friends called when I was home. It seemed that after the initial three-month crisis, they removed themselves from the situation, as often happens.

I had a friend who really thought herself to be empathetic, except that she just couldn't "deal with" hospitals. She said that they made her uncomfortable, so she wouldn't visit. I also got tired of her talking about the silver lining of the dark cloud that has been hanging over my head. I have a really hard time dealing with that.

Friends? What friends? They disappeared, family, too. No one knew what to say to us.

Evan Handler, who was diagnosed with leukemia as a young adult, wrote a powerful memoir called *Time on Fire* about his experience. In it he discussed what his parents did to keep their friends informed:

They began to distribute a newsletter describing my progress as well as the stresses they were under—I saw it as a brilliant device. The exhaustion that is unavoidable to the parents of a sick child, even an adult child, is enough to overwhelm the strongest individual. My parents were simply accepting the offers coming forth and sharing their burden in a fashion that didn't increase their already superhuman load. By revealing themselves in the newsletter, both the good news and the bad, they gave their friends the option of tuning in or out, without having to suffer the indignity of those who could not cope with what my parents coped with daily.

Additional Information

National Marrow Donor Program
3001 Broadway St. NE
Suite 500
Minneapolis, MN 55413-1753
Toll-Free: 800-627-7692
Tel: 612-627-5800
Website: www.marrow.org

The Leukemia & Lymphoma Society
1311 Mamaroneck Avenue
White Plains, NY 10605
Toll-Free: 800-955-4572
Tel: 914-949-5213
Fax: 914-949-6691
Website: www.leukemia-lymphoma.org

Part Three

Adult Leukemia

Chapter 20

Pre-Leukemia Myelodysplastic Syndrome (MDS)

What Are Myelodysplastic Syndromes?

Myelodysplastic syndromes, also called pre-leukemia or smoldering leukemia, are diseases in which the bone marrow does not function normally and not enough normal blood cells are made. The bone marrow is the spongy tissue inside the large bones in the body. The bone marrow makes red blood cells (which carry oxygen and other materials to all tissues of the body), white blood cells (which fight infection), and platelets (which make the blood clot). Normally, bone marrow cells called blasts develop (mature) into several different types of blood cells that have specific jobs in the body.

Myelodysplastic syndromes occur most often in older people, but they can occur in younger people. The most common sign is anemia, which means there are not enough mature red blood cells to carry oxygen. There may also be too few white blood cells in the blood to fight infections. If the number of platelets in the blood is lower than normal, this may cause people to bleed or bruise more easily. A doctor should be seen if a person bleeds without any reason, bruises more

PDQ® Cancer Information Summary, National Cancer Institute; Bethesda, MD, "Myelodysplastic Syndromes Treatment (PDQ®)–Patient," updated 08/2002, available at: http://cancer.gov, accessed 03/31/2002; and an excerpt from PDQ® Cancer Information Summary, National Cancer Institute; Bethesda, MD, "Myelodysplastic Syndromes Treatment (PDQ)– Health Professional," updated 08/2002, available at: http://cancer.gov, accessed 03/31/2003.

easily than normal, has an infection that won't go away, or feels tired all the time.

If there are symptoms, a doctor may order blood tests to count the number of each kind of blood cell. If the results of the blood test are not normal, the doctor may do a bone marrow biopsy. During this test, a needle is inserted into a bone and a small amount of bone marrow is taken out and looked at under the microscope. The doctor can then determine the kind of disease and plan the best treatment.

A myelodysplastic syndrome may develop following treatment with drugs or radiation therapy for other diseases, or it may develop without any known cause. The myelodysplastic syndromes may change into acute myeloid leukemia, a form of cancer in which too many white blood cells are made.

Myelodysplastic syndromes are grouped together based on how the bone marrow cells and blood cells look under a microscope. There are five types of myelodysplastic syndromes: refractory anemia, refractory anemia with ringed sideroblasts, refractory anemia with excess blasts, refractory anemia with excess blasts in transformation, and chronic myelomonocytic leukemia.

Cellular Classification

The myelodysplastic syndromes have been classified into 5 types according to the French-American-British classification. [1-3] The types have different degrees of disordered hematopoiesis, frequencies of transformation to acute leukemia, and prognoses.

Refractory Anemia (RA)

The myeloid and megakaryocytic series in the bone marrow appear normal, but megaloblastoid erythroid hyperplasia is present. Dysplasia is usually minimal. Macrocytic anemia with reticulocytopenia is present in the blood. Transformation to acute leukemia is rare, and median survival varies from 2 to 5 years in most series. This type accounts for 20% to 30% of patients.

Refractory Anemia with Ringed Sideroblasts (RAS)

The blood and marrow are identical to those in patients with RA, except that at least 15% of marrow red cell precursors are ringed sideroblasts. Only 2% to 5% of patients present with this type, and prognosis is identical to that of RA.

Refractory Anemia with Excess Blasts (RAEB)

There is significant evidence of disordered myelopoiesis and megakaryocytopoiesis in addition to abnormal erythropoiesis. The marrow contains 5% to 20% myeloid blasts, and 1% to 5% of blasts may circulate in the blood. Progression to acute leukemia occurs in approximately 40% of patients, and median survival is usually 6 to 9 months. Approximately one-third of patients present with this type.

Refractory Anemia with Excess Blasts in Transformation (RAEB-t)

This is a panmyelosis in which 20% to 30% of marrow cells are blasts and more than 5% blasts are seen in the blood. Auer rods may be seen. Sixty to 75% of patients develop overt acute leukemia, and median survival is 6 months or less. Approximately 25% of patients present with this type.

Chronic Myelomonocytic Leukemia (CMML)

The red cell precursors in the marrow appear normal, although mild anemia may be present. Mild thrombocytopenia associated with morphologically normal megakaryocytes may be present. The marrow contains 5% to 20% blasts, and the circulating monocyte count is 1000 per cubic millimeter or more. Hepatosplenomegaly may be present. Approximately 30% of patients progress to acute leukemia. Median survival is on the order of 14 to 18 months. This type accounts for approximately 15% to 20% of myelodysplastic syndromes.

Stage Information

Stages of Myelodysplastic Syndromes

There is no staging for the myelodysplastic syndromes. Treatment depends on whether or not the disease developed following other treatments, or whether the patient has been treated for the myelodysplastic syndrome. Myelodysplastic syndromes are grouped as follows:

De Novo Myelodysplastic Syndromes

De novo myelodysplastic syndromes develop without any known cause. The patient has not received radiation therapy or chemotherapy for other diseases.

Secondary Myelodysplastic Syndromes

Secondary myelodysplastic syndromes develop following treatment with radiation therapy or chemotherapy for other diseases.

Previously Treated Myelodysplastic Syndromes

Previously treated myelodysplastic syndrome means the disease has been treated but has gotten worse.

Treatment Option Overview

How Myelodysplastic Syndromes Are Treated

There are treatments for all patients with myelodysplastic syndromes. Often the main treatment is giving red blood cells or platelets by a needle in a vein (transfusion) to control anemia or bleeding. Vitamins or other drugs may also be given to treat anemia.

Chemotherapy and biological therapy are being tested in clinical trials. Chemotherapy uses drugs to treat disease. Chemotherapy may be taken by pill, or it may be put into the body by a needle in the vein or muscle. Chemotherapy is called a systemic treatment because the drug enters the bloodstream, travels through the body, and affects cells throughout the body. Biological therapy tries to get the body to fight disease. It uses materials made by the body or made in a laboratory to boost, direct, or restore the body's natural defenses against disease. Biological therapy is sometimes called biological response modifier (BRM) therapy or immunotherapy.

Bone marrow transplantation is a newer type of treatment that uses high doses of chemotherapy and/or radiation therapy (high doses of x-rays or other high-energy rays) to destroy all of the bone marrow in the body, then transplants healthy bone marrow back into the body. Healthy marrow is then taken from another person (a donor) whose tissue is the same or almost the same as the patient's. The donor may be a twin (the best match), a brother, sister, or other relative, or another person not related. The healthy marrow is given to the patient through a needle in the vein, and the marrow replaces the marrow that was destroyed. A bone marrow transplant using marrow from a relative or person not related to the patient is called an allogeneic bone marrow transplant.

Treatment by Stage

The choice of treatment depends on the type of myelodysplastic syndrome, and the patient's age and general health. Standard treatment may be considered because of its effectiveness in patients in past studies, or participation in a clinical trial may be considered. Most patients with myelodysplastic syndromes are not cured with standard therapy and some standard treatments may have more side effects than are desired. For these reasons, clinical trials are designed to find better ways to treat cancer patients and are based on the most up-to-date information. Clinical trials are ongoing in most parts of the country for patients with myelodysplastic syndromes. To learn more about clinical trials, call the Cancer Information Service at 800-4-CANCER (800-422-6237); TTY at 800-332-8615.

De Novo Myelodysplastic Syndrome

Treatment may be one of the following:

1. Treatment to relieve symptoms of the disease, such as anemia or bleeding.

2. Allogeneic bone marrow transplantation.

3. Clinical trials of chemotherapy or biological therapy.

Secondary Myelodysplastic Syndrome

Patients will probably receive treatment to relieve symptoms of the disease, such as anemia or bleeding. They may also choose to take part in a clinical trial of chemotherapy or biological therapy.

Previously Treated Myelodysplastic Syndrome

Patients will probably receive treatment to relieve symptoms of the disease, such as anemia or bleeding. They may also choose to take part in a clinical trial of chemotherapy or biological therapy.

References

1. van der Weide M, Sizoo W, Nauta JJ, et al.: Myelodysplastic syndromes: analysis of clinical and prognostic features in 96 patients. *Eur J Haematol* 41 (2): 115-22, 1988.

2. Economopoulos T, Stathakis N, Foudoulakis A, et al.: Myelodysplastic syndromes: analysis of 131 cases according to the FAB classification. *Eur J Haematol* 38 (4): 338-44, 1987.

3. Bennett JM, Catovsky D, Daniel MT, et al.: Proposals for
    the classification of the myelodysplastic syndromes. *Br J
    Haematol* 51 (2): 189-99, 1982.

Additional Information

National Cancer Institute
6166 Executive Blvd., MSC8322
Suite 3036A
Bethesda, MD 20892-8322
Toll-Free: 800-422-6237
Toll-Free TTY: 800-332-8615
Website: www.cancer.gov

Chapter 21

Acute Lymphocytic Leukemia (ALL)

About 3,800 new cases of acute lymphocytic leukemia (ALL) are diagnosed each year in the United States. It is the most common type of leukemia under the age of 15. Children are most likely to develop the disease, but it can occur at any age. Acute lymphocytic leukemia may be called by several names, including acute lymphoid leukemia and acute lymphoblastic leukemia.

ALL results from an acquired (not inherited) genetic injury to the DNA of a single cell in the bone marrow. The disease is often referred to as acute lymphoblastic leukemia because the leukemic cell that replaces the normal marrow is the (leukemic) lymphoblast. The effects are: 1) the uncontrolled and exaggerated growth and accumulation of cells called lymphoblasts or leukemic blasts, which fail to function as normal blood cells and 2) the blockade of the production of normal marrow cells, leading to a deficiency of red cells (anemia),

This chapter begins with excerpts from "Acute Lymphocytic Leukemia," © 2002 The Leukemia & Lymphoma Society, additional information available at www.leukemia-lymphoma.org, reprinted with permission. Text under "What Is Adult Acute Lymphoblastic Leukemia? is from PDQ® Cancer Information Summary, National Cancer Institute; Bethesda, MD, "Adult Acute Lymphoblastic Leukemia (PDQ®): Treatment–Patient," updated 08/2002, available at: http://cancer.gov, accessed 03/31/2003; and text under "Risks, Statistics, and Treatment Outcomes," is excerpted from PDQ® Cancer Information Summary, National Cancer Institute; Bethesda, MD, "Adult Acute Lymphoblastic Leukemia (PDQ®): Treatment–Health Professional," updated 08/2002, available at: http://cancer.gov, accessed 03/31/03.

platelets (thrombocytopenia), and normal white cells (especially neutrophils, i.e., neutropenia) in the blood.

Causes and Risk Factors

In most cases, the cause of acute lymphocytic leukemia is not evident. Few factors have been associated with an increased risk of developing the disease. Exposure to high doses of irradiation, as carefully studied in the Japanese survivors of atomic bomb detonations, is one such factor. Unlike other forms of leukemia, acute lymphocytic leukemia occurs at different rates in different locations. There are higher leukemia rates in more developed countries and in higher socioeconomic groups.

The current causes of acute lymphoblastic leukemia in children or adults are not known. Scientists continue to explore possible relationships with lifestyle or environmental factors but no firm conclusions have yet been reached. Given the amount of study, this suggests that multifaceted complex factors may be involved. It is extremely disconcerting to patients and their families to wonder what they may have done differently to avoid the disease. Unfortunately, at the present time there is no known way to prevent the disease. Acute lymphocytic leukemia occurs most often in the first decade of life but increases in frequency again in older individuals.

Subtypes of Acute Lymphocytic Leukemia

Acute lymphocytic leukemia can develop from primitive lymphocytes that are in various stages of development. The principal subtypes are uncovered by special tests on the leukemic lymphoblasts called immunophenotyping. Phenotype is the physical characteristics of the cells and these are measured using immune tools. The subclassification of cell types is important since it helps to determine the best treatment to apply in each type of leukemia. The principle subtypes are T lymphocyte and B lymphocyte types, so named because the cell has features that are similar to normal T or B lymphocytes. In addition, the B cell type can be divided into a precursor B cell type, as well. Once these features are determined the term used may be acute T lymphoblastic leukemia or acute precursor (or pre) B cell lymphoblastic leukemia. Other markers on the lymphoblasts that can be detected with immunophenotyping and may be useful to the physician include the common acute lymphoblastic leukemia antigen, cALLa, now called CD 10.

Immunophenotypes

B lymphocytic lineage subtypes. These cases are identified by finding cell surface markers on the leukemic blast cells that are identical to those that develop on normal B lymphocytes. About 85 percent of cases are of the precursor B or B cell subtype.

T lymphocytic lineage subtypes. These cases are identified by finding cell surface markers on the leukemic blast cells that are identical to those that develop in normal T lymphocytes. About 15 percent of cases are of the T cell subtype.

Chromosome Abnormalities

Injury to chromosomes can be assessed by cytogenetic methods, and the specific alteration in chromosomes aids in subclassifying acute lymphocytic leukemia, also. For example, a change in chromosome number 22, referred to as the Philadelphia or Ph chromosome, which occurs in a small percentage of children and a larger percentage of adults with acute lymphocytic leukemia, places the patient in a higher risk category. Thus, the approach to therapy would be intensified in those subsets of patients.

Examination of leukemic cells by cytogenetic techniques permits identification of chromosomes or gene abnormalities in the cells.

The immunophenotype and chromosome abnormalities in the leukemic cells are very important guides in determining the approach to treatment and the intensity of the drug combinations to be used.

Other features are important in guiding therapy including age of the patient, level of the white blood cell count, or involvement of the central nervous system or of lymph nodes, among others.

Symptoms and Signs

Most patients feel a loss of well-being. They tire more easily and may feel short of breath when physically active. They may have a pale complexion from anemia. Signs of bleeding because of a very low platelet count may be noticed. These include black-and-blue marks occurring for no reason or because of a minor injury, the appearance of pinhead-sized, red spots under the skin, called *petechiae*, or prolonged bleeding from minor cuts. Discomfort in the bones and joints may occur. Fever in the absence of an obvious cause is common. Leukemic lymphoblasts may accumulate in the lymphatic system, and the lymph nodes can become enlarged. The leukemia cells can also collect on the lining of the brain and spinal cord and lead to headache or vomiting.

Diagnosis

To diagnose the disease, the blood and marrow cells must be examined. In addition to low red cell and platelet counts, examination of the stained (dyed) blood cells with a light microscope will usually show the presence of leukemic blast cells. This is confirmed by examination of the marrow which almost always shows leukemia cells. The blood and/or marrow cells are also used for studies of the number and shape of chromosomes (cytogenetic examination), immunophenotyping, and other special studies, if required.

Childhood Versus Adult Leukemia

Acute lymphocytic leukemia has an unusual pattern of age distribution. In the other types of leukemia, older people are more likely to develop the disease. Risk of developing the disease peaks at 4 years of age and then decreases until about age 50. At age 50, the incidence increases again, especially among men. Although remission rates and

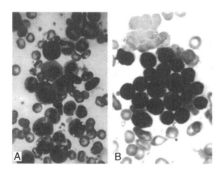

Figure 21.1. *Panel A shows a photograph of developing cells in healthy marrow which have been placed on a glass slide and stained with dyes to make the cells more distinctive. The variation in the appearance of the cells is characteristic of normal marrow. Panel B shows a photograph of marrow cells from a patient with acute lymphocytic leukemia. A monotonous appearance of leukemic blast cells is present.*

remission duration have improved in adults, current therapy has not resulted in the high rate of extended remissions (greater than five years) and cures possible for children.

What Is Adult Acute Lymphoblastic Leukemia?

Adult acute lymphoblastic leukemia (also called acute lymphocytic leukemia or ALL) is a disease in which too many infection-fighting white blood cells called lymphocytes are found in the blood and bone marrow. Lymphocytes are made by the bone marrow and by other organs of the lymph system. The bone marrow is the spongy tissue inside the large bones in the body. The bone marrow makes red blood cells (which carry oxygen and other materials to all tissues of the body), white blood cells (which fight infection), and platelets (which make the blood clot). Normally, the bone marrow makes cells called blasts that develop (mature) into several different types of blood cells that have specific jobs to do in the body.

Lymphocytes are found in the lymph which is a colorless, watery fluid present in the lymph vessels. The lymph vessels are part of the lymph system which is made up of thin tubes that branch, like blood vessels, into all parts of the body. Along the network of vessels are groups of small, bean-shaped organs called lymph nodes. Clusters of lymph nodes are found in the underarm, pelvis, neck, and abdomen. The spleen (an organ in the upper abdomen that makes lymphocytes and filters old blood cells from the blood), the thymus (a small organ beneath the breastbone), and the tonsils (an organ in the throat) are also part of the lymph system.

Lymphocytes fight infection by making substances called antibodies, which attack germs and other harmful bacteria in the body. In ALL, the developing lymphocytes do not mature and become too numerous. These immature lymphocytes are then found in the blood and the bone marrow. They also collect in the lymph tissues and make them swell. Lymphocytes may crowd out other blood cells in the blood and bone marrow. If the bone marrow cannot make enough red blood cells to carry oxygen, then anemia may develop. If the bone marrow cannot make enough platelets to make the blood clot normally, the bleeding or bruising may develop more easily. The cancerous lymphocytes can also invade other organs, the spinal cord, and the brain.

Leukemia can be acute (progressing quickly with many immature cancer cells) or chronic (progressing slowly with more mature looking leukemia cells). ALL progresses quickly and can occur in adults and children. Treatment is different for adults than it is for children.

ALL is often difficult to diagnose. The early signs may be similar to the flu or other common diseases. A doctor should be seen if the following signs or symptoms do not go away: fever, persistent weakness or tiredness, aches in the bones or joints, or swollen lymph nodes.

If there are symptoms, a doctor may order blood tests to count the number of each of the different kinds of blood cells. If the results of the blood tests are not normal, a doctor may do a bone marrow biopsy. During this test, a needle is inserted into a bone and a small amount of bone marrow is taken out and looked at under the microscope. A doctor may also do a spinal tap in which a needle is inserted through the back to take a sample of the fluid that surrounds the brain and spine. The fluid is then looked at under a microscope to see if leukemia cells are present. A doctor can then tell what kind of leukemia is present and plan the best treatment.

The chance of recovery (prognosis) depends on how the leukemia cells look under a microscope, how far the leukemia has spread, and the patient's age and general health.

Stages of Adult Acute Lymphoblastic Leukemia

There is no staging for ALL. The choice of treatment depends on whether a patient has been treated before.

Untreated

Untreated ALL means that no treatment has been given except to treat symptoms. There are too many white blood cells in the blood and bone marrow, and there may be other signs and symptoms of leukemia.

In Remission

Remission means that treatment has been given and that the number of white blood cells and other blood cells in the blood and bone marrow is normal. There are no signs or symptoms of leukemia.

Recurrent

Recurrent disease means that the leukemia has come back after going into remission. Refractory disease means that the leukemia has failed to go into remission following treatment.

Treatment Option Overview

There are treatments for all patients with ALL. The primary treatment of ALL is chemotherapy. Radiation therapy may be used in certain cases. Bone marrow transplantation is being studied in clinical trials.

Chemotherapy uses drugs to kill cancer cells. Chemotherapy may be taken by pill, or it may be put into the body by a needle in a vein or muscle. Chemotherapy is called a systemic treatment because the drug enters the blood stream, travels through the body, and can kill cancer cells throughout the body. Chemotherapy may sometimes be put into the fluid that surrounds the brain by inserting a needle in the brain or back (intrathecal chemotherapy).

Radiation therapy uses x-rays or other high-energy rays to kill cancer cells and shrink tumors. Radiation for ALL usually comes from a machine outside the body (external radiation therapy).

There are two phases of treatment for ALL. The first stage is called induction therapy. The purpose of induction therapy is to kill as many of the leukemia cells as possible and make patients go into remission. Once in remission with no signs of leukemia, patients enter a second phase of treatment (called continuation therapy), which tries to kill any remaining leukemia cells. A patient may receive chemotherapy for up to several years to stay in remission.

Radiation therapy or chemotherapy to the brain may be given to patients if leukemia cells have spread to the brain. Patients may also receive central nervous system (CNS) prophylaxis, another type of therapy, to prevent leukemia cells from growing in the brain during induction therapy and remission.

Bone marrow transplantation is used to replace bone marrow with healthy bone marrow. First, all of the bone marrow in the body is destroyed with high doses of chemotherapy with or without radiation therapy. Healthy marrow is then taken from another person (a donor) whose tissue is the same as or almost the same as the patient's. The donor may be a twin (the best match), a brother or sister, or a person who is not related. The healthy marrow from the donor is given to the patient through a needle in the vein, and the marrow replaces the marrow that was destroyed. A bone marrow transplant using marrow from a relative or person not related to the patient is called an allogeneic bone marrow transplant.

Another type of bone marrow transplant, called autologous bone marrow transplant, is being studied in clinical trials. To do this type of transplant, bone marrow is taken from the patient and treated with drugs to kill any cancer cells. The marrow is frozen to save it. Next, high-dose chemotherapy is given with or without radiation therapy to destroy all of the remaining marrow. The frozen marrow that was saved is then thawed and given to the patient through a needle in a vein to replace the marrow that was destroyed.

A greater chance for recovery occurs if the doctor chooses a hospital that does more than five bone marrow transplantations per year.

Treatment by Stage

Treatment of adult ALL depends on the type of disease, the patient's age, and overall condition.

Standard treatment may be considered based on its effectiveness in past studies, or participation in a clinical trial may be considered. Not all patients are cured with standard therapy, and some standard treatments may have more side effects than are desired. For these reasons, clinical trials are designed to find better ways to treat cancer patients and are based on the most up-to-date information. Clinical trials are ongoing in most parts of the country for most stages of ALL.

Untreated Adult Acute Lymphoblastic Leukemia

Treatment will probably be systemic chemotherapy. This may be intrathecal chemotherapy alone or combined with either radiation therapy to the brain or high doses of systemic chemotherapy to treat or prevent leukemia in the brain. Treatment may also include blood transfusions, antibiotics, and instructions to keep the body and teeth especially clean. Clinical trials are testing new drugs.

Adult Acute Lymphoblastic Leukemia in Remission

Treatment may be one of the following:

1. Clinical trials of short-term, high-dose chemotherapy followed by long-term, low-dose chemotherapy.

2. Clinical trials of allogeneic bone marrow transplantation.

3. Clinical trials of autologous bone marrow transplantation.

4. Intrathecal chemotherapy alone, or combined with either radiation to the brain or high doses of systemic chemotherapy, to prevent leukemia cells from growing in the brain (CNS prophylaxis).

Recurrent Adult Acute Lymphoblastic Leukemia

Radiation therapy may be given to reduce symptoms. Patients may also choose to take part in a clinical trial of bone marrow transplantation.

Risks, Statistics, and Treatment Outcomes

Sixty percent to 80% of adults with acute lymphoblastic leukemia (ALL) can be expected to attain complete remission status following appropriate induction therapy. Approximately 35% to 40% of adults with ALL can be expected to survive 2 years with aggressive induction combination chemotherapy and effective supportive care during induction therapy (appropriate early treatment of infection, hyperuricemia, and bleeding). A few studies that use intensive multiagent approaches suggest that a 50% 3-year survival is achievable in selected patients, but these results must be verified by other investigators.[1-4]

As in childhood ALL, adult patients with ALL are at risk of developing central nervous system (CNS) involvement during the course of their disease. This is particularly true for patients with L3 histology.[5] Both treatment and prognosis are influenced by this complication. The examination of bone marrow aspirates and/or biopsy specimens should be done by an experienced oncologist, hematologist, hematopathologist, or general pathologist who is capable of interpreting conventional and specially stained specimens. Diagnostic confusion with acute myelocytic leukemia (AML), hairy cell leukemia, and malignant lymphoma is not uncommon. Proper diagnosis is crucial because of the difference in prognosis and treatment of ALL and AML. Immunophenotypic analysis is essential because leukemias that do not express myeloperoxidase include M0 and M7 AML as well as ALL.

Appropriate initial treatment, usually consisting of a regimen that includes the combination of vincristine, prednisone, and anthracycline, with or without asparaginase, results in a complete remission rate of up to 80%. Median remission duration for the complete responders is approximately 15 months. Entry into a clinical trial is highly desirable to assure adequate patient treatment and also maximal information retrieval from the treatment of this highly responsive, but usually fatal, disease. Patients who experience a relapse after remission can be expected to succumb within 1 year, even if a second complete remission is achieved. If there are appropriate available donors and if the patient is younger than 55 years of age, bone marrow transplantation may be a consideration in the management of this disease.[6] Transplant centers performing 5 or fewer transplants annually usually have poorer results than larger centers.[7] If allogeneic transplant is considered, transfusions with blood products from a potential donor should be avoided if possible.[4,8-13]

Patients with L3 morphology have improved outcomes when treated according to specific treatment algorithms.[14,15] Age, which is a significant factor in childhood ALL and in AML, may also be an important prognostic factor in adult ALL. In one study, overall the prognosis was better in patients younger than 25 years; another study found a better prognosis in those younger than 35 years. These findings may, in part, be related to the increased incidence of the Philadelphia (Ph) chromosome in older ALL patients, a subgroup associated with poor prognosis.[1,2] Elevated B2-microglobulin is associated with a poor prognosis in adults as evidenced by lower response rate, increased incidence of CNS involvement, and significantly worse survival.[16] Patients with Ph chromosome-positive ALL are rarely cured with chemotherapy. Many patients who have molecular evidence of the bcr-abl fusion gene, which characterizes the Ph chromosome, have no evidence of the abnormal chromosome by cytogenetics. Because many patients have a different fusion protein from the one found in chronic myelogenous leukemia (p190 versus p210), the bcr-abl fusion gene may be detectable only by pulsed-field gel electrophoresis or reverse-transcriptase polymerase chain reaction (RT-PCR). These tests should be performed whenever possible in patients with ALL, especially those with B-cell lineage disease. Two other chromosomal abnormalities with poor prognoses are t(4;11), which is characterized by rearrangements of the MLL gene and may be rearranged despite normal cytogenetics, and t(9;22). In addition to t(9;22) and t(4;11), patients with deletion of chromosome 7 or trisomy 8 have been reported to have a lower probability of survival at 5 years compared to patients with a normal karyotype.[17] L3 ALL is associated with a variety of translocations which involve translocation of the c-myc proto-oncogene to the immunoglobulin gene locus (t(2;8), t(8;12), and t(8;22)).

References

1. Gaynor J, Chapman D, Little C, et al.: A cause-specific hazard rate analysis of prognostic factors among 199 adults with acute lymphoblastic leukemia: the Memorial Hospital experience since 1969. *Journal of Clinical Oncology* 6(6): 1014-1030, 1988.

2. Hoelzer D, Thiel E, Loffler H, et al.: Prognostic factors in a multicenter study for treatment of acute lymphoblastic leukemia in adults. *Blood* 71(1): 123-131, 1988.

3. Zhang MJ, Hoelzer D, Horowitz MM, et al.: Long-term follow-up of adults with acute lymphoblastic leukemia in first remission treated with chemotherapy or bone marrow transplantation. *Annals of Internal Medicine* 123(6): 428-431, 1995.

4. Larson RA, Dodge RK, Burns CP, et al.: A five-drug remission induction regimen with intensive consolidation for adults with acute lymphoblastic leukemia: Cancer and Leukemia Group B study 8811. *Blood* 85(8): 2025-2037, 1995.

5. Kantarjian HM, Walters RS, Smith TL, et al.: Identification of risk groups for development of central nervous system leukemia in adults with acute lymphocytic leukemia. *Blood* 72(5): 1784-1789, 1988.

6. Bortin MM, Horowitz MM, Gale RP, et al.: Changing trends in allogeneic bone marrow transplantation for leukemia in the 1980s. *JAMA: Journal of the American Medical Association* 268(5): 607-612, 1992.

7. Horowitz MM, Przepiorka D, Champlin RE, et al.: Should HLA-identical sibling bone marrow transplants for leukemia be restricted to large centers? *Blood* 79(10): 2771-2774, 1992.

8. Linker CA, Levitt LJ, O'Donnell M, et al.: Treatment of adult acute lymphoblastic leukemia with intensive cyclical chemotherapy: a follow-up report. *Blood* 78(11): 2814-2822, 1991.

9. Barrett AJ, Horowitz MM, Gale RP, et al.: Marrow transplantation for acute lymphoblastic leukemia: factors affecting relapse and survival. *Blood* 74(2): 862-871, 1989.

10. Dinsmore R, Kirkpatrick D, Flomenberg N, et al.: Allogeneic bone marrow transplantation for patients with acute lymphoblastic leukemia. *Blood* 62(2): 381-388, 1983.

11. Jacobs AD, Gale RP: Recent advances in the biology and treatment of acute lymphoblastic leukemia in adults. *New England Journal of Medicine* 311(19): 1219-1231, 1984.

12. Doney K, Buckner CD, Kopecky KJ, et al.: Marrow transplantation for patients with acute lymphoblastic leukemia in first

marrow remission. *Bone Marrow Transplantation* 2(4): 355-363, 1987.

13. Vernant JP, Marit G, Maraninchi D, et al.: Allogeneic bone marrow transplantation in adults with acute lymphoblastic leukemia in first complete remission. *Journal of Clinical Oncology* 6(2): 227-231, 1988.

14. Lee EJ, Petroni GR, Schiffer CA, et al.: Brief-duration high-intensity chemotherapy for patients with small noncleaved-cell lymphoma or FAB L3 acute lymphocytic leukemia: results of Cancer and Leukemia Group B study 9251. *Journal of Clinical Oncology* 19(20): 4014-4022, 2001.

15. Hoelzer D, Ludwig WD, Thiel E, et al.: Improved outcome in adult B-cell acute lymphoblastic leukemia. *Blood* 87(2): 495-508, 1996.

16. Kantarjian HM, Smith T, Estey E, et al.: Prognostic significance of elevated serum beta2-microglobulin levels in adult acute lymphocytic leukemia. *American Journal of Medicine* 93(6): 599-604, 1992.

17. Wetzler M, Dodge RK, Mrozek K, et al.: Prospective karyotype analysis in adult acute lymphoblastic leukemia: the Cancer and Leukemia Group B experience. *Blood* 93(11): 3983-3993, 1999.

Additional Information

National Cancer Institute
Cancer Information Service
6166 Executive Blvd., MSC 8322
Suite 3036A
Bethesda, MD 20892-8322
Toll-Free: 800-422-6237
TTY Toll-Free: 800-332-8615
Website: www.cancer.gov

The Leukemia & Lymphoma Society
1311 Mamaroneck Ave.
White Plains, NY 10605
Toll-Free: 800-955-4572
Tel: 914-949-5213, Fax: 914-949-6691
Website: www.leukemia-lymphoma.org

Chapter 22

Chronic Lymphocytic Leukemia (CLL)

Chronic lymphocytic leukemia (CLL) is a disease in which too many infection-fighting white blood cells called lymphocytes are found in the body. Lymphocytes are made in the bone marrow and by other organs of the lymph system. The bone marrow is the spongy tissue inside the large bones in the body. The bone marrow makes red blood cells (which carry oxygen and other materials to all tissues of the body), white blood cells (which fight infection), and platelets (which make the blood clot). Normally, bone marrow cells called blasts develop (mature) into several different types of blood cells that have specific jobs to do in the body.

The lymph system is made up of thin tubes that branch, like blood vessels, into all parts of the body. Lymph vessels carry lymph, a colorless, watery fluid that contains lymphocytes. Along the network of vessels are groups of small, bean-shaped organs called lymph nodes. Clusters of lymph nodes are found in the underarm, pelvis, neck, and abdomen. The spleen (an organ in the upper abdomen that makes lymphocytes and filters old blood cells from the blood), the thymus (a

This chapter includes PDQ® Cancer Information Summary, National Cancer Institute; Bethesda, MD, "Chronic Lymphocytic Leukemia (PDQ®): Treatment – Patient," updated 10/2002, available at http://cancer.gov, accessed 03/31/03; "Chronic Lymphocytic Leukemia: What Patients Should Know," Recorded Live: October 5, 2001, © Healthology, Inc., reprinted with permission; and "Will Targeted Therapies Work for CLL," Recorded Live: December 8, 2001, © Healthology, Inc., reprinted with permission.

small organ beneath the breastbone), and the tonsils (an organ in the throat) are also part of the lymph system.

Lymphocytes fight infection by making substances called antibodies, which attack germs and other harmful things in the body. In CLL, the developing lymphocytes do not mature correctly and too many are made. The lymphocytes may look normal, but they cannot fight infection as well as they should. These immature lymphocytes are then found in the blood and the bone marrow. They also collect in the lymph tissues and make them swell. Lymphocytes may crowd out other blood cells in the blood and bone marrow. Anemia may develop if the bone marrow cannot make enough red blood cells to carry oxygen. If the bone marrow cannot make enough platelets to make the blood clot normally, bleeding or bruising may occur easily.

Leukemia can be acute (progressing quickly with many immature cells) or chronic (progressing slowly with more mature, normal-looking cells). Chronic lymphocytic leukemia progresses slowly and usually occurs in people 60 years of age or older. In the first stages of the disease there are often no symptoms. As time goes on, more and more lymphocytes are made and symptoms begin to appear. A doctor should be seen if the lymph nodes swell, the spleen or liver becomes larger than normal, a feeling of fatigue persists, or bleeding occurs easily.

If there are symptoms, a doctor will do a physical examination and may order blood tests to count the number of each of the different kinds of blood cells. More blood tests may be done if the results of the blood tests are not normal. The doctor also may do a bone marrow biopsy. During this test, a needle is inserted into a bone and a small amount of bone marrow is taken out and looked at under the microscope. The doctor can then tell what kind of leukemia the patient has and plan the best treatment.

The chance of recovery (prognosis) depends on the stage of the disease, and the patient's age and general health.

Stage Information

Once chronic lymphocytic leukemia has been found (diagnosed), more tests may be done to find out if leukemia cells have spread to other parts of the body. This is called staging. A doctor needs to know the stage of the disease to plan treatment. The following stages are used for chronic lymphocytic leukemia:

Stage 0

There are too many lymphocytes in the blood, but there are usually no other symptoms of leukemia. Lymph nodes and the spleen and liver are not swollen and the number of red blood cells and platelets is normal.

Stage I

There are too many lymphocytes in the blood and lymph nodes are swollen. The spleen and liver are not swollen and the number of blood cells and platelets is normal.

Stage II

There are too many lymphocytes in the blood and lymph nodes and the liver and spleen are swollen.

Stage III

There are too many lymphocytes in the blood and there are too few red blood cells (anemia). Lymph nodes and the liver or spleen may be swollen.

Stage IV

There are too many lymphocytes in the blood and too few platelets, which make it hard for the blood to clot. The lymph nodes, liver, or spleen may be swollen and there may be too few red blood cells (anemia).

Refractory

Refractory means that the leukemia does not respond to treatment.

Treatment Option Overview

There are treatments for all patients with chronic lymphocytic leukemia. Three kinds of treatment are used:

- chemotherapy (using drugs to kill cancer cells)
- radiation therapy (using high dose x-rays or other high energy rays to kill cancer cells)
- treatment for complications of the leukemia, such as infection.

The use of biological therapy (using the body's immune system to fight cancer) is being tested in clinical trials. Surgery may be used in certain cases.

Chemotherapy uses drugs to kill cancer cells. Chemotherapy may be taken by pill, or it may be put into the body by a needle in the vein or muscle. Chemotherapy is called a systemic treatment because the drug enters the bloodstream, travels through the body, and can kill cancer cells throughout the body.

Radiation therapy uses x-rays or other high-energy rays to kill cancer cells and shrink tumors. Radiation for CLL usually comes from a machine outside the body (external radiation therapy).

If the spleen is swollen, a doctor may take out the spleen in an operation called a splenectomy. This is only done in rare cases.

Biological therapy tries to get the body to fight cancer. It uses materials made by the body or made in a laboratory to boost, direct, or restore the body's natural defenses against disease. Biological therapy is sometimes called biological response modifier (BRM) therapy or immunotherapy.

Because infection often occurs in patients with CLL, a special substance called immunoglobulin, which contains antibodies, may be given to prevent infections.

Sometimes a special machine is used to filter the blood to take out extra lymphocytes. This is called leukapheresis.

Bone marrow transplantation is used to replace the bone marrow with healthy bone marrow. First, all of the bone marrow in the body is destroyed with high doses of chemotherapy with or without radiation therapy. Healthy marrow is then taken from another person (a donor) whose tissue is the same as or almost the same as the patient's. The donor may be a twin (the best match), a brother or sister, or another person not related. The healthy marrow from the donor is given to the patient through a needle in the vein, and the marrow replaces the marrow that was destroyed. A bone marrow transplant using marrow from a relative or person not related to the patient is called an allogeneic bone marrow transplant.

Another type of bone marrow transplant, called autologous bone marrow transplant, is being studied in clinical trials. To do this type of transplant, bone marrow is taken from the patient and treated with drugs to kill any cancer cells. The marrow is frozen to save it. Next, the patient is given high-dose chemotherapy with or without radiation therapy to destroy all of the remaining marrow. The frozen marrow that was saved is then thawed and given back to the patient through a needle in a vein to replace the marrow that was destroyed.

Treatment by Stage

Treatment of chronic lymphocytic leukemia depends on the stage of the disease, and the patient's age and overall health. Standard treatment may be considered because of its effectiveness in patients in past studies, or participation in a clinical trial may be considered. Most patients with chronic lymphocytic leukemia are not cured with standard therapy and some standard treatments may have more side effects than are desired. For these reasons, clinical trials are designed to find better ways to treat cancer patients and are based on the most up-to-date information. Clinical trials are on going in most parts of the country for most stages of chronic lymphocytic leukemia. To know more about clinical trials, call the Cancer Information Service at 800-4-CANCER (800-422-6237); TTY at 800-332-8615.

Stage 0 Chronic Lymphocytic Leukemia

If the patient has stage 0 CLL, treatment may not be needed or chemotherapy may be given. A doctor will follow the patient closely so treatment can be started if the leukemia gets worse.

Stage I Chronic Lymphocytic Leukemia

Treatment may be one of the following:

1. If there are no symptoms, no treatment may be needed. A doctor will follow the patient closely so treatment can be started if the leukemia gets worse.

2. Chemotherapy with or without steroids.

3. Other chemotherapy drugs.

4. External radiation therapy to swollen lymph nodes.

5. Combination chemotherapy.

6. A clinical trial evaluating monoclonal antibodies.

7. A clinical trial evaluating bone marrow or peripheral stem cell transplantation.

Stage II Chronic Lymphocytic Leukemia

Treatment may be one of the following:

1. If there are few or no symptoms, no treatment may be needed. A doctor will follow the patient closely so treatment can be started if the leukemia gets worse.

2. Chemotherapy with or without steroids.

3. Other chemotherapy drugs.

4. Combination chemotherapy.

5. External radiation therapy to swollen lymph nodes.

6. External radiation therapy to the spleen to reduce symptoms caused by the enlargement of the spleen.

7. A clinical trial evaluating monoclonal antibodies.

8. A clinical trial evaluating bone marrow or peripheral stem cell transplantation.

Stage III Chronic Lymphocytic Leukemia

Treatment may be one of the following:

1. If there are few or no symptoms, no treatment may be needed. A doctor will follow the patient closely so treatment can be started if the leukemia gets worse.

2. Chemotherapy with or without steroids.

3. Other chemotherapy drugs.

4. Combination chemotherapy.

5. Surgery to remove the spleen or external radiation therapy to the spleen to reduce symptoms caused by the enlargement of the spleen.

6. A clinical trial evaluating monoclonal antibodies.

7. A clinical trial evaluating bone marrow or peripheral stem cell transplantation.

Stage IV Chronic Lymphocytic Leukemia

Treatment may be one of the following:

1. If there are few or no symptoms, no treatment may be needed. A doctor will follow the patient closely so treatment can be started if the leukemia gets worse.

2. Chemotherapy with or without steroids.

3. Other chemotherapy drugs.

4   Combination chemotherapy.

5. Surgery to remove the spleen or external radiation therapy to the spleen to reduce symptoms caused by the enlargement of the spleen.

6. A clinical trial evaluating monoclonal antibodies.

7. A clinical trial evaluating bone marrow or peripheral stem cell transplantation.

Refractory Chronic Lymphocytic Leukemia

Treatment depends on many factors; patients may wish to consider entering a clinical trial of new chemotherapy drugs and bone marrow or peripheral stem cell transplantation.

What Patients Should Know about Chronic Lymphocytic Leukemia

This section contains information about chronic lymphocytic leukemia discussed during an interview with John D. Hainsworth, MD of the Sarah Cannon Cancer Center, hosted by Maryann Bird, Nashville, TN.

Chronic lymphocytic leukemia or CLL accounts for 25% of all leukemias in the U.S., most common in adults over 50. It affects certain white blood cells called lymphocytes with serious consequences for the body's immune system.

What is chronic lymphocytic leukemia?

CLL is one kind of leukemia that's actually the most common adult leukemia in this country. It is different than the other leukemias in that it really is a chronic disease. Patients can live for quite awhile. It's a malignancy of lymphocytes of a certain type of lymphocyte called a "B" lymphocyte. And these cells are normally in the human body to fight infection. They're the cells that produce antibodies against infection.

How does CLL differ from other blood cancers like chronic myeloid leukemia and non-Hodgkin's lymphoma?

In general, these different hematologic cancers are derived from different cells.

Do we know what causes CLL?

We don't know what causes it. It's a disease that happens more frequently with increasing age. This is the only leukemia that's actually the most common in elderly patients. It's uncommon in patients younger than 50 years old.

What happens when patients get CLL?

CLL, like any kind of cancer, involves a proliferation—an abnormal proliferation of the cell that's the cancer cell. But in general, the big problems in this kind of cancer come when the bone marrow gets too full of these lymphocytes, and they start to affect the bone marrow's ability to do its normal functions, which are to produce other blood cells.

What are the signs or symptoms of this disease?

This is a disease that probably presents in one of three major ways. In this country, probably the most common way that people get diagnosed is that they go to their doctor for something else. And on a blood test, they're found to have a high white blood count level. And that leads to other tests, and then they get diagnosed. So often they're asymptomatic.

The second most common way is probably that they feel some enlarged lymph nodes. And often that's fairly diffuse. They can feel them in the neck, under the arms, in the groin.

The third way—and this is also fairly common—is that they develop fatigue. The fatigue is basically from anemia, and that's as a result of the bone marrow infiltration.

Is there a cure for CLL?

This is a leukemia that is not curable at present. On the other hand, it's one that many people who have it don't end up dying from it either. They have it and it's chronic and they live with it and then die from something else.

What are the treatment options for patients who have CLL?

For some patients, the best treatment option initially, if they're asymptomatic and are feeling fine, is actually not to treat them. So this is one kind of leukemia that often patients can be observed. When symptoms occur, that's when treatments are begun.

And typically, treatments have been able with relatively mild chemotherapy drugs, often oral drugs, to put a patient in remission. They can stay in remission for a while and off treatment. And then something—the white count starts to go up or symptoms recur. They get another treatment, get back into remission, etc. And this can go on for several years where they get different treatments.

What cutting-edge therapies are there for CLL? What's new on the horizon?

In CLL, there are several new what are called targeted therapies. Actually the two that are out there right now are antibodies, and they weren't available before and actually are highly active against CLL. These targeted drugs go directly to the abnormal B-lymphocytes that are involved in CLL and then kill those cells once they get there.

What about using the cutting-edge therapies with the traditional therapies?

The new agents—the monoclonal antibodies—are really new enough that their place in CLL has not been entirely defined yet. The two antibodies that came out recently in the last two or three years are Rituxan and Campath. They have been used by themselves but now probably the real interesting and exciting thing is that they're being used earlier in treatment, often in conjunction with our more standard chemotherapy. And already, using these antibodies plus chemotherapy have been able to give higher complete response rates in these patients.

How about bone marrow or stem cell transplantation?

Bone marrow transplants are high-dose chemotherapy with support with stem cells, [they have] not really been that useful, and I'd say probably will not play a major role in CLL in the future. Part of this is due to the fact that this is an elderly population. And that kind of treatment approach has a lot of toxicity and a lot of side effects.

Does the stage of a patient's disease impact his or her treatment?

The stage of disease in CLL is important but mostly with respect to making the decision of whether to treat the patient or not.

I imagine that some of your patients have a hard time to being told to watch and wait instead of seeking treatment.

That's true. This is one of the few cancers for which that is a reasonable option. And I think people are uncomfortable with that once they find out they have a cancer. It's difficult to convince people not to have treatment originally. But I think it's mostly a matter of just talking to them and educating them about this particular type of cancer.

Will Targeted Therapies Work for CLL?

This section contains information from an interview with Kanti Rai, MD, Long Island Jewish Hospital, New York and Joseph M. Connors, MD, FRCPC, British Columbia Cancer Agency hosted by Bret Scott, Orlando, FL.

Monoclonal antibody therapies that directly attack cancer cells are a hot topic in medicine. At the December 2001 meeting of the American Society of Hematology, several research presentations focused on the use of these therapies for chronic lymphocytic leukemia, or CLL.

Is Rituxan improving on traditional treatments for CLL? And if so, how?

Kanti Rai, MD: Rituxan is indeed improving on traditional treatment, if one considers today in year 2001, that fludarabine is the standard treatment for CLL. We get just so much of what we call remission rate with fludarabine. And we find that when we add Rituxan to fludarabine, the remission rate is practically doubled.

In terms of schedule and dose, will Rituxan be used differently to treat CLL compared with NHL?

Joseph M. Connors, MD, FRCPC: I would expect that it will. The schedule that works for a tumor-like lymphoma, where the cells are settled in one place in the body may well be different from the schedule that works best for a leukemia, where the malignant cells circulate around in the bloodstream. So I think we may expect different doses, different schedules, and even different lengths or durations of treatment.

Kanti Rai, MD: Rituxan in lymphoma is given once a week for several weeks. Four weeks, six weeks, eight weeks. And it is quite effective in those patients. But when you give Rituxan in the same manner to a person with CLL, it just does not have much activity. However, when you give Rituxan in combination with other standard chemotherapy drugs and, instead of giving it on a weekly basis, you give it once a month, the combination is a blockbuster.

Several treatment options for CLL using Rituxan were discussed at this meeting. What are the main options?

Kanti Rai, MD: The introduction of Rituxan in CLL is a relatively recent happening. So we cannot claim that we know everything as to how to use Rituxan in the most effective manner for our patients with CLL. Therefore there are lots of combinations and permutations being tried with an objective of finding out what works best for what group of patients.

How will Rituxan be used in treating younger patients versus older patients with CLL?

Joseph M. Connors, MD, FRCPC: I'm going to turn that question around a little bit, because one of the real virtues of antibody treatment—monoclonal antibody treatment—is the ability to treat older patients with it, when the toxic effects of other kinds of treatments may prevent you from doing so. I think that we will find that rituximab is used in older patients that we might not have been able to otherwise treat well. But to return to younger patients, I expect it to be combined with other still fairly intensive treatments in attempts to get rid of all of the leukemia completely. But that is moving to an era where we actually attempt to cure the disease, as opposed to control it as we might have in the past.

Campath is another monoclonal used to treat CLL. How does it differ from Rituxan and how is it used?

Joseph M. Connors, MD, FRCPC: The difference is the target. The monoclonal antibody in question is always directed at a specific surface characteristic or a small bump as I describe it on the surface of the cells. Rituximab is targeted at one that has the technical name of CD20 and is shared across many different kinds of lymphocytes, but closely restricted to lymphocytes. Campath is directed at a different surface characteristic or bump that is shared across not only lymphocytes, but other different types of blood cells. And so, although restricted to a small number of cells, the Campath antibody does have effects on some of the cells we aren't targeting it towards, and we have to allow for that affect and the possible side effects that may come with it.

What about side effects?

Kanti Rai, MD: Side effects with the rituximab are somewhat of a lesser magnitude than side effects with Campath. Campath is an antibody which kills all lymphocytes, whether they are B-cells or T-cells. In CLL, as you perhaps know, that it is the B-cells that we are trying to kill, because those are the malignant cells. But the T-cells we don't have to kill, but Campath does not discriminate between Bs and Ts, so they kill all the cells and thereby render a person's immune system much more vulnerable to opportunistic infections, such as pneumonias and blood infections.

As far as other immediate effects or concerns, both the drugs—Campath and Rituxan—do cause some degree of shaking, chills and fever, and drop in blood pressure when a patient's body first is exposed to either one of these drugs. But with continued use, the body gets adjusted to this, and in subsequent use that problem is reduced markedly.

Does adding chemotherapy to these targeted approaches increase the side effects?

Joseph M. Connors, MD, FRCPC: It's an exciting area of research to add these together, because the antibodies and the chemotherapy can interact with each other and boost the effectiveness of each other. As we do this, we monitor patients carefully to see if any new or unexpected side effects or toxicity develops. So far, that hasn't been a problem in large part because the antibodies have different kinds of side effects than traditional chemotherapy, and patients can actually tolerate the combination of these two side effects without them adding together.

What is the ultimate goal of these targeted approaches? Can they cure CLL?

Kanti Rai, MD: That is our aim, and that is our objective, but I would be overstating the case that these combinations will get us to that endpoint. But, in my view, the combination of both of these antibodies along with chemotherapy, in some form or another—as time goes on, we will find out—will aid us in significantly better overall treatment for CLL patients than we have been able to deliver to those patients for the last three or four decades.

Joseph M. Connors, MD, FRCPC: We continue to work, I think, in an increasingly exciting era of the treatment of cancers. Understanding the basic biology, identifying specific targets that cancer cells uniquely express, and developing the therapeutic—the treatment tools to go after these cancer cells with these specifically targeted treatments is a change compared to the first twenty years I spent in this field. It adds to the excitement and the anticipation that these treatments will be gradually turning into effective curative ways of getting rid of the cancer.

Additional Information

National Cancer Institute
6166 Executive Blvd., MSC 8322
Suite 3036A
Bethesda, MD 20892-8322
Toll-Free: 800-4-CANCER (800-422-6237)
Toll-Free TTY: 800-332-8615
Website: www.cancer.gov

Chapter 23

Acute Myelogenous Leukemia (AML)

About 10,000 new cases of acute myelogenous leukemia are diagnosed each year in the United States. Acute myelogenous leukemia may be called by several names, including acute myelocytic leukemia, acute myeloblastic leukemia, acute granulocytic leukemia, or acute nonlymphocytic leukemia.

The earliest observations of patients who had marked elevation of their white blood cells by European physicians in the 19th century led to their coining the term *weisses blut* or white blood as a designation for the disorder. Later, the term leukemia, which is derived from the Greek words *leukos* meaning white and *haima* meaning blood, was used to indicate the disease.

The major forms of leukemia are divided into four categories: myelogenous and lymphocytic, each having an acute or chronic form. The terms myelogenous or lymphocytic denote the cell type involved. Acute leukemia is a rapidly progressing disease that affects principally cells that are unformed or primitive (not yet fully developed or differentiated). These immature cells cannot carry out their normal functions. Chronic leukemia progresses slowly and permits the growth of greater

Excerpts from "Acute Myelogenous Leukemia (AML)," © 10/01 The Leukemia & Lymphoma Society, additional information is available at www.leukemia-lymphoma.org, reprinted with permission. Text under "Remission Rates, Prognosis, and Relapse," is excerpted from PDQ® Cancer Information summary, National Cancer Institute; Bethesda, MD, "Adult Acute Myeloid Leukemia (PDQ®): Treatment–Health Professional," updated 08/2002, available at: http://cancer.gov, accessed 03/31/2003.

numbers of more developed cells. In general, these more mature cells can carry out some of their normal functions. Thus, the four major types of leukemia are acute or chronic myelogenous and acute or chronic lymphocytic leukemia.

The ability to measure specific features of cells has led to further subclassification of the major categories of leukemia. The categories and subsets allow the physician to decide what treatment works best for the cell type and how quickly the disease may develop.

Acute myelogenous leukemia (AML) results from acquired (not inherited) genetic damage to the DNA of developing cells in the bone marrow. The effects are 1) the uncontrolled, exaggerated growth and accumulation of cells called leukemic blasts, which fail to function as normal blood cells and 2) the blockade of the production of normal marrow cells, leading to a deficiency of red cells (anemia), and platelets (thrombocytopenia) and normal white cells (especially neutrophils, i.e. neutropenia) in the blood.

Causes and Risk Factors

In most cases the cause of acute myelogenous leukemia is not evident. Several factors have been associated with an increased risk of disease. These include exposure to very high doses of irradiation, as carefully studied in the Japanese survivors of atomic bomb detonations, exposure to the chemical benzene, usually in the work place, and exposure to chemotherapy used to treat cancers such as breast cancer, cancer of the ovary, or the lymphomas. Acute myelogenous leukemia is not contagious and is not inherited. Uncommon genetic disorders such as Fanconi anemia, Down syndrome, and others are associated with an increased risk of AML. About 15 percent of childhood leukemia cases are of acute myelogenous leukemia. Older people are more likely to develop the disease. The risk increases about tenfold from age 30 (about 1 case per 100,000 people) to age 70 (about 1 case per 10,000 people) (see Figure 23.1).

Subtypes of Acute Myelogenous Leukemia

Leukemia is a malignant disease (cancer) of the bone marrow and blood. Acute myelogenous leukemia can occur in a variety of ways—different types of cells may be seen by the physician in blood or marrow. Since most patients have one of eight different patterns of blood cell involvement, these patterns have formed a subclassification which is shown in Table 23.1.

Myeloblasts are undeveloped cells. If they are the dominant leukemia cells in the marrow at the time of diagnosis the leukemia is referred to as myeloblastic type. If there are many myeloblasts, but there are some cells developing towards fully formed blood cells, the added designation *with maturation* is used. If there are cells that are developing features of monocytes (monocytic type) or red cells (erythroleukemia type), these designations are used and so forth.

Even though the leukemia cells look somewhat like blood cells, the process of their formation is incomplete. Normal, healthy blood cells are insufficient in quantity (see Figure 23.1).

The subclassification of the disease is important. Different types of therapy may be used and the course of the disease may be different. Additional features may be important in guiding the choice of therapy including abnormalities of chromosomes, the cell immunophenotype, the age and the general health of the patient, and others.

Symptoms and Signs

Most patients feel a loss of well-being. They tire more easily, may feel short of breath when physically active. They may have a pale complexion from anemia. Several signs of bleeding caused by a very low platelet count may be noticed. They include black and blue marks or bruises occurring for no reason or because of a minor injury, the appearance of pinhead sized spots under the skin, called petechiae, or prolonged bleeding from minor cuts. Mild fever, swollen gums, frequent

Table 23.1. Acute Myelogenous Leukemia

Designation	Cell Subtype
M0	Myeloblastic, on special analysis
M1	Myeloblastic, without maturation
M2	Myeloblastic, with maturation
M3	Promyelocytic
M4	Myelomonocytic
M5	Monocytic
M6	Erythroleukemia
M7	Megakaryocytic

minor infections like pustules or perianal sores, slow healing of cuts, or discomfort in bones or joints may occur.

Diagnosis

To diagnose the disease, the blood and marrow cells must be examined. In addition to low red cell and platelet counts, examination of the stained (dyed) blood cells with a microscope usually will show the presence of leukemic blast cells. This is confirmed by examination of the marrow, which invariably shows leukemic blast cells. The blood and/or marrow cells are also used for studies of the number and shape of chromosomes (cytogenetic examination), immunopheno-typing, and other special studies, if required.

Treatment

Nearly all patients with acute myelogenous leukemia require treatment as soon after diagnosis as possible. The principal goal of treatment is to bring about a remission in which there is no evidence of

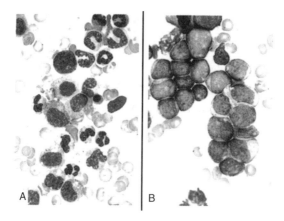

Figure 23.1. Panel A (on left) shows a photograph taken through a microscope of normal marrow cells. The differences in appearance among the cells reflect their different developmental stages. Panel B (on right) shows a photograph taken through a microscope of acute myelogenous leukemia blast cells. The monotonous appearance of these cells, which are "frozen" in an earlier stage of development, is in contrast to the normal cells in panel A.

leukemic blast cells in the blood or marrow. Normal blood cell production is restored and blood cell counts return to normal levels.

In most patients intensive chemotherapy is required to achieve complete remission. At least two drugs are combined to treat patients initially. Approaches to treatment are undergoing intensive study throughout the world; there are variations on the general descriptions given here. Thus, a patient may receive either a different number of drugs, sequence of drugs, or types of drugs than described here, and may be receiving appropriate and effective treatment. It is, however, important to seek treatment in a center where physicians are experienced in the care of patients with acute leukemia.

In order to prepare the patient for treatment, an indwelling catheter is placed in a vein in the upper chest to allow ready access for infusion of drugs, blood cells, and the removal of blood samples for cell counts and chemical tests. In some patients, if the white cell count is very high, a drug called allopurinol is given to minimize the build up of blood uric acid. Uric acid is a breakdown product of cells. It enters the blood and is excreted in the urine. If many cells are killed simultaneously by therapy, the amount of uric acid in the urine can be so high that uric acid kidney stones can form which may seriously interfere with the flow of urine.

Chemotherapy

Induction Therapy

This is the initial phase of specific treatment. In most cases an anthracycline antibiotic (e.g. daunorubicin, doxorubicin, or idarubicin) is combined with cytarabine (syn. cytosine arabinoside, ara-C). Both drugs act in different ways to prevent DNA synthesis of leukemia cells, stopping their growth, and leading to their death. The anthracycline antibiotic is given, usually, in the first three days of treatment. Cytarabine is started at the same time, but is given for seven to 10 days of treatment. Both drugs are dissolved in fluids and injected into a vein. The goal of induction therapy is to rid the blood and marrow of visible leukemic blast cells. If blast cells are still evident, a second course of chemotherapy may be required to rid the marrow of blasts. Usually the same drugs are used for each course.

When chemotherapy is effective, developing blood cells as well as leukemia cells are eliminated from the marrow, resulting in a severe deficiency of red cells (anemia), phagocytes (neutropenia and monocytopenia), and platelets (thrombocytopenia) in the blood. Transfusion of red cells and, often, platelets may be required. The deficiency of phagocytes (microbe-eating cells) permits bacteria and fungi, normally present on skin, in the nose, mouth, or large bowel (colon), or transferred from other persons or the environment, to establish infection during this period. Because of this, antibiotic therapy frequently is required.

In most patients, after several weeks normal blood cell production will return and transfusion of cells and antibiotics no longer will be needed. Blood cell counts gradually approach normal, well-being returns and leukemia cells cannot be identified in blood or marrow. This is a remission. In this state, residual leukemic cells are inactive. They do not interfere with normal blood cell development but have the potential to regrow and cause a relapse of the leukemia. For this reason, additional therapy in the form of chemotherapy with or without autologous stem cell infusion or allogeneic stem cell transplantation usually is advised.

One exception to this pattern is the treatment of the acute promyelocytic subtype of AML. In this subtype, the cells that accumulate in the marrow can be identified as promyelocytes, the next step in blood cell formation after the myeloblast. They also have a specific chromosome abnormality involving chromosome number 15, usually in conjunction with chromosome 17. As a part of the expression of this form of AML, the leukemia cells are stalled at this stage of development. A derivative of vitamin A, all-trans retinoic acid, often abbreviated as ATRA, is administered with chemotherapy. Retinoic acid is capable of inducing the leukemic promyelocytes to develop into mature cells (neutrophils). It markedly decreases the concentration of leukemic blast cells in the marrow and a remission frequently ensues. For the remission to be long lasting, chemotherapy must follow or be concurrent. But retinoic acid often minimizes the side effects of chemotherapy because blood cell counts may be improved and the number of primitive leukemia cells is decreased as chemotherapy is started.

Arsenic trioxide, like retinoic acid, can induce remission of acute promyelocytic leukemia. This agent has been approved for use in patients who have relapsed or are resistant to treatment. Studies are in progress to learn how best to use these drugs in combination with chemotherapy.

Some Drugs Used in the Treatment of Acute Myelogenous Leukemia

Most anti-leukemic drugs interact with the genetic material in the cell (the DNA or deoxyribonucleic acid).

254

Antitumor Antibiotics: These drugs interact directly with the DNA in the nucleus of cells interfering with cell survival.

- daunorubicin (daunomycin, rubidomycin, Cerubidine)
- doxorubicin (Adriamycin, Rubex)
- mitoxantrone (Novantrone)
- idarubicin (Idamycin)

Antimetabolites: These are chemicals that are very similar to natural building blocks of DNA or RNA, but they are changed sufficiently from the natural chemical. When they substitute for it, they block the cell's ability to form RNA or DNA, preventing the cell from growing.

- 5-azacytidine (Mylosar)
- cytarabine (cytosine arabinoside, Ara-C, Cytosar)
- cladribine (Leustatin)
- fludarabine (Fludara)
- hydroxyurea (Hydrea)
- 6-mercaptopurine (Purinethol)
- methotrexate (Mexate)
- 6-thioguanine (Thioguanine)

DNA Repair Enzyme Inhibitors: These drugs act on certain proteins (enzymes) which help to repair injury to DNA. These drugs prevent the enzymes from working and make the DNA more susceptible to injury.

- etoposide (VP-16, VePesid, Etopophos, Toposar)
- teniposide (VM-26, Vumon)
- topotecan (Hycamtin)

DNA Synthesis Inhibitors: The drug reacts with DNA to alter it chemically and keep it from permitting cell growth.

- carboplatin (Paraplatin)

Cell Maturing Agents

- all-trans retinoic acid
- arsenic trioxide

Monoclonal Antibodies

- gemtuzumab ozogamicin (Mylotarg)

Post-Remission Therapy

Since residual leukemic cells that cannot be detected by the blood or marrow examination remain after a remission, the optimal treatment of AML usually requires additional intensive therapy after remission has been achieved. There is no consensus as to the best approach, in part, because individual factors such as age of the patient, the ability to tolerate intensive treatment, cytogenetic findings, the availability of a stem cell donor, and others may influence the approach used. If chemotherapy is to be used, the best results occur if intensive treatment is applied. One current approach is to use very high doses of cytarabine given intravenously soon after remission occurs.

Therapy can be further intensified in patients who do not have a histocompatible donor by giving very intensive chemotherapy and reinfusing the patient's own marrow to restore blood cell production, which otherwise would be profoundly impaired by this amount of chemotherapy. The marrow is harvested from the patient shortly after remission is induced and frozen (cryopreserved) until it is thawed for use. Special techniques are required to keep marrow cells from being damaged during the freezing and thawing process.

Patients between the age of approximately 1 and 50 years who are in remission and have a histocompatible donor are candidates for allogeneic stem cell transplantation. The decision to do a transplant depends on the features of the leukemia, the age of the patient, and the patient's understanding of the potential benefits and risks. For example, a younger patient with cytogenetic findings that are associated with a higher probability of relapse would be a candidate for allogeneic stem cell transplantation.

Older Patients

Acute myelogenous leukemia occurs more frequently with advancing age. At least half the patients are over 65 years of age when the disease occurs. At this time other medical problems including heart disease, lung disease, diabetes mellitus, or others may be present. The intensity of treatment requires consideration of these factors and the drugs, doses, and frequency of treatment are often individualized to consider the features of the leukemia, the health of the patient, and the patient's anticipated tolerance of therapy. Older patients are more resistant to treatment on average, and this adds to the complexity of management.

Side Effects of Treatment and Their Management

Acute myelogenous leukemia decreases the production of normal blood cells, but the levels are further decreased by the added effects of chemotherapy. The intensity of chemotherapy required to destroy sufficient leukemia cells to permit a remission leads to even more severe decreases in red cells, phagocytes, and platelets. Severe anemia, the risk of bleeding from a low platelet count, and a high likelihood of infection result. Red cell and platelet transfusions are usually effective in providing sufficient amounts of those cells until the beneficial effects of treatment occur several weeks later and blood cell counts return toward normal. Practical methods for transfusion of phagocytes are not currently available, except in infants and very small children, and antibiotic therapy is used when the earliest signs of infection develop.

A rise in temperature or chills may be the only signs of infection in a patient with a very low white blood cell concentration. In this setting, persistent coughing, tenderness at a site prone to infection like the area surrounding the anus or facial sinuses, sore throat, pain on urination, or frequent loose stools also may be signs of an infection. Efforts to decrease the risk of infection by vigorous hand washing by all visitors and medical personnel and meticulous care of indwelling catheter sites are important. Care of the gums, a site of bacterial accumulation, also is an important area of infection prevention.

The use of blood cell growth factors that stimulate the production of phagocytes can shorten the period during which the white cell count is low. Those used most frequently are granulocyte-colony stimulating factor (G-CSF) and granulocyte-macrophage colony stimulating factor (GM-CSF).

Chemotherapy affects tissues that require a high rate of cell birth (cell division) to keep them functional. The lining of the mouth, the lining of the intestines, the skin, and the hair follicles are such tissues. This explains why mouth ulcers, diarrhea, and hair loss are common after chemotherapy. Skin rashes also may occur.

Nausea and vomiting can be distressing features of chemotherapy. The causes can be complex. The effects are the result of actions on the intestines and on centers of the brain which, when triggered, lead to vomiting. Fortunately, drugs that counteract the nausea and vomiting can relieve these distressing side effects in most cases, if they occur.

Refractory Leukemia and Relapsed Leukemia

Some patients, even after intensive treatment, have residual leukemic cells in their marrow. This circumstance is referred to as refractory leukemia. Other patients, who have had a remission of leukemia after therapy, have a return of leukemia cells in the marrow and a decrease in normal blood cells. This situation is referred to as relapse. In the case of refractory leukemia, different approaches, such as drugs not used in the first course of treatment or stem cell transplantation, may be used in an effort to induce remission. In patients who relapse, the duration of the remission, their age, and the cytogenetic findings in the leukemia cells influence the approach to therapy. Drugs similar to those administered initially, different drugs, or stem cell transplantation may be used to treat the leukemia. A monoclonal antibody that is coupled to a potent cell-killing agent that targets myelogenous leukemia blast cells has been approved for treatment of older patients who have relapsed AML. This agent is also being studied in combination with other drugs to treat this very difficult situation.

Remission Rates, Prognosis, and Relapse

Advances in the treatment of adult acute myeloid leukemia (AML; also called acute nonlymphocytic leukemia or ANLL) have resulted in substantially improved complete remission rates.[1-5] Treatment should be sufficiently aggressive to achieve complete remission because partial remission offers no substantial survival benefit. Approximately 60% to 70% of adults with AML can be expected to attain complete remission status following appropriate induction therapy. More than 15% of adults with AML (about 25% of those who attain complete remission) can be expected to survive 3 or more years and may be cured. Remission rates in adult AML are inversely related to age, with an expected remission rate of greater than 65% for those younger than 60 years of age. Data suggest that once attained, duration of remission may be shorter in older patients. Increased morbidity and mortality during induction appear to be directly related to age. Other adverse prognostic factors include central nervous system involvement with leukemia, systemic infection at diagnosis, elevated white blood cell count (>100,000 per cubic millimeter), treatment-induced

AML, and history of myelodysplastic syndrome. Leukemias that express the progenitor cell antigen CD34 and/or the P-glycoprotein (MDR1 gene product) have an inferior outcome.[6-8] Expression of the bcl-2 oncoprotein, which inhibits programmed cell death, has been shown to predict poor survival.[9]

Cytogenetic analysis provides some of the strongest prognostic information available, predicting outcome of both remission induction and post-remission therapy.[10] Cytogenetic abnormalities which indicate a good prognosis include t(8;21), inv(16), and t(15;17). Normal cytogenetics portend average-risk AML. Patients with AML that is characterized by deletions of the long arms or monosomies of chromosomes 5 or 7; by translocations or inversions of chromosome 3, t(6;9), t(9;22); or by abnormalities of chromosome 11q23 have particularly poor prognoses with chemotherapy. These cytogenetic subgroups predict clinical outcome in elderly patients with AML as well as in younger patients.[11] The fusion genes formed in t(8;21) and inv(16) can be detected by reverse-transcriptase polymerase chain reaction (RT-PCR), which will indicate the presence of these genetic alterations in some patients in whom standard cytogenetics was technically inadequate. RT-PCR does not appear to identify significant numbers of patients with good risk fusion genes who have normal cytogenetics.[12] Abnormalities of the MLL gene (chromosome 11q23) can also be detected using RT-PCR and may be detected in some cases of leukemia with normal cytogenetics. These molecular diagnostic techniques are not readily available.[1-4,13,14]

Allogeneic bone marrow transplantation can be considered in patients younger than 60 years of age in first remission if a histocompatible sibling is available as a potential donor. Although data have shown that partially matched donors can also be used in some circumstances, the incidence of severe graft-versus-host disease, delayed engraftment, and graft rejection is significantly increased. Transfusion of blood products from potential donors should be avoided, and histocompatibility testing should be done at the earliest possible time. Although some data suggest that transplantation in patients during their first remission may improve long-term survival, these data need to be confirmed. In some studies, results from chemotherapy alone or high-dose chemotherapy with autologous bone marrow transplantation [15-25] appear to be comparable to those of allogeneic transplantation.[24,25]

As a generalization, most studies demonstrate that the rate of leukemic relapse is decreased following allogeneic bone marrow transplantation in first remission compared with chemotherapy alone.

Because of the higher initial mortality with bone marrow transplantation caused by graft-versus-host disease and interstitial pneumonia, however, comparative analyses of the two approaches demonstrate similar overall survivals. An analysis of bone marrow transplant results has also suggested that the same factors that predict for shorter response durations with chemotherapy (i.e., high initial white blood cell count, monocytic morphology, and age) may also result in shorter remission duration following transplantation. Allogeneic bone marrow transplantation has yielded a high rate of complete response in patients for whom initial induction therapy failed,[28] and autologous bone marrow transplantation may produce long-term leukemia-free survival in approximately one-third of patients in either first relapse or second complete remission.[29] Results of allogeneic bone marrow transplantation have modestly improved since 1980, largely because of a reduction in transplant-related mortality;[30] further follow-up of these and other studies is needed before firm recommendations can be made.[22,31] It should be noted that transplant centers performing five or fewer transplants annually usually have poorer results than larger centers.[32]

Long-term follow-up of 30 patients with AML in remission for at least 10 years has demonstrated a 13% incidence of secondary malignancies. Of 31 long-term female survivors of AML or acute lymphoblastic leukemia under 40 years of age, 26 resumed normal menstruation following completion of therapy. Among 36 live offspring of survivors, 2 congenital problems occurred.[33]

Cytogenetic studies should be performed at the time of diagnosis.[34] As noted, there is increasing evidence of nonrandom chromosomal rearrangements in some of the subtypes in the French-American-British classification, which have important prognostic significance.[35]

The differentiation of AML from acute lymphocytic leukemia has important therapeutic implications. Histochemical stains, TdT determinations, and cell surface antigen determinations aid in discrimination.

References

1. Yates J, Glidewell O, Wiernik P, et al.: Cytosine arabinoside with daunorubicin or Adriamycin for therapy of acute myelocytic leukemia: a CALGB study. *Blood* 60(2): 454-462, 1982.

2. Champlin R, Gale RP: Acute myelogenous leukemia: recent advances in therapy. *Blood* 69(6): 1551-1562, 1987.

3. Keating MJ, McCredie KB, Bodey GP, et al.: Improved prospects for long-term survival in adults with acute myelogenous leukemia. *JAMA: Journal of the American Medical Association* 248(19): 2481-2486, 1982.

4. Weinstein HJ, Mayer RJ, Rosenthal DS, et al.: Chemotherapy for acute myelogenous leukemia in children and adults: VAPA update. *Blood* 62(2): 315-319, 1983.

5. Preisler HD, Anderson K, Rai K, et al.: The frequency of long-term remission in patients with acute myelogenous leukemia treated with conventional maintenance chemotherapy: a study of 760 patients with a minimal follow-up time of 6 years. *British Journal of Haematology* 71(2): 189-194, 1989.

6. Myint H, Lucie NP: The prognostic significance of the CD34 antigen in acute myeloid leukaemia. *Leukemia and Lymphoma* 7(5-6): 425-429, 1992.

7. Geller RB, Zahurak M, Hurwitz CA, et al.: Prognostic importance of immunophenotyping in adults with acute myelocytic leukaemia: the significance of the stem-cell glycoprotein CD34 (My10). *British Journal of Haematology* 76(3): 340-347, 1990.

8. Campos L, Guyotat D, Archimbaud E, et al.: Clinical significance of multidrug resistance P-glycoprotein expression on acute nonlymphoblastic leukemia cells at diagnosis. *Blood* 79(2): 473-476, 1992.

9. Campos L, Rouault JP, Sabido O, et al.: High expression of bcl-2 protein in acute myeloid leukemia cells is associated with poor response to chemotherapy. *Blood* 81(11): 3091-3096, 1993.

10. Slovac ML, Kopecky KJ, Cassileth PA, et al.: Karyotypic analysis predicts outcome of preremission and postremission therapy in adult acute myeloid leukemia: a Southwest Oncology Group/Eastern Cooperative Oncology Group study. *Blood* 96(13): 4075-4083, 2000.

11. Grimwade D, Walker H, Harrison G, et al.: The predictive value of hierarchical cytogenetic classification in older adults with acute myeloid leukemia (AML): analysis of 1065 patients entered into the United Kingdom Medical Research Council AML11 trial. *Blood* 98(5): 1312-1320, 2001.

12. Mrozek K, Prior TW, Edwards C, et al.: Comparison of cytogenetic and molecular genetic detection of t(8;21) and inv(16) in a prospective series of adults with de novo acute myeloid leukemia: a Cancer and Leukemia Group B study. *Journal of Clinical Oncology* 19(9): 2482-2492, 2001.

13. Holmes R, Keating MJ, Cork A, et al.: A unique pattern of central nervous system leukemia in acute myelomonocytic leukemia associated with inv(16)(p13q22). *Blood* 65(5): 1071-1078, 1985.

14. Dutcher JP, Schiffer CA, Wiernik PH: Hyperleukocytosis in adult acute nonlymphocytic leukemia: impact on remission rate and duration, and survival. *Journal of Clinical Oncology* 5(9): 1364-1372, 1987.

15. Tallman MS, Kopecky KJ, Amos D, et al.: Analysis of prognostic factors for the outcome of marrow transplantation or further chemotherapy for patients with acute nonlymphocytic leukemia in first remission. *Journal of Clinical Oncology* 7(3): 326-337, 1989.

16. Appelbaum FR, Fisher LD, Thomas ED: Chemotherapy vs marrow transplantation for adults with acute nonlymphocytic leukemia: a five-year follow-up. *Blood* 72(1): 179-184, 1988.

17. Geller RB, Saral R, Piantadosi S, et al.: Allogeneic bone marrow transplantation after high-dose busulfan and cyclophosphamide in patients with acute nonlymphocytic leukemia. *Blood* 73(8): 2209-2218, 1989.

18. Clift RA, Buckner CD, Thomas ED, et al.: The treatment of acute non-lymphoblastic leukemia by allogeneic marrow transplantation. *Bone Marrow Transplantation* 2(3): 243-258, 1987.

19. Cassileth PA, Andersen J, Lazarus HM, et al.: Autologous bone marrow transplant in acute myeloid leukemia in first remission. *Journal of Clinical Oncology* 11(2): 314-319, 1993.

20. Beatty PG, Clift RA, Mickelson EM, et al.: Marrow transplantation from related donors other than HLA-identical siblings. *New England Journal of Medicine* 313(13): 765-771, 1985.

21. Rees JKH, Swirsky D, Gray RG, et al.: Principal results of the Medical Research Council's 8th acute myeloid leukaemia trial. *Lancet* 2(8518): 1236-1241, 1986.

22. Dutcher JP, Wiernik PH, Markus S, et al.: Intensive maintenance therapy improves survival in adult acute nonlymphocytic leukemia: an eight-year follow-up. *Leukemia* 2(7): 413-419, 1988.

23. Transplant or chemotherapy in acute myelogenous leukaemia. International Bone Marrow Transplant Registry. *Lancet* 1(8647): 1119-1122, 1989.

24. McMillan AK, Goldstone AH, Linch DC, et al.: High-dose chemotherapy and autologous bone marrow transplantation in acute myeloid leukemia. *Blood* 76(3): 480-488, 1990.

25. Champlin R, Gajewski J, Nimer S, et al.: Postremission chemotherapy for adults with acute myelogenous leukemia: improved survival with high-dose cytarabine and daunorubicin consolidation treatment. *Journal of Clinical Oncology* 8(7): 1199-1206, 1990.

26. Cassileth PA, Lynch E, Hines JD, et al.: Varying intensity of postremission therapy in acute myeloid leukemia. *Blood* 79(8): 1924-1930, 1992.

27. Biggs JC, Horowitz MM, Gale RP, et al.: Bone marrow transplants may cure patients with acute leukemia never achieving remission with chemotherapy. *Blood* 80(4): 1090-1093, 1992.

28. Petersen FB, Lynch MH, Clift RA, et al.: Autologous marrow transplantation for patients with acute myeloid leukemia in untreated first relapse or in second complete remission. *Journal of Clinical Oncology* 11(7): 1353-1360, 1993.

29. Bortin MM, Horowitz MM, Gale RP, et al.: Changing trends in allogeneic bone marrow transplantation for leukemia in the 1980s. *JAMA: Journal of the American Medical Association* 268(5): 607-612, 1992.

30. McGlave PB, Haake RJ, Bostrom BC, et al.: Allogeneic bone marrow transplantation for acute nonlymphocytic leukemia in first remission. *Blood* 72(5): 1512-1517, 1988.

31. Horowitz MM, Przepiorka D, Champlin RE, et al.: Should HLA-identical sibling bone marrow transplants for leukemia be restricted to large centers? *Blood* 79(10): 2771-2774, 1992.

32. Larson RA, Le Beau MM, Vardiman JW, et al.: The predictive value of initial cytogenetic studies in 148 adults with acute

nonlymphocytic leukemia: a 12-year study (1970-1982). *Cancer Genetics and Cytogenetics* 10(3): 219-236, 1983.

33. Micallef IN, Rohatiner AZ, Carter M, et al.: Long-term outcome of patients surviving for more than ten years following treatment for acute leukaemia. *Br J Haematol* 113 (2): 443-5, 2001.

34. Keating MJ, Smith TL, Kantarjian H, et al.: Cytogenetic pattern in acute myelogenous leukemia: a major reproducible determinant of outcome. *Leukemia* 2(7): 403-412, 1988.

35. Bloomfield CD, de la Chapelle A: Chromosome abnormalities in acute nonlymphocytic leukemia: clinical and biologic significance. *Seminars in Oncology* 14(4): 372-383, 1987.

Chapter 24

Chronic Myelogenous Leukemia (CML)

What Is Chronic Myelogenous Leukemia?

Chronic myelogenous leukemia (also called CML or chronic granulocytic leukemia) is a disease in which too many white blood cells are made in the bone marrow. The bone marrow is the spongy tissue inside the large bones in the body. The bone marrow makes red blood cells (which carry oxygen and other materials to all tissues of the body), white blood cells (which fight infection), and platelets (which make the blood clot).

Normally, bone marrow cells called blasts develop (mature) into several different types of blood cells that have specific jobs to do in the body. CML affects the blasts that are developing into white blood cells called granulocytes. The blasts do not mature and become too numerous. These immature blast cells are then found in the blood and the bone marrow. In most people with CML, the genetic material (chromosomes) in the leukemia cells have a feature that is not normal

This chapter includes PDQ® Cancer Information Summary, National Cancer Institute; Bethesda, MD, "Chronic Myelogenous Leukemia (PDQ®): Treatment – Patient," updated 08/2002, available at: http://cancer.gov, accessed 3/31/03; "How Is Chronic Myeloid Leukemia Treated?" April 20 2001, © Healthology, Inc., reprinted with permission; "Choosing an Initial Treatment for CML," May 31, 2002, © Healthology, Inc., reprinted with permission; and "Facts to Know while Undergoing Therapy for CML," May 31, 2002, © Healthology, Inc., reprinted with permission.

called a Philadelphia chromosome. This chromosome usually doesn't go away, even after treatment.

Leukemia can be acute (progressing quickly with many immature blasts) or chronic (progressing slowly with more mature-looking cancer cells). Chronic myelogenous leukemia progresses slowly and usually occurs in people who are middle-aged or older, although it also can occur in children. In the first stages of CML, most people don't have any symptoms of cancer. A doctor should be seen if any of the following symptoms appear:

- tiredness that won't go away,
- a feeling of no energy,
- fever,
- not feeling hungry, or
- night sweats.

Also, the spleen (the organ in the upper abdomen that makes other types of white blood cells and filters old blood cells from the blood) may be swollen.

If there are symptoms, a doctor may order blood tests to count the number of each of the different kinds of blood cells. If the results of the blood test are not normal, the doctor may order more blood tests. A bone marrow biopsy also may be done. During this test, a needle is inserted into a bone and a small amount of bone marrow is taken out and looked at under the microscope. The doctor can then tell what kind of leukemia the patient has and plan the best treatment.

Stages of Chronic Myelogenous Leukemia

Once chronic myelogenous leukemia (CML) has been found (diagnosed), more tests may be done to find out if leukemia cells have spread into other parts of the body such as the brain. This is called staging. CML progresses through different phases and these phases are the stages used to plan treatment. The following stages are used for chronic myelogenous leukemia.

Chronic Phase

There are few blast cells in the blood and bone marrow and there may be no symptoms of leukemia. This phase may last from several months to several years.

Accelerated Phase

There are more blast cells in the blood and bone marrow, and fewer normal cells.

Blastic Phase

More than 30% of the cells in the blood or bone marrow are blast cells. The blast phase of CML is sometimes called blast crisis. Sometimes blast cells will form tumors outside of the bone marrow in places such as the bone or lymph nodes. Lymph nodes are small bean-shaped structures that are found throughout the body. They produce and store infection-fighting cells.

Relapsing

Leukemia cells do not decrease even though treatment is given.

Treatment Option Overview

There are treatments for all patients with chronic myelogenous leukemia. Three kinds of treatment are used:

- Chemotherapy (using drugs to kill cancer cells)
- Radiation therapy (using high-dose x-rays or other high-energy rays to kill cancer cells)
- Bone marrow transplantation (killing the bone marrow and replacing it with healthy marrow).

The use of biological therapy (using the body's immune system to fight cancer) is being tested in clinical trials. Surgery may be used in certain cases to relieve symptoms.

Chemotherapy uses drugs to kill cancer cells. Chemotherapy may be taken by pill, or it may be put into the body by a needle in the vein or muscle. Chemotherapy is called a systemic treatment because the drug enters the bloodstream, travels through the body, and can kill cancer cells throughout the body. Chemotherapy also can be put directly into the fluid around the brain and spinal cord through a tube inserted into the brain or back. This is called intrathecal chemotherapy.

Radiation therapy uses x-rays or other high-energy rays to kill cancer cells and shrink tumors. Radiation for CML usually comes from a machine outside the body (external radiation therapy) and is sometimes used to relieve symptoms or as part of therapy given before a bone marrow transplant.

Bone marrow transplantation is used to replace the patient's bone marrow with healthy bone marrow. First, all of the bone marrow in the body is destroyed with high doses of chemotherapy with or without radiation therapy. Healthy marrow is then taken from another person (a donor) whose tissue is the same as or almost the same as the patient's. The donor may be a twin (the best match), a brother or sister, or another person not related. The healthy marrow from the donor is given to the patient through a needle in the vein, and the marrow replaces the marrow that was destroyed. A bone marrow transplant using marrow from a relative or person not related to the patient is called an allogeneic bone marrow transplant.

Another type of bone marrow transplant, called autologous bone marrow transplant, is being tested in clinical trials. To do this type of transplant, bone marrow is taken from the patient and treated with drugs to kill any cancer cells. The marrow is then frozen to save it. The patient is given high-dose chemotherapy with or without radiation therapy to destroy all of the remaining marrow. The frozen marrow that was saved is then thawed and given back to the patient through a needle in a vein to replace the marrow that was destroyed.

A greater chance for recovery occurs if a doctor chooses a hospital which does more than 5 bone marrow transplantations per year.

Biological therapy tries to get the body to fight cancer. It uses materials made by the body or made in a laboratory to boost, direct, or restore the body's natural defenses against disease. Biological therapy is sometimes called biological response modifier (BRM) therapy or immunotherapy.

If the spleen is swollen, a doctor may take out the spleen in an operation called a splenectomy.

Treatment by Stage

Standard treatment may be considered because of its effectiveness in patients in past studies, or participation in a clinical trial may be considered. Most patients are not cured with standard therapy and some standard treatments may have more side effects than are desired. For these reasons, clinical trials are designed to find better ways to treat cancer patients and are based on the most up-to-date information. Clinical trials are on going in most parts of the country for patients with CML of any phase. To know more about clinical trials, call the Cancer Information Service at 800-4-CANCER (800-422-6237); TTY at 800-332-8615.

Chronic Phase Chronic Myelogenous Leukemia

Treatment may be one of the following:

1. High-dose chemotherapy with radiation therapy followed by bone marrow transplantation.

2. Biological therapy.

3. Imatinib mesylate (STI157).

4. Chemotherapy to lower the number of white blood cells.

5. Surgery to remove the spleen (splenectomy).

Accelerated Phase Chronic Myelogenous Leukemia

Treatment may be one of the following:

1. Bone marrow transplantation.

2. Imatinib mesylate (STI157).

3. Biologic therapy.

4. High-dose chemotherapy.

5. Chemotherapy to lower the number of white blood cells.

6. Other chemotherapy drugs.

7. Transfusions of blood or blood products to relieve symptoms.

Blastic Phase Chronic Myelogenous Leukemia

Treatment may be one of the following:

1. Imatinib mesylate (STI157).

2. Chemotherapy.

3. Bone marrow transplantation.

4. Chemotherapy to relieve symptoms associated with the cancer.

5. High-dose chemotherapy.

Relapsing Chronic Myelogenous Leukemia

Treatment may be one of the following:

1. Imatinib mesylate (STI157).

2. Biologic therapy or white blood cells given into a vein for patients relapsing after bone marrow transplantation.

3. A clinical trial evaluating new combinations of chemotherapy drugs for patients unable to tolerate biologic therapy.

How Is Chronic Myeloid Leukemia Treated?

This section is from a radio statement given May 31, 2002 by Hagop Kantarjian, MD, Chairman of the Leukemia Department at M.D. Anderson Cancer Center.

Our department sees about 1,500 new patients with leukemia, including about 300 patients with CML. With the traditional treatments that we've used in the past, such as hydrouria or busulfan, the prognosis of patients with chronic myeloid leukemia was very poor, and their average lifespan was about three to five years.

When we introduced the new treatments, such as interferon and it's combinations, the average survival increased to about seven years and at 10 years we have about 20% of the patients who continue on interferon therapy without evidence of the disease.

Another modality used to treat chronic myeloid leukemia is allogeneic bone marrow transplantation, which refers to taking the bone marrow from a person who matches the patient, wiping out the sick bone marrow of the patient, and then re-infusing the bone marrow stem cells from the donor into the patient so that the patient now lives with the bone marrow of the donor.

The cure fraction in chronic myeloid leukemia with allogeneic bone marrow transplantation can range anywhere from 30%-80%, and that cure fraction depends on the age of the patient and the compatibility of the donor with the patient, as well as some other minor factors. But this procedure has a high treatment-associated mortality, which can vary anywhere from 5%-50% in the first year. So it's a risky modality which can lead to the potential of a cure.

Gleevec™ is the new kid on the block. Gleevec™ is probably, in my opinion, the most active treatment against chronic myeloid leukemia. The reason we believe it is so is, when we take patients who are resistant to interferon therapy, we're able to induce the complete hematologic remission, which means normalization of the counts in over 95% of the patients. Another reason why we believe that STI therapy is superior to interferon is, it works in phases where the interferon therapy does not work, like the accelerated and blastic phases.

Even in the blastic phase, we can get marrow-complete remissions, meaning that the blasts in the bone marrow are under 5%, in about 40% of the patients, which is amazing compared to what we get with either intensive combination chemotherapy or with interferon therapy.

In my opinion, Gleevec™ therapy has now become the front line standard of care for patients with newly diagnosed chronic phase CML. In patients who are in accelerated or blastic phase, there is no doubt that we should offer them allogeneic bone marrow transplantation as the preferred option because we do not know the results of Gleevec™ therapy in those phases, and we also know that the responses in the blastic phase with single agents are short lasting.

However, there's controversy as to whether Gleevec™ therapy should be offered to all or some of the patients who are diagnosed in chronic phase CML. In my opinion, Gleevec™ therapy should be offered to all patients with newly diagnosed CML, and allogeneic bone marrow transplantation offered only in patients who fail Gleevec™ therapy in the chronic phase. However, other investigators still argue that allogeneic bone marrow transplantation should be offered to younger patients where the one year mortality is still less than 20%, and the reason behind this argument is that allogeneic bone marrow transplantation has a track record for a cure, while Gleevec™ therapy has not been used long enough for us to ensure that we can produce a high cure fraction in these patients.

Choosing an Initial Treatment for CML

This section presents information discussed in a radio interview May 31, 2002 by Stephen O'Brien, MBChB, PhD, University of Newcastle, UK; Gwen L. Nichols, MD, Columbia University College of Physicians and Surgeons, New York, NY; Steve MacKinnon, MD, University College London; and Judy Orem, patient.

When a patient is diagnosed with chronic myeloid leukemia or CML, he or she quickly learns that choosing an initial therapy will not be easy.

Stephen O'Brien, MD, Ph.D: "The key factor is the informed choice of the patient. And neither myself nor any other doctor in the

271

world at the moment has all the answers for the best therapy for patients with newly diagnosed CML. The traditional accepted curative therapy for CML is a bone marrow transplant from another individual—either from a sibling (a brother or a sister) or from an unrelated donor. The concerns about that procedure are that it's risky. There is a chance that the patient might not even make it through the transplant. If you're 20 and you had a related donor that matched very well and you were fit and healthy I suspect myself and most other doctors would recommend a bone marrow transplant. If you're 60, I think the risks of transplant are excessive perhaps and then drug therapy would clearly be indicated."

Several drugs, including a chemotherapy agent called hydroxyurea, are effective in restoring white blood cell counts to normal, what's called a good hematologic response. This can eliminate early symptoms of the disease—including fatigue, loss of appetite, weight loss, and night sweats. Another drug, interferon, may be even more effective, and has been shown to delay the progression of CML, but interferon is not a good option for all patients.

Stephen O'Brien, MD, Ph.D: "One has to inject oneself everyday, much like a diabetic would. And the side effects for the drug are really quite frequent and quite troublesome."

Gwen Nichols, MD: "Early, patients often experience flu-like symptoms—achiness, fatigue, fevers. Most of these symptoms go away after several weeks of therapy, but some of them can continue. And fatigue, in particular, is very difficult."

Judy Orem, patient: "I had no energy. I would take naps. I got so I could take a two-hour nap in the morning, take a two-hour nap in the afternoon, and still sleep all night long."

Gwen Nichols, MD: "Interferon can also be associated with later neurologic symptoms, with depression, [and] with irritability."

Gleevec™

Patients have yet another option a drug called imatinib, sold under the brand name Gleevec™. It has few, mild, and generally well-tolerated side effects. Gleevec™ has been approved only for patients who do not respond well to interferon. But a new study shows Gleevec™ may be effective for newly diagnosed patients as well.

Stephen O'Brien, MD, Ph.D: "Those data very much support the use of imatinib as first-line therapy for patients in whom a bone marrow transplant is not thought appropriate."

Success in Therapy for CML Is Measured by Three Yardsticks

Steve Mackinnon, MD: "There's what's called the hematologic response; that is when the blood counts return to normal and the patient feels normal. The second type of response is called a cytogenetic response; that is where the abnormal chromosome that's in the malignant leukemia cells disappears. The third type of response is what's called a molecular response. This is a much more sensitive test; it can pick out one leukemic cell and a million normal cells."

A good hematological response is important for a patient's day-to-day well being. But a therapy is likely to prolong life only when tests show blood cells with normal chromosomes are replacing the cancerous ones.

Steve Mackinnon, MD: "With the arrival of Gleevec™ and the new randomized trial comparing Gleevec™ head-to-head with interferon, Gleevec™ clearly gives you superior response rate, not just in terms of the blood counts returning to normal, but also the underlying genetic defect."

Gwen Nichols, MD: "There are a large number—maybe 40 percent of patients—who get a chromosome response to Gleevec™, We don't know how long those will last, but some of them seem to be quite stable."

Judy Orem, patient: "There's like this feeling of I'm not looking at a three to five year life sentence anymore. And actually, I passed that a long time ago."

Steven O'Brien, MD, Ph.D: "Historically the experience shows that improved cytogenetic response equates to improved survival. And it seems reasonable to expect that of new drug therapies, particularly imatinib or Gleevec™."

No one yet knows whether Gleevec™ will prolong survival for CML patients. But clearly it expands the treatment options for patients newly diagnosed with the disease.

Facts to Know while Undergoing Therapy for CML

This section presents information discussed in a radio interview May 31, 2002 by Stephen O'Brien, MBChB, PhD, University of Newcastle, UK; Stephen Nimer, MD, Memorial Sloan-Kettering Cancer Center; Richard Stone, MD, Dana-Farber Cancer Institute; Gwen L. Nichols, MD, Columbia University College of Physicians and Surgeons, New York, NY; Steve MacKinnon, MD, University College London; and Judy Orem, patient.

Patients with chronic myeloid leukemia or CML face many decisions over the course of their treatment. Doctors don't have all the answers. So CML patients must collaborate in decision-making. That means patients must become well educated about their disease and understand how their body responds to therapy.

Stephen O'Brien, MD, PhD: "It's very important for patients to know the nature or the natural history of chronic myeloid leukemia because that must inform decision-making."

A patient must understand how CML, a cancer of the white blood cells may progress. In the early, or chronic phase of CML, the disease is stable, and the patient may experience no, or only mild symptoms, like fatigue. But later, low platelet counts may lead to uncontrolled bleeding. Too few normal white blood cells may lead to serious infection.

Stephen Nimer, MD: "As the disease progresses, it becomes more difficult to treat and ultimately becomes untreatable. And so patients die not in the chronic phase of their disease, but from accelerated phase or blast phase disease."

Stephen O'Brien, MD: "Well, clearly the most desirable treatment goal is to cure the patient with chronic myeloid leukemia. At the moment, the only know curative therapy is a bone marrow transplant."

CML patients must learn the factors that determine eligibility for transplant—age, overall health, tolerance for risk, and the quality of a potential donor match.

Stephen Nimer, MD: "And really, only about a third of patients will have a suitable donor for the transplant, which leaves the other two-thirds of the patients for whom transplantation is not really an option."

So most patients discover their best goal in therapy falls short of cure.

Richard Stone, MD: "In general the goal of treatment of CML should be to lengthen life, lengthen good quality of life. In other words, the idea is to prolong the stable phase as long as possible."

A patient undergoing drug therapy for CML must understand how his body's response is measured. There are three different kinds of tests, tracking hematologic, cytogenetic, and molecular responses.

Gwen Nichols, MD: "When we see that that the medicine treats the blood counts, we call this a hematologic response. When it returns the blood counts to what we consider a normal range."

Some drugs, like interferon, have a deeper impact, reducing the number of cancerous cells containing the abnormal chromosome at the heart of the disease, the so-called Philadelphia chromosome.

Stephen Nimer, MD: "And if more than two-thirds of the bone marrow, or the peripheral blood are in fact normal cells and not the CML cells, we would call that a major cytogenetic response. Now if we find no CML cells when we do the chromosome analysis, that's call a complete cytogenetic response."

CML patients learn that doctors can also monitor the response to treatment at the molecular level, testing for signs of an aberrant gene called BCR-able which is found on the Philadelphia chromosome.

Richard Stone, MD: "It's good to have a hematologic response. It's better to have a chromosome response. It's better still to have a molecular response."

CML patients and their doctors follow the results of these tests closely. Good responses at the chromosome and molecular levels correlate to longer survival.

Stephen O'Brien, MD, PhD: "The goal of medical therapy is as far as possible to reduce the Philadelphia chromosome, the hallmark of chronic myeloid leukemia, as much as possible. Because previous studies with medical therapy have shown that survival of patients with a low level or with no detectable Philadelphia chromosome is considerably better than for those who have not had the Philadelphia chromosome reduced or eliminated."

Patients must understand there can be setbacks, that drugs sometimes loose their efficacy.

Judy Orem, patient: "And I'd taken interferon for two years, and they said that it really wasn't working very well. It had made some progress getting rid of the Philadelphia chromosome, but not a lot."

Judy Orem entered a clinical trial for the drug imatinib, and she responded well. In three weeks, her hematologic tests were normal. In nine months, she was showing a good cytogenetic response. Imatinib, known also by the brand name Gleevec™ blocks a protein in the leukemia cells, preventing them from multiplying. The drug has been approved only for treatment of CML when other therapies have failed. But a recent trial shows Gleevec™ is very effective for newly diagnosed patients as well.

Steve Mackinnon, MD: "The hematological response rates are greater than 90 percent and the complete cytogenetic response rates are between 60 and 70 percent in the treatment. And this is much better than any of the previous therapies that have been used for CML."

CML patients quickly learn different drugs have different impact on their quality of life. Interferon requires daily injections and often brings about aches, fever, and fatigue. Gleevec™ is taken as a pill, and generally has easily tolerated side effects, like weight gain, and puffiness around the eyes.

Judy Orem, patient: "Now, those side effects are basically nothing by comparison. I have the energy. You know, I feel good. I don't sleep as much as I used to, but then I get more done."

Steven O'Brien, MD, PhD: "One of the most striking things I've seen over the last few years in patients who are coming into my clinic who have been on interferon, for example and who are now on imatinib, is that they are transformed in many cases—going back to work, feeling well, going on holiday whereas they wouldn't have been doing those sorts of things on interferon."

There are many effective therapies for chronic myeloid leukemia. Choosing among them is often difficult. Experience shows a patient does best when she understands the disease and collaborates with her doctor on treatment decisions.

Additional Information

National Cancer Institute
Cancer Information Service
6166 Executive Blvd., MSC 8322
Suite 3036A
Bethesda, MD 20892-8322
Toll-Free: 800-4-CANCER (800-422-6237)
Toll-Free TTY: 800-332-8615
Website: www.cancer.gov

Chapter 25

Hairy Cell Leukemia

What Is Hairy Cell Leukemia?

Hairy cell leukemia is a disease in which cancer (malignant) cells are found in the blood and bone marrow. The disease is called hairy cell leukemia because the cancer cells look hairy when examined under a microscope.

Hairy cell leukemia affects white blood cells called lymphocytes. Lymphocytes are made in the bone marrow and other organs. The bone marrow is the spongy tissue inside the large bones in the body. The bone marrow makes red blood cells (which carry oxygen and other materials to all tissues of the body), white blood cells (which fight infection), and platelets (which make the blood clot). Lymphocytes also are made in the spleen (an organ in the upper abdomen that makes lymphocytes and filters old blood cells from the blood), the lymph nodes (small bean-shaped organs throughout the body), and other organs.

When hairy cell leukemia develops, the leukemia cells may collect in the spleen, and the spleen swells. There also may be too few normal white blood cells in the blood because the leukemia cells invade the bone marrow, and the marrow cannot produce enough normal

This chapter includes PDQ® Cancer Information Summary, National Cancer Institute; Bethesda, MD, "Hairy Cell Leukemia (PDQ®): Treatment–Patient," updated 08/2002, available at: http://cancer.gov, accessed 04/01/03; and "Scientists Report Complete Remissions in Early Leukemia Trial," National Cancer Institute (NCI), July 25, 2001.

white blood cells. This may result in an infection. A doctor should be seen if the following symptoms occur:

- Constant tiredness.
- The spleen is larger than normal.
- The development of an infection that won't go away.

If there are symptoms, a doctor will order blood tests to count the number of each of the different types of blood cells. If the results of the blood tests are not normal, more blood tests may have to be done. The doctor may also do a bone marrow biopsy. During this test, a needle is inserted into a bone and a small amount of bone marrow is taken out and looked at under the microscope. The doctor can then tell what kind of leukemia the patient has and plan the best treatment.

The chance of recovery (prognosis) depends on how many cancer cells are in the blood and bone marrow, the patient's age, and general health.

Stage Information

Stages of Hairy Cell Leukemia

There is no staging system for hairy cell leukemia. Patients are grouped together based on whether or not they have been treated for their leukemia.

Untreated Hairy Cell Leukemia

No treatment has been given for the leukemia. Treatment may have been given for infections or other side effects of the leukemia.

Progressive Hairy Cell Leukemia

Splenectomy (surgery to remove the spleen) has been done or systemic therapy (treatment that uses substances that travel through the bloodstream, reaching and affecting cells all over the body) has been given, but the leukemia is getting worse.

Refractory Hairy Cell Leukemia

The leukemia has been treated but no longer responds to the treatment.

Treatment Option Overview

Some people with hairy cell leukemia have few symptoms and may not need treatment right away. There are treatments for all patients with hairy cell leukemia that is causing symptoms. Three kinds of treatment are used:

- Surgery.
- Chemotherapy (using drugs to kill cancer cells).
- Biological therapy (using the body's immune system to fight cancer).

Bone marrow transplants are being tested in clinical trials.

If the spleen is swollen, the doctor may take out the spleen in an operation called a **splenectomy**.

Chemotherapy uses drugs to kill cancer cells. Chemotherapy may be taken by pill, or it may be put into the body by a needle in the vein, muscle, or under the skin. Chemotherapy is called a systemic treatment because the drug enters the bloodstream, travels through the body, and can kill cancer cells throughout the body.

Biological therapy tries to get the body to fight the cancer. It uses materials made by the body or made in a laboratory to boost, direct, or restore the body's natural defenses against disease. Biological therapy is sometimes called biological response modifier (BRM) therapy or immunotherapy. Interferon, a substance made by the body to fight off foreign materials, is often used to treat hairy cell leukemia.

Bone marrow transplantation is used to replace the bone marrow with healthy bone marrow. First, all of the bone marrow in the body is destroyed with high doses of chemotherapy with or without radiation therapy. Healthy marrow is then taken from another person (a donor) whose tissue is the same as or almost the same as the patient's. The donor may be a twin (the best match), a brother or sister, or another unrelated person. The healthy marrow from the donor is given to the patient through a needle in the vein, and the marrow replaces the marrow that was destroyed. Bone marrow transplants using marrow from a relative or unrelated person is called an allogeneic bone marrow transplant.

Treatment by Stage

Standard treatment may be considered because of its effectiveness in patients in past studies, or participation in a clinical trial may be considered. Not all patients are cured with standard therapy and some standard treatments may have more side effects than are desired. For these reasons, clinical trials are designed to find better ways to treat cancer patients and are based on the most up-to-date information. Clinical trials are ongoing in most parts of the country for patients with hairy cell leukemia. To learn more about clinical trials, call the Cancer Information Service at 800-4-CANCER (800-422-6237); TTY at 800-332-8615.

Untreated Hairy Cell Leukemia

Treatment may be one of the following:

1. If there are no symptoms, treatment may not be needed. The doctor will follow the patient closely so treatment can be started if the leukemia gets worse.

2. Biological therapy.

3. Chemotherapy.

4. Surgery to remove the spleen (splenectomy).

Refractory Hairy Cell Leukemia

If the patient has not responded to biological therapy, chemotherapy may be given. The patient may also wish to take part in a clinical trial of new chemotherapy drugs.

Scientists Report Complete Remissions in Early Leukemia Trial

Scientists reported in the July 26, 2001 issue of the *New England Journal of Medicine** that 11 of 13 patients with hairy cell leukemia, a cancer of the immune system, had complete remissions after receiving adequate treatment with the recombinant immunotoxin BL22. A recombinant immunotoxin is an antibody that has been bioengineered to recognize and directly deliver a deadly toxin to tumors, in this case, hairy cell leukemia cells.

According to the authors, these results are particularly impressive because the patients, all of whom failed previous chemotherapy, were treated in a Phase I clinical trial, an early study designed primarily to determine how to administer a drug, not cure the disease. Pastan said the two other patients in the study who received adequate treatment had partial remissions, and they continue to receive BL22.

"We expected that some patients would respond to the treatment," said Ira Pastan, MD, a senior author on the paper and leader of the National Cancer Institute's immunotoxin therapy group. "But we didn't imagine in our wildest dreams that almost all of the patients would go into complete remission. Half of the patients went into complete remission after a single cycle of treatment, and that was exciting to see."

Pastan said BL22, developed in the laboratory jointly with NCI scientists Robert J. Kreitman, MD, and David J. FitzGerald, Ph.D., was licensed over a year ago to AlbaPharm, Inc., of Rockville, MD. The company, in collaboration with Pastan's group, is now planning a larger clinical trial with the immunotoxin that will involve hairy cell leukemia patients from throughout the country. Hairy cell leukemia, or HCL, is diagnosed in about 700 Americans each year, accounting for about 2 percent of all leukemias.

These results were highlighted in April 2001 during a presentation at the annual meeting of the American Association for Cancer Research.

According to Kreitman, the principal investigator of the clinical trial and a senior author on the paper, BL22 is made by cloning portions of antibodies to portions of a toxin secreted by the bacteria Pseudomonas aeruginosa. "Recombinant DNA techniques allow cloning part of the antibody and part of the toxin to make a smaller recombinant immunotoxin that gets into the tumor faster and reduces the toxicity to the body," said Kreitman.

The antibody portion of BL22 specifically binds to the CD22 receptor, which is found in abundance on the surface of many types of leukemia cells. CD22 is also found, in lower amounts, on the surface of normal B cells. Therefore, it seems likely that BL22 would bind to and destroy both leukemic cells and normal B cells. Because stem cells—the progenitors of normal B cells—do not have CD22, any B cells lost in the short-term treatment should be replaced by the patient's untouched stem cells. And, in fact, Kreitman and his colleagues did not detect a decrease in normal B cells of patients.

Kreitman added, "Malignant stem cells—the progenitors of the leukemic cells—may be CD22-positive as well and be lost, too. But only further follow-up will determine if this is correct." Therefore, it is thought that this treatment may not only clear the body of malignant circulating cells but may remove the source of the cells, the malignant stem cells.

The most serious side effect of BL22 immunotoxin treatment was a decrease in platelet and red blood cell counts. This decrease was associated with the clotting and breaking up of red blood cells in the kidney, which can cause kidney failure. However, both patients experiencing the side effect completely recovered and had complete remissions of HCL. Using a modified method of BL22 administration, this side effect was not detected in many patients treated later in the study.

It is possible that the BL22 immunotoxin will prove to be useful in treating more than just hairy cell leukemia. The Phase I trial includes patients with other types of leukemia and, while Kreitman and his colleagues saw the most dramatic response in HCL, a significant benefit was seen in chronic lymphocytic leukemia. These leads are being followed-up by the researchers. "The hairy cell leukemia cells have more CD22 receptors and therefore respond faster and more thoroughly than the other cancers being investigated," Kreitman explained.

*The article is titled, "High Complete Remission Rate in Chemotherapy-Resistant Classic or Variant Hairy Cell Leukemia Induced by the Anti-CD22 Recombinant Immunotoxin BL22," published in the July 26, 2001, issue of the *New England Journal of Medicine.* The authors are: Robert J. Kreitman, Wyndham H. Wilson, Karen Bergeron, Miranda Raggio, Maryalice Stetler-Stevenson, David FitzGerald, and Ira Pastan.

Additional Information

National Cancer Institute
Cancer Information Service
6166 Executive Blvd., MSC 8322
Suite 3036A
Bethesda, MD 20892-8322
Toll-Free: 800-422-6237
TTY Toll-Free: 800-322-8615
Website: www.cancer.gov

Part Four

Leukemia Treatments

Chapter 26

Understanding Drug Therapy and Managing Side Effects

Drug Therapy

The number of persons living in the United States who will be diagnosed with blood-related cancers—leukemia, Hodgkin and non-Hodgkin lymphoma, and myeloma—each year is approximately 106,300. Leukemia and lymphoma are among the most curable forms of cancer, so for many patients, the application of drug therapy may result in a cure or a significant prolongation of active life.

Today's treatments generally include radiation therapy, drug therapy (sometimes in combination with a stem cell transplantation), and immunotherapy. The dramatic progress in treatment and survival for patients with blood-related cancers is due to the development of new drugs over the last 50 years. Understanding how drugs fight leukemia, lymphoma, and myeloma makes it easier to understand how side effects occur. This chapter discusses drug therapy, explaining some of the side effects and how to manage them.

The number of agents available has soared since their first usage in the late 1940s. Today, numerous drugs are used, either alone or in combination with one another, to achieve maximum cancer cell-killing ability.

Drug Use

Chemotherapy is the use of drugs or chemicals, often in combinations, to kill or damage cancer cells in the body. This is why these drugs may be referred to as anticancer agents.

Normal cells divide and grow in a patterned behavior. Moreover, normal cells may not divide if replacement cells are not needed. Cancer cells, on the other hand, often accumulate uncontrollably. There is no purpose to their multiplication, unlike the case in normal cells in which spent cells are being replaced. Cancer cells may accumulate because the rate of cell growth is too rapid or the rate of cell death is too slow or a combination of both. Drug therapy can accelerate cancer cell death in these two circumstances: too many cells are being made or too many cells are living too long.

The goal of drug therapy is either to eliminate cancer cells so there is no longer any sign of illness and to permit normal cells to restore their function (called remission), or to damage or kill cancer cells to the point that the progress of the disease is slowed. Today, acute leukemia and lymphoma occurring in children have high cure rates, as do some types of leukemia and lymphoma in adults. As leukemias and lymphomas are now more accurately defined by the genetic changes that occur within the cancer cells, drugs are being developed that can target the specific molecular abnormalities in the type of disease under treatment. Such therapy may work better and have fewer side effects. Current drug therapy can produce long-term remission or outright cure for many persons, depending on the specific type and extent of the cancer.

Drug Action

Chemotherapy drugs interfere with cancer cells' ability to grow (multiply) or to survive. Different groups of drugs act in different ways on the cell's ability to grow or survive. Identification of the type of disease is important because certain drugs are given only for certain disease types. For example, a patient with acute myelogenous leukemia is treated with different agents than one with acute lymphocytic leukemia or Hodgkin lymphoma. Even patients with the same disease are sometimes treated with different agents depending on what the physician believes will be most effective for an individual at a given stage of disease.

Types of drugs: More drugs that act to kill cancer cells by different methods continue to result from research progress. Following is a brief description of several examples of drug types that are used to fight cancer.

Some Drugs Used in the Treatment of Leukemia, Lymphoma, or Myeloma

DNA Damaging Drugs

These drugs react with DNA to alter it chemically and keep it from permitting cell growth.

- busulfan (Myleran)
- carboplatin (Paraplatin)
- carmustine (BiCNU)
- chlorambucil (Leukeran)
- cisplatin (Platinol)
- cyclophosphamide (Cytoxan, Neosar)
- dacarbazine (DTIC)
- ifosfamide (Ifex)
- lomustine (CCNU)
- mechlorethamine (nitrogen mustard, Mustargen)
- melphalan (Alkeran)
- procarbazine

Antitumor Antibiotics

These drugs interact directly with DNA in the nucleus of cells, interfering with cell survival.

- bleomycin (Blenoxane)
- daunorubicin (daunomycin, Rubidomycin, Cerubidine)
- doxorubicin (Adriamycin, Rubex)
- idarubicin (Idamycin)
- mitoxantrone (Novantrone)

Antimetabolites

These are chemicals that are very similar to the building blocks of DNA or RNA. They are changed from the natural chemical sufficiently so that when they substitute for it, they block the cells' ability to form RNA or DNA, preventing cell growth.

- 5-azacytadine (AZA-CR)
- cladribine (chlorodeoxyadenosine, Leustatin)
- cytarabine (cytosine arabinoside, Ara-C, Cytosar)
- fludarabine (Fludara)
- hydroxyurea (Hydrea)
- 6-mercaptopurine (Purinethol)
- methotrexate (Folex, Mexate)
- 6-thioguanine (Thioguanine)

DNA Repair Enzyme Inhibitors

These drugs act on certain proteins (enzymes) in the cell nucleus that normally repair injury to DNA. These drugs prevent the enzymes from working and make the DNA more susceptible to injury.

- etoposide (VP-16, VePesid)
- teniposide (VM-26, Vumon)
- topotecan (Hycamtin)

Drugs That Prevent Cells from Dividing by Blocking Mitosis

These drugs impair structures in the cell that are required for cells to divide into two daughter cells.

- vinblastine (Velban, Velsar)
- vincristine (Oncovin, Vincasar)
- paclitaxel (Taxol)

Hormones That Can Kill Lymphocytes

In high doses these synthetic hormones, relatives of the natural hormone, cortisol, can kill malignant lymphocytes.

- dexamethasone (Decadron)
- methylprednisolone (Medrol)
- prednisone (Deltasone)

Cell Maturing Agents

Drugs that act on a type of leukemia to induce maturation of leukemic cells.

- All-trans retinoic acid (ATRA)
- Arsenic trioxide

Biomodifiers

Drugs that are based on natural products and which exact mechanism of action are unclear. They may impair DNA or act in other ways.

- Interferon-alpha (Roferon A, Intron)

Monoclonal Antibodies

A class of agents for treatment of lymphoma and leukemia, monoclonal antibodies target and destroy cancer cells with fewer side effects than conventional chemotherapy.

- Rituximab (Rituxan)
- Gemtuzumab ozogamicin (Mylotarg)

Drugs with Specific Molecular Targets

These agents are designed to block the specific mutant protein that initiates the malignant cell transformation.

- Imatinib mesylate (Gleevec™)

This list does not include every drug being used or studied in clinical trials. Combinations of these drugs and drug groups often form the basis of treatment. Certain of these drugs have been found to be more or less active in a particular subtype of leukemia or lymphoma.

Many drugs act against cancer cells by interacting with DNA or RNA of the cancer cell. This interaction damages DNA such that the cancer cell is killed or is prevented from growing and producing more cancer cells. Four of the chemotherapy drug types that act directly to impair the DNA in cancer cells are the DNA-damaging agents: antitumor antibiotics; antimetabolites; and DNA-repair enzyme inhibitors.

DNA-damaging agents, such as chlorambucil, cyclophosphamide, or melphalan, are referred to collectively as alkylating agents. These agents damage the DNA so severely that the cancer cell is killed.

Other DNA-damaging agents, such as carboplatin, attach to the DNA and prevent the cancer cell from growing.

Antitumor antibiotics, such as daunorubicin, doxorubicin, idarubicin, and mitoxantrone, insert themselves into the DNA of the cancer cell, prevent the DNA from functioning normally, and often kill the cancer cell.

Antimetabolites, such as methotrexate, fludarabine, and cytarabine, are drugs that mimic substances that the cancer cell needs to build DNA and RNA. When the cancer cell uses the antimetabolite instead of the natural substances, it cannot produce normal DNA or RNA, and the cell dies.

DNA-repair enzyme inhibitors, such as etoposide or topotecan, attack the cancer cell proteins that normally repair any damage to the cell DNA. Repair of DNA damage is a normal and vital process in the cell. Without this repair process, the cancer cell is much more susceptible to damage and is prevented from growing.

High doses of a certain class of hormone, which includes prednisone and dexamethasone, can kill lymphoma or lymphocytic leukemia cells.

Another type of chemotherapy drug, such as vincristine or vinblastine, damages cancer cells by blocking a process called mitosis (cell division), preventing the cancer cells from dividing and multiplying.

A group of agents consists of antibodies that are made specifically to attach to the surface of cancer cells. Once these antibodies attach to the cancer cells, they may interfere with the cell's function and kill the cell. In addition, some antibodies are linked to a toxin or radioactive substance. When the antibody attaches to the cancer cell, the antibody and the toxin or radioactive substance work to kill the cell. In the case of a toxin, the cell must internalize the antibody. In the case of a radioactive substance, the antibody need only attach to the cell.

Resistance: Sometimes cancer cells may be resistant to the initial drugs used or may become resistant to these drugs later, causing the cancer to return. In this case, the doctor may prescribe different drugs to fight the cancer cells.

Today, doctors have access to more anticancer drugs to use in initial therapy or for subsequent therapy. This progress has resulted in an increased frequency of very long-term remissions or cures.

Effect on normal cells: Unfortunately, most drugs used in chemotherapy affect normal cells as well as cancer cells. Normal cells most affected are those that most rapidly divide, including those of the hair follicles, lining of the gastrointestinal tract, and bone marrow. This is why hair loss, nausea, diarrhea, and low blood cell counts are common side effects of most intensive chemotherapy programs. These side effects may, however, vary greatly among different patients because they depend on the specific drug(s) used; the dose of drug(s) used; how long the therapy lasts; and the overall health of the patient, including the condition of his or her bone marrow and other susceptible organs before the chemotherapy.

Methods of Drug Administration

Drugs are often given in combination with each other and can be given in different ways. The four most common methods are; intravenous, oral, intramuscular, and intrathecal. The method is based on the actual disease diagnosed and the agent's effectiveness.

A very common way of giving medicine is directly into a vein, referred to as the intravenous route, or IV. A small plastic needle is inserted into one of the veins in the lower arm. There is some discomfort during insertion because a needle stick is required to get into the vein. After that, administration of the medication is almost painless. Chemotherapy flows from a plastic bag, through tubing, into the bloodstream. Sometimes a syringe is used to push the chemotherapy through the tubing. This method is especially useful for delivering drugs that might damage tissues if given by mouth or by injection.

The oral method takes the form of a pill, capsule, or liquid taken by mouth. This is the easiest and most convenient method since it can be done at home.

The term intramuscular means that the drug is injected into the muscle. There is a slight pinch as the needle is placed through the skin and into the muscle of the arm, thigh, or buttocks. However, the procedure lasts only a few seconds. Some chemotherapy drugs may be given by injection into the tissue under the skin, rather than into the muscle. This is referred to as a subcutaneous injection.

Certain types of leukemia and lymphoma have a tendency to spread to the nervous system. To prevent or to treat this event, doctors may perform a spinal tap and inject a chemotherapy drug into the spinal fluid to destroy any cancer cells. This is known as an intrathecal method of administration. If many treatments are needed, doctors may place a permanent device, called an Ommaya reservoir, under the scalp. Once the Ommaya reservoir is inserted, chemotherapy treatments can be given through this device and the patient will no longer need spinal taps. The patient can go home with the Ommaya reservoir in place.

Permanent catheter: Some patients have small veins and some have very few veins, making IV insertions difficult. Frequent IV insertions and too small or too few veins may prompt the doctor to recommend a permanent type of IV catheter. Permanent catheters allow patients to go home and receive chemotherapy without needing to have other IVs inserted. Along with receiving drug therapy and IV fluids through this catheter, patients can receive blood products and have blood drawn without painful needle sticks.

These types of catheters are called permanent because they can remain in place from months to years. These catheters are commonly called tunneled catheters because a rubber tube is tunneled through surface skin tissue between the neck and shoulder to another separate incision, usually on the chest wall. This placement requires a surgical procedure under general or local anesthesia.

The entrance site will have stitches and a small bandage to facilitate healing. The exit site for the catheter is easy to see and care for since patients should change their dressings three times a week to prevent infection. The catheters should be flushed with a medication to prevent blood from clotting in the catheter. Patients and family members may learn to care for their catheters while in the hospital.

Another type of permanent catheter to a central vein is known as the implanted port. It is round in shape and surgically inserted under the skin surface on the chest wall between the neck and shoulder area. A nurse inserts a needle through the top skin surface to gain access to the vein. The chemotherapy can then be given through the catheter as if it were an IV in the arm. As with the tunneled catheter, blood can be removed and received through this device. There is no home care required.

Temporary catheters: There is a temporary access device for administering therapy that works in the same way as the tunneled catheter, but it is removed before discharge from the hospital. This is called the multilumen catheter because there are usually three IV lines in one plastic catheter tube. Insertion is performed in the patient's room, with local numbing medication injected around the insertion sites. Located near the neck, the site is kept covered with a dressing. Often, the dressing is removed before discharge from the hospital.

Drug therapy regimens for most patients with cancer include the use of several chemotherapy drugs. Usually these drugs differ in how strong or potent they are and in the way that they attack the cancer cells. This combination approach allows the chemotherapy drugs to attack the cancer cells at different critical points in their cell growth cycles, thereby making the therapy more effective and reducing the chance for cancer cells to become resistant to the therapy.

Side Effects

The goal of therapy is to destroy cancer cells. Although most of the effect of chemotherapy drugs does amount to the injury or death of cancer cells, the drugs also affect normal cells, causing certain side effects. The side effects of different chemotherapy drugs are known from previously conducted clinical trials or research studies. These expected side effects are different depending on which drugs are being used, the route drugs are being given (oral, IV, injection), and for how long the drug is being given.

A patient's decision to proceed with treatment includes a decision of benefit versus risk. The benefits of drug therapy must be weighed against the risks of not receiving it at all. The side effects of treatment can be unpleasant, but they must be measured against the medicine's ability to destroy the disease. Most side effects are temporary and subside once the chemotherapy is completed. Each day, healthy new cells begin to grow and develop. The most common side effects of drugs involve three main types of tissue in the body: the lining of the gastrointestinal tract, the skin and scalp (hair follicles), and the bone marrow. Each of these areas depends on the rapid growth of new cells to perform its normal functions in the body.

Effects of Drug Therapy on the Gastrointestinal Tract

The lining of the mouth, esophagus, stomach, and intestines contain rapidly dividing cells. If these cells are destroyed by chemotherapy, sores (called ulcers) and other difficulties, such as vomiting or diarrhea, can develop.

Mouth and throat symptoms: If mouth sores develop from inflammation, a patient may experience a burning sensation or pain in the mouth or throat. This is a condition called stomatitis. With some chemotherapy drugs, the amount of saliva in the mouth may decrease early on and increase later. The tongue may also be red and swollen. A stinging sensation in the throat may develop and lead to difficulty swallowing or a sensation that food becomes caught in the throat, a condition called dysphagia. In addition, some persons may develop a white shiny coating or white patches on their tongue, inside of the cheeks, or floor of the mouth. This symptom indicates a yeast infection, also called thrush or oral candidiasis.

If any of these symptoms or other changes in the mouth or throat are experienced, the doctor can prescribe medications and make recommendations to improve comfort. Following are just a few ways the doctor might help to manage uncomfortable side effects:

- If time permits, doctors often recommend that patients see their dentist before beginning chemotherapy. In addition, maintenance of good dental and oral hygiene may help prevent gum disease, infection, and some other side effects.

- If the patient is at risk for developing a yeast infection, the doctor may prescribe a medication to be swished around in the mouth and swallowed to prevent or to treat this side effect.

- If pain is associated with a yeast infection or other side effect, the doctor may prescribe a pain medication for relief.

The mouth should be inspected daily to detect problems early. The healthcare team can then be notified for suggestions on oral hygiene or proper diet that might reduce or relieve discomfort.

Diarrhea and constipation: Diarrhea can be a side effect of some chemotherapy drugs. Caused by the destruction of normal, dividing cells of the gastrointestinal tract, diarrhea varies from patient to patient but it is better treated if detected early. It is important to notify the doctor or nurse if cramping, gas, or loose stools begin. Constipation too can be a side effect of chemotherapy. If constipation is a problem to begin with, some chemotherapy drugs will intensify it. Older persons and those with low-fiber diets are also at a greater risk. Like other side effects, however, some patients experience constipation with chemotherapy while others do not. It is most helpful to watch daily habits to reduce the risk of constipation. If diarrhea, constipation, or other bowel symptoms are experienced, the doctor and nurse should be alerted promptly so that they can help to manage these symptoms.

Nausea and vomiting: Nausea and vomiting are side effects that involve the gastrointestinal tract, but also stimulation of the area of the brain that induces such effects. Individuals often connect nausea and vomiting with chemotherapy treatment. However, there are many chemotherapy drugs that do not always cause these disturbing side effects. When nausea and vomiting do occur, these are drug and dose dependent side effects that vary from patient to patient. Sometimes, nausea and vomiting subside as a person adjusts to the treatment.

For people who are experiencing nausea or vomiting, there are a number of antinausea drugs, also called antiemetic drugs, that the doctor can prescribe to prevent or minimize this troublesome side effect.

Effects of Drug Therapy on the Skin and Hair

Skin rashes: Chemotherapy drugs can affect the skin in several ways, and skin rashes ranging from dry skin to redness to more severe lesions can occur during or after treatment with some drugs. If skin changes are noticed, it is important to alert the doctor promptly.

Hair loss: Some chemotherapy drugs can also cause scalp hair loss by blocking the growth of cells in the hair follicle that normally replace hair. However, hair growth resumes when the drugs are stopped or are decreased in dose. In the meantime, some suggestions for helping with hair loss may be useful:

- Wash hair and scalp every few days, using a mild, moisturizing shampoo.

- Comb hair during hair loss to prevent knots and tangles. Once the drugs affect the hair shaft, hair will fall out whether it is combed or not. Sometimes persons with long hair get a short haircut before hair loss begins.

- If planning to buy a wig, cut a portion of hair prior to hair loss so color and texture can be matched more easily.

- Some persons who have severe hair loss choose not to cover their heads. Bandannas, hats, or scarves may be worn to keep the head warm. Apply mineral oil if the scalp is dry or flaking.

Effects of Drug Therapy on Blood Cell Formation

Bone marrow: The bone marrow is found at the center of the bones, especially in areas of the skull, sternum, ribs, backbone, and pelvis. The function of the bone marrow is to produce blood cells and send them out into the blood to circulate throughout the body. Young cells in the bone marrow, called stem cells, mature into the three types of blood cells the body needs: white blood cells, red blood cells, and platelets. White blood cells have several functions, but one of the most important is to prevent and fight infection. Red blood cells carry oxygen to all parts of the body. Platelets help to make the blood clot if a blood vessel is injured. Developing blood cells remain in the bone marrow until they are mature enough to perform these vital functions and then are released into the circulation.

Chemotherapy effects: Because the cells in the marrow are rapidly dividing and multiplying, many chemotherapy drugs will act upon these cells, decreasing the bone marrow's ability to produce and deliver new cells to the circulating blood for a time after treatment. For this reason, persons undergoing chemotherapy may experience low blood cell counts. The white blood cell counts decrease most quickly, followed by the platelets, and then red blood cells.

This effect can be compared to a bathtub filled with water, in which the level of water represents the normal level of cells in the circulating blood. Water coming through the spout represents new cells being delivered from the bone marrow to the circulating blood. The open drain through which the water empties represents the normal loss of cells from the blood. To maintain the level of the water in the tub constant, the running spout restores water at the same rate that water escapes out of the drain; thus, the level of the water in the tub remains steady. If the spout is partially closed and the open drain remains unchanged, the water level will fall. The more the spout is closed, the lower the level of the water in the tub becomes. In most persons receiving chemotherapy, the loss of blood cells (the drain) remains normal or is slightly increased. Hence, the blood cell level in the circulating blood after chemotherapy is a function of how much damage the drugs do to the marrow's ability to deliver new cells (the spout) to the circulating blood (the tub).

The degree of the effect of chemotherapy on the marrow depends on several factors, including whether the marrow is already damaged by the cancer before treatment begins as well as the type and duration of the drugs used. Some chemotherapy drugs have little or no damaging effect on the marrow, while others have definite effects that can be reversed quickly once the therapy is stopped. Still other chemotherapy drugs have effects on the marrow that can last for several weeks.

Measuring blood cell counts: Because of the effect that many chemotherapy drugs have on the marrow, doctors usually measure the patient's blood cell counts periodically. These measurements tell whether the red blood cells, white blood cells, or platelets are decreased. The level of the blood counts will help the doctor decide how well the chemotherapy is working, whether the dose needs adjusting, or whether the patient may need a transfusion of new blood cells during the treatment.

During the course of undergoing treatment and blood cell measurements, the term nadir may be used. This refers to the point when the cells in the blood are at their lowest number. This is a point that can be approximated, based on the chemotherapy drug used. One drug may have a nadir of 7 to 14 days. This means that 7 to 14 days after beginning chemotherapy, the white blood cells, red blood cells, and platelets will be at their lowest point. Once this period is over, the blood counts will begin to rise back to normal.

Risk of infection: The white blood cells help the body to fight infections. When chemotherapy is introduced into the body, it may destroy both the cancerous cells and the healthy, infection-fighting cells, thereby decreasing the body's ability to fight off infection. The degree to which a patient is more susceptible to infection depends on how low the white blood cell count is and how long it remains low. Moderate decreases in white blood cells, especially if they return toward normal within a short period of time, create little increased risk and do not require special precautions. However, a severe or prolonged low white blood cell count may occur in some persons, especially after intensive chemotherapy in the hospital and may increase the risk of developing an infection.

Signs of infection should be reported to the doctor immediately. The doctor can then examine the patient and prescribe antibiotics to fight any infection. The following are a few ways that infection can be prevented:

- When receiving chemotherapy on an outpatient basis, patients should ask the doctor or nurse whether very low white blood cell counts are expected and whether there are any special precautions needed to avoid infection.

- When in the hospital, hospital staff will take special precautions to avoid exposing the patient to bacteria, viruses, and other infection-causing organisms.

- When in the hospital, the hospital staff will wash their hands frequently using special soaps and vigorous techniques. They may also wear masks, gowns, and gloves in some cases.

- Patients may also reduce the risk of developing an infection by washing their hands frequently and thoroughly.

- If patients in the hospital have a catheter, the hospital staff will be meticulous in cleaning and caring for the catheter, as bacteria can otherwise be introduced through this device.

- If the very low white blood cell count is likely to persist for a time, more stringent measures, such as avoiding uncooked fruits and vegetables, may be needed.

Risk of anemia: Red blood cells contain hemoglobin, which carries oxygen to the muscles and organs in the body, helping them to function normally. In some cases, chemotherapy drugs destroy developing red blood cells in the marrow, causing a decrease in red blood cell count. Persons who have a low red blood cell count are said to have anemia. Persons who have anemia may have several side effects, depending on the severity of the anemia and how rapidly it develops, including:

- Being easily fatigued, especially upon physical activity;
- Having pale skin;
- Feeling light headed;
- Feeling short of breath, especially with physical activity;
- Having limited ability to exercise or perform physical activities.

Many persons who have a mild or moderate decrease in red blood cells, especially if the decrease is gradual, will not realize that they have anemia. If any of the symptoms of anemia are noticed, it is important to alert the doctor promptly. In some cases, the doctor may prescribe a medicine or, if severe enough, a blood transfusion to help restore the red blood cells to a higher level.

Risk of bleeding: Platelets are small cells, about one-tenth the size of red blood cells. If a blood vessel is cut or injured, platelets help to prevent excessive bleeding by forming a plug at this site. In some cases, chemotherapy drugs damage the marrow, causing a decrease in the platelet formation. While a mild or moderate decrease in the platelet count usually does not cause any bleeding, persons with a severely low platelet count can experience the following side effects:

- An increased risk of excessive bleeding from cuts or bruises;
- Pinhead-sized bleeding points in the skin, called petechiae, especially on the lower leg and ankles;
- Black and blue spots in the skin with minor bumps or in the absence of any injury.

Once the chemotherapy is stopped and the platelet count is restored to a sufficient level these side effects rapidly fade. However, if a patient needs to receive additional chemotherapy and the platelet count remains very low, the transfusions of platelets may be required.

Improving blood cell counts: The body naturally makes substances, or hormones, that stimulate blood cell production. These natural substances, called cytokines, have been identified in the laboratory, and drugs have been made to resemble them. These drugs, or synthetically manufactured cytokines, can be administered to patients to help increase specific types of blood cells. Three of these drugs include:

- Erythropoietin (also called Procrit®), which helps stimulate red blood cell production;

- Darbepoetin Alfa (also called Aranesp™), a long-acting form of erythropoietin that also helps stimulate red blood production but requires less frequent injections;

- Granulocyte colony stimulating factor (also called G-CSF, filgrastim, or Neupogen®), which helps stimulate white blood cell production;

- Granulocyte-monocyte colony-stimulating factor (also called GM-CSF, sargramostim, Leukine®, or Prokine®), which also helps stimulate white blood cell production.

In some persons, these cytokine drugs can help blood cell counts to recover more rapidly than they would on their own. Often in persons with leukemia, lymphoma, or myeloma, marrow injury from their disease, complicated by damage from intensive drug therapy, makes this approach of only modest usefulness. Cytokines to improve the recovery of platelet counts are being studied for their potential usefulness.

Fatigue: Many individuals who undergo chemotherapy for leukemia, lymphoma, or myeloma say that they feel unusually tired or fatigued. If the patient is experiencing this extreme fatigue, he or she may have any of the following signs and symptoms:

- Having only a limited ability to perform physical activities, concentrate for long periods of time, or deal with emotions.

- Lacking the energy to take care of him or herself, home or family, or work.

- Lacking the energy or desire to participate in social or intimate relationships.

- Feeling out of sorts.

Excessive fatigue in persons with leukemia, lymphoma, or myeloma may be due to any of several factors. First, the disease itself often causes fatigue. Secondly, chemotherapy can sometimes cause anemia, in which case the feeling of fatigue may be even more intense. So too radiation therapy, sometimes used with chemotherapy, can cause fatigue.

The cancer and the effects of treatment may also cause other side effects, all of which can diminish a person's sense of well being. This, together with the emotional stress of being diagnosed with a life-threatening illness, making treatment decisions, undergoing treatment, and worrying about personal and work responsibilities, may add to a person's level of fatigue.

Other Possible Side Effects of Drug Therapy

A number of other side effects can occur during or after drug therapy for leukemia, lymphoma, or myeloma. These side effects vary depending on the drug and dose of the drug used. Occasionally, unexpected side effects occur; however, often side effects can be predicted because some chemotherapy drugs are more likely than others to affect certain body tissues, such as the nervous system, kidney, bladder, heart, or other areas.

It is important to ask the doctor which side effects to expect with chemotherapy treatments, and to alert the doctor of any expected or unexpected side effects that occur. The doctor can determine if the side effect is from the chemotherapy drug or another source and can alter the treatment plan accordingly.

Social and Emotional Effects

"Why me?" is a common question patients ask. It is a normal reaction to a diagnosis of cancer and the need for treatment. During this time, many different emotions surface. The need for chemotherapy and the realization that it will make some changes in a person's life can prompt a range of feelings. Denial, fear, hopelessness, and depression are just a few of the emotions common for many persons diagnosed with leukemia, lymphoma, or myeloma.

Persons newly diagnosed with cancer face the uncertainty of what comes next. Together, the patient, family, doctors, and other healthcare providers can address these concerns in a clear and straightforward manner. Often, the beginning of treatment and chance for remission bring emotional relief as the patient focuses on the treatment journey ahead and the prospect of recovery.

Children's concerns: Like adults with cancer, children with cancer may feel frightened and helpless but may be too young to fully understand the nature of the problem. As part of adjusting to their illness and treatment, they will have to reconcile lost schooling, separation from friends, and an inability to participate in outdoor activities such as sports at least for a time. Children with cancer may direct their feelings toward the healthcare staff for hurting them or toward their parents for allowing them to become ill. Re-engaging the child in as many activities as possible is one of the best ways to soothe and reassure the child and minimize disruptions in the child's development.

Siblings of the child with cancer also may require special attention. They may fear the disease will strike them, feel guilt about their brother or sister's illness, and receive less time from parents who devote extra time to their ill child.

The parents of a child with cancer are often confused, angry, and fearful. To complicate matters, disciplining a child with cancer or the time commitment and financial burdens of the child's illness may cause disagreements within the family. It is important for parents of a child with cancer to ask the doctors, nurses, and social workers for help and guidance in addressing not only the medical concerns of the child with cancer but also the emotional issues of the child with cancer, siblings, and parents.

Treatment choices: Sometimes having to make choices about chemotherapy and other treatment options can cause a great deal of anxiety. Often, if patients with cancer ask their doctor about the medical questions they have, it provides some sense of relief in making these choices. In addition, the patient's nurses, social workers, and other health professionals understand the complexity of the emotions and special ongoing needs of those undergoing chemotherapy. They are available to spend time with the patient, answer questions, lend emotional support, and provide referrals to other useful resources.

Family and friends: The support of family and friends can contribute to a patient's ability to cope with what lies ahead. Many doctors and nurses recommend that a friend or family member accompany a patient during chemotherapy treatments, especially for the first several treatments. The presence of a friend or family member may help to ease anxiety. In addition, this person can act as an advocate, asking questions for the patient and listening to and retaining treatment information. Often, patients with cancer become acquainted with one another, and these friendships too can provide a support system.

Lifestyle changes: A change in lifestyle will occur for a patient with cancer and his or her family. Whether an inpatient or outpatient, routines of daily living may have to be adjusted to accommodate treatment schedules. However, many individuals are able to carry out their day-to-day routines with few or no changes.

Stress and side effects associated with the diagnosis of cancer and its treatment often will cause a person to question his or her self-worth, identity, and appearance. These feelings are common and may affect one's relationships, including sexual relationships. Recognition that these feelings are normal, and that many side effects are temporary, may be reassuring. Open, honest communications regarding fears and concerns can be very helpful. Together, doctors and nurses work toward minimizing any discomforts of chemotherapy administration. If during treatment there are any questions or concerns related to emotional or social issues, doctors, nurses, and social workers can help provide the answers and can often refer patients to available support groups, counseling services, or community programs.

Drugs Used with Chemotherapy

Glucocorticoids

Dexamethasone

Pronunciation: Dex-a-METH-a-zone.

Brand name: a commonly used brand name is Decadron®.

Dexamethasone is taken by mouth.

Hydrocortisone

Pronunciation: Hi-dro-KOR-ti-zone.

Brand names: commonly used brand names are Cortef®, Hydrocortone®, Solu-Cortef®.

Hydrocortisone is given by intravenous (IV), intramuscular (IM) or subcutaneous (SC) injection, or taken by mouth.

Prednisone

Pronunciation: PRED-ni-sone.

Brand names: commonly used brand names are Deltasone®, Meticorten®, Orasone®.

Prednisone is taken by mouth.

Special precautions: the doctor may want the patient to follow a low salt and/or high potassium diet while using these agents. Before having any kind of surgery (including dental surgery) or emergency treatment, the doctor in charge should be told that the patient is taking a glucocorticoid agent. Take with meals to reduce stomach upset. Stomach problems are more likely to occur if patient drinks alcoholic beverages or smokes while taking this medicine. Check with the doctor before drinking alcoholic beverages or smoking. Diabetic patients: this medicine may decrease the effectiveness of insulin and can affect blood sugar levels. If a change in the results of a urine sugar test is noticed or if there are questions about diabetes, check with the doctor. The body may need time to adjust after stopping use of this medicine. Do not stop taking this medicine suddenly.

Side effects needing medical attention as soon as possible: swelling of feet and ankles; muscle weakness; ulcers or stomach pain or burning; easy bruising; wounds that are slow to heal; dizziness; severe headaches; menstrual problems; blood-sugar problems; blurred or decreased vision or seeing halos around lights; sore throat and fever; depression; mood or mental changes.

Side effects needing medical attention, although not on an emergency basis: indigestion; mild euphoria; sleeplessness; nervousness or restlessness; weight gain or increased appetite.

Pamidronate

Pronunciation: Pam-ih-DRO-nate.

Brand name: a commonly used brand name is Aredia®.

Pamidronate is given by intravenous (IV) infusion.

Side effects needing medical attention as soon as possible: fever; unusual tiredness or fatigue; difficulty breathing; shortness of breath; coughing; swelling; pain; injection site reactions (redness or swelling).

Side effects needing medical attention, although not on an emergency basis: nausea; abdominal cramping; diarrhea; constipation; headache; loss of appetite; vomiting.

Thalidomide

Pronunciation: tha-LI-doe-mide.

Brand name: commonly used brand name is Thalomid.

Thalidomide is given by mouth.

Special precaution: *For women of childbearing age:* if you are able to bear children, you must have a pregnancy test within 24 hours of starting thalidomide treatment, once a week during the first month of treatment, and every 2 to 4 weeks after that. Also, you must not have sexual contact unless you use two effective birth control methods at the same time for at least 1 month before starting thalidomide treatment, during treatment, and for at least 1 month after you stop taking thalidomide. Patients noticing peripheral neuropathy (tingling, burning, numbness, or pain in the hands or feet) must stop taking medication and call their doctor immediately.

Side effects needing immediate medical attention: muscle weakness; tingling, burning, numbness, or pain in the hands, arms, feet, or legs; blood in urine; decreased urination; fever, alone or with chills and sore throat; irregular heartbeat; low blood pressure; skin rash.

Side effects needing medical attention, although not on an emergency basis: constipation; diarrhea; dizziness; drowsiness; nausea; stomach pain; dryness of mouth; dry skin; headache; increased appetite; mood changes; swelling in the legs.

Other Drugs

Leucovorin

Pronunciation: Loo-koh-VOR-in.

Brand name: Wellcovorin®.

Also commonly referred to as folinic acid. Leucovorin is given by intravenous (IV) or intramuscular (IM) injection, or taken by mouth.

Special precautions: drug interactions have been reported between leucovorin and certain anticonvulsant agents (e.g., phenytoin, phenobarbital, primidone), resulting in decreased efficacy of the anticonvulsant. The doctor should be informed if the patient is taking any of these drugs.

Side effects needing medical attention as soon as possible: hives; allergic-like reactions; fatigue; weakness.

Side effects needing medical attention, although not on an emergency basis: nausea; vomiting; diarrhea; constipation; loss of appetite.

Further Readings

Leukemia & Lymphoma Society Patient Booklets

Acute Lymphocytic Leukemia. The Leukemia & Lymphoma Society, 2002.

Acute Myelogenous Leukemia. The Leukemia & Lymphoma Society, 2001.

Chronic Lymphocytic Leukemia. The Leukemia & Lymphoma Society, 2002.

Chronic Myelogenous Leukemia. The Leukemia & Lymphoma Society, 2002.

The Lymphomas. The Leukemia & Lymphoma Society, 2002.

Myeloma. The Leukemia & Lymphoma Society, 2000.

Blood and Marrow Stem Cell Transplantation. The Leukemia & Lymphoma Society, 2002.

Complementary and Alternative Therapies For Leukemia, Lymphoma, Hodgkin's Disease, and Myeloma Fact Sheet. The Leukemia & Lymphoma Society, 1999.

Coping with Survival. The Leukemia & Lymphoma Society, 2000.

Cancer Clinical Trials Fact Sheet. The Leukemia & Lymphoma Society, 2002.

Fatigue Fact Sheet. The Leukemia & Lymphoma Society, 1999.

Understanding Blood Cell Counts Fact Sheet. The Leukemia & Lymphoma Society, 1999.

Nontechnical Resources

Childhood Leukemia. 3rd Edition, N. Keene. Sebastopol, CA: O'Reilly and Associates, 2002.

The Chemotherapy Survival Guide. J. Mckay RN and N. Hirano, RN, MSN. Oakland, CA: New Harbinger Publications, Inc., 1999.

Non-Hodgkin's Lymphoma. L. Johnson. Sebastopol, CA: O'Reilly and Associates, 1999.

Technical Sources

Handbook of Cancer Chemotherapy. Fifth edition, Skeel, Ronald, T. Lippincott Williams & Wilkins. 1999.

Oncology Pocket Guide to Chemotherapy. Third edition, Berkery, R. RN, Baltzer Cheri, L. RN, and A Skarin, MD. Mosby-Wolf Medical Communications, 1997.

USP DI, Volume I, *Drug Information for the Healthcare Professional*, 19th Edition, 2002.

USP DI, Volume II, *Advice for the Patient: Drug Information in Lay Language*, 19th Edition, 2002.

Additional Information

The Leukemia and Lymphoma Society
1311 Mamaroneck Ave.
White Plains, NY 10605
Toll-Free: 800-955-4572
Tel: 914-949-5213
Fax: 914-949-6691
Website: www.leukemia-lymphoma.org

Chapter 27

Radiation Therapy for Cancer Treatment

Fast Facts about Radiation Therapy

- Radiation treatments are painless.
- External radiation treatment does not make you radioactive.
- Treatments are usually scheduled every day except Saturday and Sunday.
- You need to allow 30 minutes for each treatment session although the treatment itself takes only a few minutes.
- It's important to get plenty of rest and to eat a well-balanced diet during the course of your radiation therapy.
- Skin in the treated area may become sensitive and easily irritated.
- Side effects of radiation treatment are usually temporary and they vary depending on the area of the body that is being treated.

What Is Radiation Therapy?

Radiation therapy (sometimes called radiotherapy, x-ray therapy, or irradiation) is the treatment of disease using penetrating beams

"Radiation Therapy and You: A Guide to Self-Help during Cancer Treatment," National Cancer Institute (NCI), revised September 22, 1999.

of high energy waves or streams of particles called radiation. Many years ago doctors learned how to use this energy to see inside the body and find disease. You've probably seen a chest x-ray or x-ray pictures of your teeth or your bones. At high doses (many times those used for x-ray exams) radiation is used to treat cancer and other illnesses. The radiation used for cancer treatment comes from special machines or from radioactive substances. Radiation therapy equipment aims specific amounts of the radiation at tumors or areas of the body where there is disease.

How Does Radiation Therapy Work?

Radiation in high doses kills cells or keeps them from growing and dividing. Because cancer cells grow and divide more rapidly than most of the normal cells around them, radiation therapy can successfully treat many kinds of cancer. Normal cells are also affected by radiation, but unlike cancer cells, most of them recover from the effects of radiation.

To protect normal cells, doctors carefully limit the doses of radiation and spread the treatment out over time. They also shield as much normal tissue as possible while they aim the radiation at the site of the cancer.

What Are the Goals and Benefits of Radiation Therapy?

The goal of radiation therapy is to kill the cancer cells with as little risk as possible to normal cells. Radiation therapy can be used to treat many kinds of cancer in almost any part of the body. In fact, more than half of all people with cancer are treated with some form of radiation. For many cancer patients, radiation is the only kind of treatment they need. Thousands of people who have had radiation therapy alone or in combination with other types of cancer treatment are free of cancer.

Radiation treatment, like surgery, is a local treatment—it affects the cancer cells only in a specific area of the body. Sometimes doctors add radiation therapy to treatments that reach all parts of the body (systemic treatment) such as chemotherapy, or biological therapy to improve treatment results. You may hear your doctor use the term, adjuvant therapy, for a treatment that is added to, and given after, the primary therapy.

Radiation therapy is often used with surgery to treat cancer. Doctors may use radiation before surgery to shrink a tumor. This makes it easier to remove the cancerous tissue and may allow the surgeon to perform less radical surgery. Radiation therapy may be used after surgery to stop the growth of cancer cells that may remain. Your doctor may choose to use radiation therapy and surgery at the same time. This procedure is known as intraoperative radiation.

In some cases, instead of surgery, doctors use radiation along with anticancer drugs (chemotherapy) to destroy the cancer. Radiation may be given before, during, or after chemotherapy. Doctors carefully tailor this combination treatment to each patient's needs depending on the type of cancer, its location, and its size. The purpose of radiation treatment before or during chemotherapy is to make the tumor smaller and thus improve the effectiveness of the anticancer drugs. Doctors sometimes recommend that a patient complete chemotherapy and then have radiation treatment to kill any cancer cells that might remain.

When curing the cancer is not possible, radiation therapy can be used to shrink tumors and reduce pressure, pain, and other symptoms of cancer. This is called palliative care or palliation. Many cancer patients find that they have a better quality of life when radiation is used for this purpose.

What Are the Risks of Radiation Therapy?

The brief high doses of radiation that damage or destroy cancer cells can also injure or kill normal cells. These effects of radiation on normal cells cause treatment side effects. Most side effects of radiation treatment are well known, and with the help of your doctor and nurse are easily treated.

The risk of side effects is usually less than the benefit of killing cancer cells. Your doctor will not advise you to have any treatment unless the benefits—control of disease and relief from symptoms—are greater than the known risks.

How Is Radiation Therapy Given?

Radiation therapy can be given in one of two ways: external or internal. Some patients have both, one after the other. Most people who receive radiation therapy for cancer have external radiation. It is usually given during outpatient visits to a hospital or treatment center. In external radiation therapy, a machine directs the high-energy rays at the cancer and a small margin of normal tissue surrounding it.

The various machines used for external radiation work in slightly different ways. Some are better for treating cancers near the skin surface; others work best on cancers deeper in the body. The most common type of machine used for radiation therapy is called a linear accelerator. Some radiation machines use a variety of radioactive substances (such as cobalt-60, for example) as the source of high-energy rays. Your doctor decides which type of radiation therapy machine is best for you.

When internal radiation therapy is used, the radiation source is placed inside the body. This method of radiation treatment is called brachytherapy or implant therapy. The source of the radiation (such as radioactive iodine, for example) sealed in a small holder is called an implant. Implants may be thin wires, plastic tubes (catheters), capsules, or seeds. An implant may be placed directly into a tumor or inserted into a body cavity. Sometimes, after a tumor has been removed by surgery, the implant is placed in the tumor bed (the area from which the tumor was removed) to kill any tumor cells that may remain. Another type of internal radiation therapy uses unsealed radioactive materials which may be taken by mouth or injected into the body. If you have this type of treatment, you may need to stay in the hospital for several days.

Who Gives Radiation Treatments?

A doctor who specializes in using radiation to treat cancer—a radiation oncologist—will prescribe the type and amount of treatment that is right for you. The radiation oncologist is the person referred to as your doctor throughout this chapter. The radiation oncologist works closely with the other doctors and health care professionals involved in your care. This highly trained health care team may include:

- The radiation physicist, who makes sure that the equipment is working properly and that the machines deliver the right dose of radiation. The physicist also works closely with your doctor to plan your treatment.

- The dosimetrist, who works under the direction of your doctor and the radiation physicist and helps carry out your treatment plan by calculating the amount of radiation to be delivered to the cancer and normal tissues that are nearby.

- The radiation therapist, who positions you for your treatments and runs the equipment that delivers the radiation.

- The radiation nurse, who will coordinate your care, help you learn about treatment, and tell you how to manage side effects.

The nurse can also answer questions you or family members may have about your treatment.

Your health care team also may include a physician assistant, radiologist, dietitian, radiation oncologist, physical therapist, social worker, or other health care professional.

Is Radiation Treatment Expensive?

Treatment of cancer with radiation can be costly. It requires very complex equipment and the services of many health care professionals. The exact cost of your radiation therapy will depend on the type and number of treatments you need.

Most health insurance policies, including Part B of Medicare, cover charges for radiation therapy. It's a good idea to talk with your doctor's office staff or the hospital business office about your policy and how expected costs will be paid.

In some states, the Medicaid program may help you pay for treatments. You can find out from the office that handles social services in your city or county whether you are eligible for Medicaid and whether your radiation therapy is a covered expense.

If you need financial aid, contact the hospital social service office or the National Cancer Institute's (NCI) Cancer Information Service at 800-4-CANCER. They may be able to direct you to sources of help. Additional sources of cancer information are described in the resource directories at the end of this book.

External Radiation Therapy: What to Expect

How Does the Doctor Plan My Treatment?

The high energy rays used for radiation therapy can come from a variety of sources. Your doctor may choose to use x-rays, an electron beam, or cobalt-60 gamma rays. Some cancer treatment centers have special equipment that produces beams of protons or neutrons for radiation therapy. The type of radiation your doctor decides to use depends on what kind of cancer you have and how far into your body the radiation should go. High-energy radiation is used to treat many types of cancer. Low-energy x-rays are used to treat some kinds of skin diseases.

After a physical exam and a review of your medical history, the doctor plans your treatment. In a process called simulation, you will be asked to lie very still on an examining table while the radiation therapist uses a special x-ray machine to define your treatment port or field. This is the exact place on your body where the radiation will be aimed. Depending on the location of your cancer, you may have more than one treatment port.

Simulation may also involve CT scans or other imaging studies to plan how to direct the radiation. Depending on the type of treatment you will be receiving, body molds or other devices that keep you from moving during treatment (immobilization devices) may be made at this time. They will be used each time you have treatment to be sure that you are positioned correctly. Simulation may take from a half hour to about 2 hours.

The radiation therapist often will mark the treatment port on your skin with tattoos or tiny dots of colored, permanent ink. It's important that the radiation be targeted at the same area each time. If the dots appear to be fading, tell your radiation therapist who will darken them so that they can be seen easily.

Once simulation has been done, your doctor will meet with the radiation physicist and the dosimetrist. Based on the results of your medical history, lab tests, x-rays, other treatments you may have had, and the location and kind of cancer you have, they will decide how much radiation is needed, what kind of machine to use to deliver it, and how many treatments you should have.

After you have started the treatments, your doctor and the other members of your health care team will follow your progress by checking your response to treatment and how you are feeling at least once a week. When necessary, your doctor may revise the treatment plan by changing the radiation dose or the number and length of your remaining radiation sessions.

Your nurse will be available daily to discuss your concerns and answer any questions you may have. Be sure to tell your nurse if you are having any side effects or if you notice any unusual symptoms.

How Long Does the Treatment Take?

For most types of cancer, radiation therapy usually is given 5 days a week for 6 or 7 weeks. (When radiation is used for palliative care, the course of treatment is shorter, usually 2 to 3 weeks.) The total dose of radiation and the number of treatments you need will depend on the size, location, and kind of cancer you have, your general health, and other medical treatments you may be receiving.

Using many small doses of daily radiation rather than a few large doses helps protect normal body tissues in the treatment area. Weekend rest breaks allow normal cells to recover.

It's very important that you have all of your scheduled treatments to get the most benefit from your therapy. Missing or delaying treatments can lessen the effectiveness of your radiation treatment.

What Happens during the Treatment Visits?

Before each treatment, you may need to change into a hospital gown or robe. It's best to wear clothing that is easy to take off and put on again.

In the treatment room, the radiation therapist will use the marks on your skin to locate the treatment area and to position you correctly. You may sit in a special chair or lie down on a treatment table. For each external radiation therapy session, you will be in the treatment room about 15 to 30 minutes, but you will be getting radiation for only about 1 to 5 minutes of that time. Receiving external radiation treatments is painless, just like having an x-ray taken. You will not hear, see, or smell the radiation.

The radiation therapist may put special shields (or blocks) between the machine and certain parts of your body to help protect normal tissues and organs. There might also be plastic or plaster forms that help you stay in exactly the right place. You need to remain very still during the treatment so that the radiation reaches only the area where it's needed and the same area is treated each time. You don't have to hold your breath—just breathe normally.

The radiation therapist will leave the treatment room before your treatment begins. The radiation machine is controlled from a nearby area. You will be watched on a television screen or through a window in the control room. Although you may feel alone, keep in mind that the therapist can see and hear you and even talk with you using an intercom in the treatment room. If you should feel ill or very uncomfortable during the treatment, tell your therapist at once. The machine can be stopped at any time.

The machines used for radiation treatments are very large, and they make noises as they move around your body to aim at the treatment area from different angles. Their size and motion may be frightening at first. Remember that the machines are being moved and controlled by your radiation therapist. They are checked constantly to be sure they're working right. If you have concerns about anything that happens in the treatment room, discuss these concerns with the radiation therapist.

What Are the Side Effects of Treatment?

External radiation therapy does not cause your body to become radioactive. There is no need to avoid being with other people because you are undergoing treatment. Even hugging, kissing, or having sexual relations with others poses no risk of radiation exposure.

Most side effects of radiation therapy are related to the area that is being treated. Many patients have no side effects at all. Your doctor and nurse will tell you about the possible side effects you might expect and how you should deal with them. You should contact your doctor or nurse if you have any unusual symptoms during your treatment, such as coughing, sweating, fever, or pain.

The side effects of radiation therapy, although unpleasant, are usually not serious and can be controlled with medication or diet. They usually go away within a few weeks after treatment ends, although some side effects can last longer. Always check with your doctor or nurse about how you should deal with side effects.

Throughout your treatment, your doctor will regularly check on the effects of the treatment. You may not be aware of changes in the cancer, but you probably will notice decreases in pain, bleeding, or other discomfort. You may continue to notice further improvement after your treatment is completed.

Your doctor may recommend periodic tests and physical exams to be sure that the radiation is causing as little damage to normal cells as possible. Depending on the area being treated, you may have routine blood tests to check the levels of red blood cells, white blood cells, and platelets; radiation treatment can cause decreases in the levels of different blood cells.

What Can I Do to Take Care of Myself during Therapy?

Each patient's body responds to radiation therapy in its own way. That's why your doctor must plan, and sometimes adjust, your treatment. In addition, your doctor or nurse will give you suggestions for caring for yourself at home that are specific for your treatment and the possible side effects.

Nearly all cancer patients receiving radiation therapy need to take special care of themselves to protect their health and to help the treatment succeed. Some guidelines to remember follow:

- Before starting treatment, be sure your doctor knows about any medicines you are taking and if you have any allergies. Do not start taking any medicine (whether prescription or over-the-counter) during your radiation therapy without first telling your doctor or nurse.

- Fatigue is common during radiation therapy. Your body will use a lot of extra energy over the course of your treatment, and you may feel very tired. Be sure to get plenty of rest and sleep as often as you feel the need. It's common for fatigue to last for 4 to 6 weeks after your treatment has been completed.

- Good nutrition is very important. Try to eat a balanced diet that will prevent weight loss.

- Check with your doctor before taking vitamin supplements or herbal preparations during treatment.

- Avoid wearing tight clothes such as girdles or close-fitting collars over the treatment area.

- Be extra kind to your skin in the treatment area:
  - Ask your doctor or nurse if you may use soaps, lotions, deodorants, sun blocks, medicines, perfumes, cosmetics, talcum powder, or other substances in the treated area.
  - Wear loose, soft cotton clothing over the treated area.
  - Do not wear starched or stiff clothing over the treated area.
  - Do not scratch, rub, or scrub treated skin.
  - Do not use adhesive tape on treated skin. If bandaging is necessary, use paper tape and apply it outside of the treatment area. Your nurse can help you place dressings so that you can avoid irritating the treated area.
  - Do not apply heat or cold (heating pad, ice pack, etc.) to the treated area. Use only lukewarm water for bathing the area.
  - Use an electric shaver if you must shave the treated area but only after checking with your doctor or nurse. Do not use a preshave lotion or hair removal products on the treated area.
  - Protect the treatment area from the sun. Do not apply sunscreens just before a radiation treatment. If possible, cover treated skin (with light clothing) before going outside. Ask

your doctor if you should use a sunscreen or a sunblock product. If so, select one with a protection factor of at least 15 and reapply it often. Ask your doctor or nurse how long after your treatments are completed you should continue to protect the treated skin from sunlight.

- If you have questions, ask your doctor or nurse. They are the only ones who can properly advise you about your treatment, its side effects, home care, and any other medical concerns you may have.

Managing Side Effects

Are Side Effects the Same for Everyone?

The side effects of radiation treatment vary from patient to patient. You may have no side effects or only a few mild ones through your course of treatment. Some people do experience serious side effects, however. The side effects that you have depend mostly on the radiation dose and the part of your body that is treated. Your general health also can affect how your body reacts to radiation therapy and whether you have side effects. Before beginning your treatment, your doctor and nurse will discuss the side effects you might experience, how long they might last, and how serious they might be.

Side effects may be acute or chronic. Acute side effects are sometimes referred to as early side effects. They occur soon after the treatment begins and usually are gone within a few weeks of finishing therapy. Chronic side effects, sometimes called late side effects, may take months or years to develop and usually are permanent.

The most common early side effects of radiation therapy are fatigue and skin changes. They can result from radiation to any treatment site. Other side effects are related to treatment of specific areas. For example, temporary or permanent hair loss may be a side effect of radiation treatment to the head. Appetite can be altered if treatment affects the mouth, stomach, or intestine.

Fortunately, most side effects will go away in time. In the meantime, there are ways to reduce discomfort. If you have a side effect that is especially severe, the doctor may prescribe a break in your treatments or change your treatment in some way.

Be sure to tell your doctor, nurse, or radiation therapist about any side effects that you notice. They can help you treat the problems and tell you how to lessen the chances that the side effects will come back. The information in this booklet can serve as a guide to handling some side effects, but it cannot take the place of talking with the members of your health care team.

Will Side Effects Limit My Activity?

Not necessarily. It will depend on which side effects you have and how severe they are. Many patients are able to work, prepare meals, and enjoy their usual leisure activities while they are having radiation therapy. Others find that they need more rest than usual and therefore cannot do as much. Try to continue doing the things you enjoy as long as you don't become too tired.

Your doctor may suggest that you limit activities that might irritate the area being treated. In most cases, you can have sexual relations if you wish. You may find that your desire for physical intimacy is lower because radiation therapy may cause you to feel more tired than usual. For most patients, these feelings are temporary.

What Causes Fatigue?

Fatigue, feeling tired and lacking energy, is the most common symptom reported by cancer patients. The exact cause is not always known. It may be due to the disease itself or to treatment. It may also result from lowered blood counts, lack of sleep, pain, and poor appetite.

Most people begin to feel tired after a few weeks of radiation therapy. During radiation therapy, the body uses a lot of energy for healing. You also may be tired because of stress related to your illness, daily trips for treatment, and the effects of radiation on normal cells. Feelings of weakness or weariness will go away gradually after your treatment has been completed.

You can help yourself during radiation therapy by not trying to do too much. If you do feel tired, limit your activities and use your leisure time in a restful way. Save your energy for doing the things that you feel are most important. Do not feel that you have to do everything you normally do. Try to get more sleep at night, and plan your day so that you have time to rest if you need it. Several short naps or breaks may be more helpful than a long rest period.

Sometimes, light exercise such as walking may combat fatigue. Talk with your doctor or nurse about how much exercise you may do while you are having therapy. Talking with other cancer patients in a support group may also help you learn how to deal with fatigue.

If you have a full-time job, you may want to try to continue to work your normal schedule. However, some patients prefer to take time off while they're receiving radiation therapy; others work a reduced number of hours. Speak frankly with your employer about your needs and wishes during this time. A part-time schedule may be possible or perhaps you can do some work at home. Ask your doctor's office or the radiation therapy department to help by trying to schedule treatments with your workday in mind.

Whether you're going to work or not, it's a good idea to ask family members or friends to help with daily chores, shopping, child care, housework, or driving. Neighbors may be able to help by picking up groceries for you when they do their own shopping. You also could ask someone to drive you to and from your treatment visits to help conserve your energy.

How Are Skin Problems Treated?

You may notice that your skin in the treatment area is red or irritated. It may look as if it is sunburned, or tanned. After a few weeks your skin may be very dry from the therapy. Ask your doctor or nurse for advice on how to relieve itching or discomfort.

With some kinds of radiation therapy, treated skin may develop a moist reaction, especially in areas where there are skin folds. When this happens, the skin is wet and it may become very sore. It's important to notify your doctor or nurse if your skin develops a moist reaction. They can give you suggestions on how to care for these areas and prevent them from becoming infected.

During radiation therapy you will need to be very gentle with the skin in the treatment area. The following suggestions may be helpful:

- Avoid irritating treated skin.

- When you wash, use only lukewarm water and mild soap; pat dry.

- Do not wear tight clothing over the area.

- Do not rub, scrub, or scratch the skin in the treatment area.

- Avoid putting anything that is hot or cold, such as heating pads or ice packs, on your treated skin.

- Ask your doctor or nurse to recommend skin care products that will not cause skin irritation. Do not use any powders, creams, perfumes, deodorants, body oils, ointments, lotions, or home remedies in the treatment area while you're being treated and for several weeks afterward unless approved by your doctor or nurse.

• Do not apply any skin lotions within 2 hours of a treatment.

• Avoid exposing the radiated area to the sun during treatment. If you expect to be in the sun for more than a few minutes you will need to be very careful. Wear protective clothing (such as a hat with a broad brim and a shirt with long sleeves) and use a sunscreen. Ask your doctor or nurse about using sunblock lotions. After your treatment is over, ask your doctor or nurse how long you should continue to take extra precautions in the sun.

The majority of skin reactions to radiation therapy go away a few weeks after treatment is completed. In some cases, though, the treated skin will remain slightly darker than it was before and it may continue to be more sensitive to sun exposure.

What Can Be Done about Hair Loss?

Radiation therapy can cause hair loss, also known as alopecia, but only in the area being treated. For example, if you are receiving treatment to your hip, you will not lose the hair from your head. Radiation of your head may cause you to lose some or all of the hair on your scalp. Many patients find that their hair grows back again after the treatments are finished. The amount of hair that grows back will depend on how much and what kind of radiation you receive. You may notice that your hair has a slightly different texture or color when it grows back. Other types of cancer treatment, such as chemotherapy, also can affect how your hair grows back.

Although your scalp may be tender after the hair is lost, it's a good idea to cover your head with a hat, turban, or scarf. You should wear a protective cap or scarf when you're in the sun or outdoors in cold weather. If you prefer a wig or toupee, be sure the lining does not irritate your scalp. The cost of a hairpiece that you need because of cancer treatment is a tax-deductible expense and may be covered in part by your health insurance. If you plan to buy a wig, it's a good idea to select it early in your treatment if you want to match the color and style to your own hair.

How Are Side Effects of the Blood Managed?

Radiation therapy can cause low levels of white blood cells and platelets. These blood cells normally help your body fight infection and prevent bleeding. If large areas of active bone marrow are treated, your red blood cell count may be low as well. If your blood tests show these side effects, your doctor may wait until your blood counts increase to continue treatments. Your doctor will check your blood counts regularly and change your treatment schedule if it is necessary.

Will Eating Be a Problem?

Sometimes radiation treatment causes loss of appetite and interferes with eating, digesting, and absorbing food. Try to eat enough to help damaged tissues rebuild themselves. It is not unusual to lose 1 or 2 pounds a week during radiation therapy. You will be weighed weekly to monitor your weight.

It is very important to eat a balanced diet. You may find it helpful to eat small meals often and to try to eat a variety of different foods. Your doctor or nurse can tell you whether you should eat a special diet, and a dietitian will have some ideas that will help you maintain your weight.

Coping with short-term diet problems may be easier than you expect. There are a number of diet guides and recipe booklets for patients who need help with eating problems. A National Cancer Institute booklet, "Eating Hints for Cancer Patients" explains how to get more calories and protein without eating more food. It also has many tips that should help you enjoy eating. The recipes it contains can be used for the whole family and are marked for people with special concerns, such as low-salt diets.

If it's painful to chew and swallow, your doctor may advise you to use a powdered or liquid diet supplement. Many of these products are available at drugstores and supermarkets and come in a variety of flavors. They are tasty when used alone or combined with other foods such as pureed fruit, or added to milkshakes. Some of the companies that make these diet supplements have recipe booklets to help you increase your nutrient intake. Ask your nurse, dietitian, or pharmacist for further information.

You may lose interest in food during your treatment. Fatigue from your treatments can cause loss of appetite. Some people just don't feel like eating because of stress from their illness and treatment or because the treatment changes the way food tastes. Even if you're not very hungry, it's important to keep your protein and calorie intake high. Doctors have found that patients who eat well can better cope with having cancer and with the side effects of treatment. Medications for appetite enhancement are now available; ask your doctor or nurse about them.

The following list suggests ways to perk up your appetite when it's poor and to make the most of it when you do feel like eating.

- Eat when you are hungry, even if it is not mealtime.

- Eat several small meals during the day rather than three large ones.

- Use soft lighting, quiet music, brightly colored table settings, or whatever helps you feel good while eating.

- Vary your diet and try new recipes. If you enjoy company while eating, try to have meals with family or friends. It may be helpful to have the radio or television on while you eat.

- Ask your doctor or nurse whether you can have a glass of wine or beer with your meal to increase your appetite. Keep in mind that, in some cases, alcohol may not be allowed because it could worsen the side effects of treatment. This may be especially true if you are receiving radiation therapy for cancer of the head, neck, or upper chest area including the esophagus.

- Keep simple meals in the freezer to use when you feel hungry.

- If other people offer to cook for you, let them. Don't be shy about telling them what you'd like to eat.

- Keep healthy snacks close by for nibbling when you get the urge.

- If you live alone, you might want to arrange for Meals on Wheels to bring food to you. Ask your doctor, nurse, social worker, or local social service agencies about Meals on Wheels. This service is available in most large communities.

If you are able to eat only small amounts of food, you can increase the calories per serving by:

- Adding butter or margarine.

- Mixing canned cream soups with milk or half-and-half rather than water.

- Drinking eggnog, milkshakes, or prepared liquid supplements between meals.

- Adding cream sauce or melted cheese to your favorite vegetables.

Some people find they can drink large amounts of liquids even when they don't feel like eating solid foods. If this is the case for you, try to get the most from each glassful by making drinks enriched with powdered milk, yogurt, honey, or prepared liquid supplements.

Will Radiation Therapy Affect Me Emotionally?

Nearly all patients being treated for cancer report feeling emotionally upset at different times during their therapy. It's not unusual to feel anxious, depressed, afraid, angry, frustrated, alone, or helpless. Radiation therapy may affect your emotions indirectly through fatigue or changes in hormone balance, but the treatment itself is not a direct cause of mental distress.

You may find that it's helpful to talk about your feelings with a close friend, family member, chaplain, nurse, social worker, or psychologist with whom you feel at ease. You may want to ask your doctor or nurse about meditation or relaxation exercises that might help you unwind and feel calmer.

Nationwide support programs can help cancer patients to meet others who share common problems and concerns. Some medical centers have formed peer support groups so that patients can meet to discuss their feelings and inspire each other.

Sexual Relations

With most types of radiation therapy, neither men nor women are likely to notice any change in their ability to enjoy sex. Both sexes, however, may notice a decrease in their level of desire. This is more likely to be due to the stress of having cancer than to the effects of radiation therapy. Once the treatment ends, sexual desire is likely to return to previous levels.

When Should I Call the Doctor?

After treatment for cancer, you're likely to be more aware of your body and to notice even slight changes in how you feel from day to day. The doctor will want to know if you are having any unusual symptoms. Promptly tell your doctor about:

- A pain that doesn't go away, especially if it's always in the same place.

- New or unusual lumps, bumps, or swelling.

- Nausea, vomiting, diarrhea, or loss of appetite.

- Unexplained weight loss.

- A fever or cough that doesn't go away.

- Unusual rashes, bruises, or bleeding.

- Any symptoms that you are concerned about.

- Any other warning signs mentioned by your doctor or nurse.

What about Returning to Work?

Many people find that they can continue to work during radiation therapy because treatment appointments are short. If you have stopped working, you can return to your job as soon as you feel up to it. If your job requires lifting or heavy physical activity, you may need a change in your work responsibilities until you have regained your strength. Check with your employer to see if a *return to work* release from your doctor is required.

When you are ready to return to work, it is important to learn about your rights regarding your job and health insurance. If you have any questions about employment issues, contact the Cancer Information Service (CIS). CIS staff can help you find local agencies that can help you deal with problems regarding employment and insurance rights that are sometimes faced by cancer survivors.

Chapter 28

Transplantation Therapy for Leukemia

Chapter Contents

Section 28.1

Peripheral Blood Stem Cell and Marrow Transplantation

"Blood and Marrow Stem Cell Transplantation: Leukemia, Lymphoma, and Myeloma," 4/2002 © The Leukemia & Lymphoma Society, reprinted with permission. For additional information visit www.leukemia-lymphoma. org. Information on minitransplants is an excerpt from "Bone Marrow Transplantation and Peripheral Blood Stem Cell Transplantation: Questions and Answers," Fact Sheet 7.41, National Cancer Institute (NCI), reviewed 8/22/2000.

Normal Blood and Marrow

Blood is composed of plasma and cells suspended in plasma. The plasma is largely made up of water in which many chemicals are dissolved. These chemicals include proteins (e.g., albumin), hormones (e.g., thyroid hormone), minerals (e.g., iron), vitamins (e.g., folic acid), and antibodies, including those we develop from our immunizations (e.g., polio virus antibodies). The cells include red blood cells, platelets, neutrophils, monocytes, eosinophils, basophils, and lymphocytes.

The red cells make up half the volume of the blood. They are filled with hemoglobin, the protein that picks up oxygen in the lungs and delivers oxygen to the tissues. The platelets are small cells (one-tenth the size of red cells) that help stop bleeding if one is injured. For example, when one has a cut, the blood vessels that carry blood are torn open. Platelets stick to the torn surface of the vessel, clump together, and plug up the bleeding site. The vessel wall then heals at the site of the clot and returns to its normal state.

The neutrophils and monocytes are white blood cells. They are phagocytes (or eating-cells) because they can ingest bacteria or fungi and kill them. Unlike the red cells and platelets, the white cells leave the blood and move into the tissues where they can ingest invading bacteria or fungi and help cure an infection. Eosinophils and basophils are two additional types of white cells that participate in allergic responses.

Most lymphocytes, another type of white blood cell, are in the lymph nodes, spleen, and lymphatic channels, but some enter the blood. There are three major types of lymphocytes: T cells, B cells, and natural killer (NK) cells.

Bone marrow is the spongy tissue where blood cell development takes place. It occupies the central cavity of bone. All bones have active marrow at birth. By the time a person reaches young adulthood, the bones of the hands, feet, arms, and legs no longer have functioning marrow. The back bones (vertebrae), hip and shoulder bones, ribs, breast bone, and skull contain marrow that is actively making blood cells.

The process of blood cell formation is called hematopoiesis. A small group of cells, the stem cells, are responsible for making all the blood cells in the marrow. The stem cells eventually develop into the specific blood cells by a process of differentiation (see Figure 28.1).

In healthy individuals, there are sufficient stem cells to keep producing new blood cells continuously. Some stem cells enter the blood and circulate. They are present in such small numbers that they cannot be counted or identified in the usual type of blood counts. Their presence in the blood is important, because they can be collected by special techniques and transplanted into a recipient if enough stem cells are harvested from a compatible donor. This stem cell circulation from marrow to blood and back occurs in the fetus as well. That is why, after birth, the placental and umbilical cord blood can be used as a source of stem cells for transplantation.

In summary, blood cells are made in the marrow and when the cells are fully formed and able to function, they leave the marrow and enter the blood. The red cells and the platelets perform their respective functions of delivering oxygen and plugging up injured blood vessels in the circulation. The neutrophils, eosinophils, basophils, monocytes and lymphocytes, which are collectively the white blood cells, move into the tissues of the lungs, for example, and can combat infection, such as pneumonia, and perform their other functions.

Figure 28.1 depicts an abbreviated diagram of the process of hematopoiesis. This process involves the development of functional blood and lymphatic cells from stem cells.

Origins of Transplantation

In the mid-19th century, Italian scientists proposed that the marrow was the source of blood cells. The idea that a factor in the blood-forming tissues from one individual might restore the injured marrow

Blood Cell and Lymphocyte Development

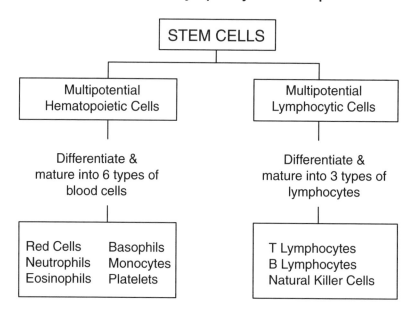

Figure 28.1. Blood Cell and Lymphocyte Development

of another individual was considered a century ago. Some thought this factor was a chemical that could be transferred by eating the marrow. At the turn of the 20th century, scientists began to formulate the idea that a small number of cells in the marrow might be responsible for the development of all blood cells. They began to refer to them as stem cells. Attempts to use the marrow cells of a healthy individual to restore the lost marrow function of an ill patient are at least 60 years old. Early attempts at human marrow transplantation were largely unsuccessful because the scientific basis for success was not yet known.

Marrow transplantation as a form of treatment began to be explored scientifically at the end of World War II. The stem cells of marrow are very sensitive to irradiation injury. Thus, marrow injury was an important and potentially lethal side effect of exposure to the atomic bomb or to industrial accidents in the atomic weapons industry. In the late 1940s, studies of marrow transplantation as a means

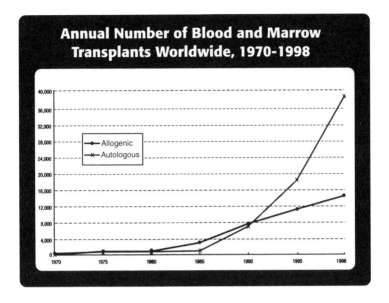

Figure 28.2. *Annual Number of Blood and Marrow Transplants Worldwide, 1970-1998*

of treating radiation-exposed combatants or civilians was spurred by the Atomic Energy Commission's concern about the spread of nuclear technology and weapons.

The idea that medical disorders that affect blood cell or immune cell formation could be cured by marrow transplantation encouraged research by civilian scientists as well. Their research efforts led to the current success of stem cell transplantation as a means of medical treatment and its increased availability to patients (see Figure 28.2).

Figure 28.2 shows the number of allogeneic and autologous transplants performed each year as reported to the International Bone Marrow Transplant Registry. Improvement in techniques of transplantation in the 1980s and after have led to a marked increase in the application of this approach. Reporting is voluntary so this probably is an underestimation of the number of transplants performed worldwide. (Kindly provided by the International Bone Marrow Transplantation Registry)

Reasons for Using Transplantation

The rationale for stem cell transplantation is based on the fact that all blood cells (e.g., red cells, phagocytes, and platelets) and immune cells (lymphocytes) arise from the stem cells, which are present in the marrow. Stem cells circulate in the blood in very small numbers. Drugs are available that increase the numbers of stem cells in the blood by drawing them out of the marrow. Sufficient quantities of these stem cells for transplantation are recovered by circulating large volumes of blood through a hemapheresis machine and skimming off a population of cells that contains stem cells.

Blood is an increasingly frequent source of stem cells for transplantation. Thus, bone marrow transplantation, or BMT, as a generic term for the procedure has been modified to mean blood or marrow transplantation, permitting the continued use of the familiar acronym, BMT. In many cases, the more specific term stem cell transplantation (or SCT) is now used.

Treating Leukemia, Lymphoma, Myeloma with Stem Cell Transplantation

Acute leukemia, lymphoma, and myeloma have remission and cure rates that increase in relationship to the amount of chemotherapy given to the patient. Large doses of chemotherapy and/or radiation are required to destroy the disease cells. These intensive therapies can destroy normal cells in the marrow as well. The capability of the marrow to make healthy blood cells is so severely impaired after very high-dose chemotherapy and radiation therapy required to treat refractory or relapsed disease that few patients would survive such treatment. They would succumb as a result of infections (because of the absence of white cells) or hemorrhage (because of the absence of blood platelets).

In order to administer larger doses of chemotherapy or radiation therapy, transplant physicians developed stem cell transplantation as a method to restore normal blood cell production in a timely fashion. With the infusion of sufficient stem cells from a closely matched donor, such as a sibling, marrow function and blood cell production are restored rapidly enough to allow recovery from the intensive treatment. After several decades of research, discovery, and clinical trials, allogeneic stem cell transplantation can be used successfully to cure patients who are at high risk of relapse, who do not respond fully to treatment, or who relapse after prior successful treatment. In some circumstances autologous stem cells (obtained from the blood and marrow of the patient) can be used.

The age, medical condition, likelihood of response of the malignancy to the conditioning regimen, and the availability of an HLA-matched donor are considerations in the decision to use allogeneic transplantation.

Thus, leukemia, lymphoma, or myeloma, if poorly responsive to standard therapy, or if biological features are present that are known to predict for a poor response to chemotherapy, may be treated with very intensive chemotherapy and/or radiotherapy, which requires complementary stem cell transplantation.

Deciding to Use Stem Cell Transplantation for Leukemia, Lymphoma, or Myeloma

Two central questions should be answered when considering a transplant for a patient in remission: Does the current evidence indicate that stem cell transplantation will be more likely to cure the disease than other forms of therapy? Is there a compatible donor available as a source of stem cells? Other important factors that influence the decision include the patient's age, the specific disease being treated, biologic features at the time of diagnosis that indicate a poor prognosis, and the presence of complicating medical conditions.

The age of the patient is a compelling factor in the decision to do a transplant. About three-quarters of individuals who develop leukemia, lymphoma, or myeloma are over 50 years of age. Patients over that age are less likely to have a favorable outcome after transplantation.

Indeed, the results of transplantation are best in children and become less favorable with each advancing decade. Older individuals are:

1. more susceptible to graft versus host disease;

2. more likely to have complicating medical problems; and

3. more likely to have a decreased tolerance for the accumulated effects of the prior intensive chemotherapy and the conditioning treatments required for transplantation.

These are generalizations and allogeneic transplantation can be used in older individuals when judgment favors that decision. Moreover, new techniques that require less harsh conditioning therapy are being explored for certain types of leukemia and lymphoma.

Although the risks of allogeneic transplantation have decreased with each succeeding decade of experience, the procedure requires careful analysis of the circumstances and in-depth and thoughtful discussions with the patient. Continued research may further change the risk-to-benefit equation in favor of transplantation. Alternatively, new drugs and new modalities may do the reverse.

Testing Donor Compatibility

When a transplant is under consideration, the patient and his or her siblings will be tested to determine their tissue type or human leukocyte antigen (HLA) type.

The tissue type of an individual is determined by proteins on the surface of cells. Like other tissue cells, the leukocytes contain these surface proteins. By testing the leukocytes obtained from a blood sample, transplant physicians can determine the HLA type of the patient and potential donors. The immune reactions that occur when nonidentical individuals receive a transplant are governed largely by these cell surface proteins. The lymphocytes of the recipient can sense the foreignness of the donor's cells and attempt to kill (reject) them. The donor's immune cells can sense the foreignness of the patient's cells and attack them.

The degree of disparity between donor and recipient is the major determinant of the intensity of host versus graft or graft versus host disease. These reactions do not happen if the recipient and donor are identical twins but do happen in nonidentical siblings, even if they are matched by tissue typing. The latter observation indicates that HLA testing does not examine all relevant tissue type factors. This expectation requires that two methods be used to permit a successful transplant: suppression of the immune system of the recipient before transplant and suppression of the donor's immune cells in the recipient after transplant.

A person's HLA type is governed by genes that reside on chromosome number 6 in tissue cells. Every human nucleated cell has 46 chromosomes: a pair of each chromosome numbered from 1 to 22 plus the two sex chromosomes (either XX in a female or XY in a male). The genes that determine tissue or HLA type are transmitted to a child. One of each pair is inherited from one's mother and the other of the pair from one's father. The genes on one chromosome 6, of the pair AB from mother and on one chromosome 6 of the pair CD from father, determine the HLA type. Each parent's contribution is referred to as a haplotype. Thus, the term haploidentical indicates that the person being typed shares half the tissue type of the potential recipient.

This pattern of inheritance explains why parents usually are not sufficiently tissue-type compatible to be donors.

On average, a person has one chance in four of having the same HLA antigens as his or her sibling. Since the average family in the United States has about two children, many patients will not have a sibling of the same tissue type.

The HLA system is broken down into two groups of cell surface antigens: Class I and Class II. Class I antigens are determined by genes referred to as A, B, and C. Class II antigens are determined by genes referred to as D. In populations, these genetic loci A through D have many variations called alleles which give each individual uniqueness. For example, one person may have A1, another A2, and another A3, and so on. In families, these variations are minimized and provide the opportunity to find a sibling that is matched, making transplantation possible, if immune system suppression is also used.

Until recently, HLA typing had been done by a procedure called serological typing. In this procedure, the white blood cells of the recipient and prospective donor are tested to see if their tissue types are identical. This procedure was very useful but less refined than the new method of molecular typing. In the latter technique, the DNA of the recipient and prospective donor are characterized to identify specific genes that direct the formation of the HLA antigens on the surface of cells. Defining the genotype of the individual gives more specific results than serological testing. This requirement is particularly important when searching for a match among unrelated donors.

Since the probability of finding a match among siblings is only one in four, efforts are being made to develop methods to permit transplantation between individuals who are only partially matched. For example, the ability to transplant from parent to child would make the availability of transplantation nearly universal for childhood disorders. Such experiments are being conducted. Children are more tolerant of such deviations from ideal matching, and hope exists that with better control of the immune reactions involved, moderately mismatched transplants may be feasible.

Sources of Stem Cells

Marrow

Obtaining marrow stem cells for transplantation requires that a compatible donor receives a thorough health examination, which includes an electrocardiogram, chest x-ray, blood chemistry evaluation, and confirmation that blood cell counts are normal. The donor is tested to insure that the hepatitis virus and human immunodeficiency virus (HIV) are not present in the blood. The presence of a positive test for cytomegalovirus (CMV) does not necessarily preclude one from being a donor. If all is in order, the donor is given anesthesia in an operating room suite. The transplant physicians use a special wide bore needle attached to a large syringe to suck out samples of marrow from the top edge of the pelvic bones. This area can be easily felt under the skin of the sides and back just below the waist. The insertion of the needle through the skin and into the rim of the pelvic bone is repeated until several pints of marrow are removed. The entire process takes place under sterile conditions.

The amount of marrow removed is related to the size of the recipient. For the transplanted stem cells to engraft, a large adult requires more marrow cells than does a small child. The marrow is filtered to remove fragments of bone or tissue, passed through a screen to break up cell aggregates, and placed in a plastic bag from which it can be infused into the recipient's vein. The infusion of a suspension of cells containing the stem cells into the recipient's vein is similar to a blood transfusion. This type of administration is used whether the source of stem cells is marrow or blood.

The harvested marrow is administered to the recipient usually within a few hours (in most cases, less than 24 hours). The donor usually remains in the hospital for about 12 hours before going home. During this time, the donor recovers from anesthesia and the pain at the needle insertion sites. If necessary, the harvested marrow cells can be frozen and stored for later use. The marrow can be frozen for years and remain suitable for stem cell transplantation. For example, freezing is commonplace in anticipation of autologous marrow infusion. In this circumstance, the patient is the source of the marrow during a period of disease remission following treatment and may be the recipient if a relapse occurs later and very intensive treatment is required.

Blood

The technique of human transplantation began with the supposition that the principal source of blood cell-forming stem cells is the marrow since this is the sole location for blood cell production after birth. It had been known that the stem cells leave the marrow, circulate in the blood, and re-enter the marrow. The rarity of these cells in the blood, however, made it seem an improbable source for transplantation.

Methods were developed to move stem cells from the marrow into the blood in sufficient numbers to be harvested and used for transplantation. This procedure requires that a donor be treated with a drug that mobilizes stem cells into the blood. In some cases of autologous transplantation, stem cells can be mobilized by a combination of chemotherapy used to treat the underlying disease and stem cell-releasing cytokines. Then the cells are removed from the donor by a process called hemapheresis. In this process, the donor is linked to a special type of refrigerated centrifuge. The blood of the donor is pumped through the instrument which separates the blood into four components: red cells, plasma, white cells, and platelets. The latter two fractions are harvested because they contain the stem cells. The red cells and plasma are returned to the donor. Hemapheresis permits blood to be recirculated through the machine for several hours. The procedure may be repeated at a later time, after which the collections are pooled. It generally takes two or more sessions to collect an adequate amount of stem cells from the bloodstream.

In this way, ample stem cells may be recovered to insure a successful transplant. The procedure avoids the general or spinal anesthesia required to harvest marrow stem cells from the donor and the day or two of discomfort from the pelvic bone needle insertions required to recover marrow stem cells.

Umbilical Cord and Placental Blood

Stem cells circulate in the blood of the fetus as well as in children and adults. In the fetal circulation, the concentration and growth potential of blood cell-forming stem cells is even greater than in the blood of adults. At the time of delivery, the umbilical cord is severed and discarded as the afterbirth along with the attached placenta. Instead of being discarded, the blood can be carefully drained into a sterile plastic container. The suspension of cells containing stem cells can then be frozen and used for transplantation at a later date. When used as a transplant product, it is referred to as cord blood cells.

Banks are being developed that contain the frozen donated samples from placental and cord blood. Since there are millions of healthy births each year, even a small proportion of these afterbirth specimens can provide a potential source of stem cells for recipients who do not have a sibling with a similar tissue type. The number of stem cells from the cord and placenta may be insufficient to transplant large recipients successfully. Children and small-and medium-sized adults usually can be treated from this source of stem cells.

There are several important considerations in using cord stem cells. The possibility that the newborn's blood carries an infectious agent or that the newborn carries gene mutations that will lead to a serious inherited blood cell disease are examples of issues that are particular to cord blood stem cells. These and other considerations are being studied as this source of stem cells becomes more prevalent.

T Lymphocyte Depletion

T lymphocytes in a donor's marrow or blood cause graft versus host disease. In order to minimize this harmful reaction, the marrow or blood cell collection to be used for transplant can be treated with agents that can decrease the number of T lymphocytes infused with the stem cells. This technique reduces the incidence and severity of graft versus host disease. The procedure is known as T lymphocyte depletion.

The T lymphocytes are beneficial as well. They help the donated stem cells take hold and grow in the recipient's marrow. In some cases, T lymphocytes attack the leukemia cells, enhancing the suppressing effects of treatment. Known as *graft versus leukemia*, this effect can be seen mostly in myelogenous leukemia. The attack on the residual tumor cells makes it less likely that the malignancy will return after transplant. Thus, transplant physicians must be careful about how many T cells are removed during this procedure.

Stem Cell Selection Procedure

When an allogeneic donor's marrow or blood is collected, the stem cells are mixed with many other cells that are present in those sites. Lymphocytes are among the other cell types present. There are specific features on the outer coat of stem cells that permit them to be removed selectively from a mixture of cells and then recovered. When this selection procedure is done, it results in a cell population that is enriched in stem cells and has many fewer other cells, including lymphocytes. By reducing the number of T lymphocytes, the frequency or severity of the graft versus host immune reaction can be decreased.

Types of Stem Cell Transplantation

Syngeneic Transplantation

Syngeneic transplantation is the term for a transplant in which the donor and recipient are identical twins and have an identical tissue type since their genetic make-up is the same. In such a transplant the donor cells would not be rejected and the recipient's tissues would not be attacked by the donor's immune cells (lymphocytes).

Allogeneic Transplantation

Allogeneic transplantation is the technical term for a transplant between two individuals of the same species. In practice, the term also implies that the donor was chosen because his or her tissue type very closely matched the recipient's. The donor who matches the prospective recipient most closely is the sibling of the patient since both received their genetic composition from the same parents. This fact does not insure compatibility but greatly increases its probability.

Transplant physicians can test to determine the degree of compatibility before a decision is made to use the donor. Compatibility is assessed by laboratory tests that identify the tissue type of donor and recipient. There are two types of allogeneic donors: related, usually sibling donors and unrelated, usually found from very large pools of volunteers and matched to a tissue type that is the same as the patient's. Transplantation from matched unrelated donors is sometimes referred to by the acronym MUD (matched unrelated donors).

Allogeneic transplantation, whether from a related or unrelated donor, differs from either syngeneic or autologous transplantation in that the potential exists for immune rejection of the donated stem cells by the recipient (host versus graft effect) and the immune reaction by the donor's cells against the tissues of the recipient (graft versus host disease). The immune rejection is usually prevented by intensive treatment of the recipient before the transplant (conditioning) to suppress the immune system. The immune reaction is combated by giving drugs to the recipient after the transplant to reduce the ability of the donated immune cells to attack and injure the patient's tissues.

Minitransplants

A minitransplant is a type of allogeneic transplant that is being studied in clinical trials for the treatment of several types of cancer, including leukemia, lymphoma, multiple myeloma, melanoma, and kidney cancer.

A minitransplant uses lower, less toxic doses of chemotherapy and/or total body irradiation (TBI—radiation therapy to the entire body) to prepare the patient for an allogeneic transplant. The use of low doses of anticancer drugs and TBI eliminates some, but not all, of the patient's bone marrow. It also reduces the number of cancer cells and suppresses the patient's immune system to prevent rejection of the transplant.

Unlike traditional BMT or peripheral blood stem cell transplant (PBSCT), bone marrow cells from both the donor and the patient may exist in the patient's body for some time after a minitransplant. Once the bone marrow cells from the donor begin to engraft, they may cause what is called a *graft versus tumor effect* and may work to destroy the cancer cells that were not eliminated by the anticancer drugs and/or TBI. To boost the graft versus tumor effect, the patient may be given an injection of their donor's white blood cells. This procedure is called a donor lymphocyte infusion.

Source: "Bone Marrow Transplantation and Peripheral Blood Stem Cell Transplantation: Questions and Answers," National Cancer Institute Fact Sheet 7.41, reviewed 8/22/2000.

Autologous Transplantation

Autologous stem cell transplantation is an important therapy. But, strictly speaking, it is not transplantation; rather it is a technique of obtaining stem cells from blood or marrow and returning them to the same individual. Therefore, immunologic transplantation barriers do not exist. Nonetheless, the procedure is usually conducted in a transplant facility, is supervised by transplant specialists, and is usually referred to as autologous blood or marrow stem cell transplantation. To be feasible, the procedure requires that an individual has sufficient numbers of healthy stem cells in marrow or blood despite the disease for which he or she is being treated. For example, in patients with acute leukemia, remission is usually achieved before the patient's marrow or blood is harvested and frozen for later use.

The patient's marrow may contain small but significant numbers of residual malignant cells that are not apparent when a marrow sample is microscopically examined. Purging may selectively rid the marrow of these unwanted cells. Autologous blood or marrow transplantation does not carry the risk of either graft rejection or graft versus host disease and thus does not require conditioning treatment or immunosuppressive treatment. However, the patient does receive very intensive cytotoxic therapy to kill residual leukemia, lymphoma, or myeloma cells. The autologous stem cells are used to restore blood cell production, thereby making the treatment tolerable.

The principal concerns in autologous transplantation are: 1) that the amount of stem cells harvested is adequate to engraft when returned to the patient and 2) that tumor cells in the cell suspension used for transplant are removed or made incapable of re-establishing the tumor. The use of autologous stem cells to restore blood cell production after intensive radiation and/or chemotherapy has been expanded to the treatment of pediatric and adult patients with a variety of cancers other than leukemia, lymphoma, or myeloma.

Purging Autologous Marrow

When autologous marrow or blood stem cells are the source of the transplant, the possibility that the patient's tumor cells (e.g., leukemia, lymphoma or myeloma cells) are reintroduced after intensive therapy is a concern. For example, if a patient with acute myelogenous leukemia in remission is to be heavily treated and transplanted with stem cells harvested from his or her own marrow (during that remission), the risk exists of reintroducing residual, inapparent leukemia cells. To avoid this, the marrow may be treated after it is harvested to rid it of tumor cells before it is frozen. Several techniques are being studied to determine the best method for purging tumor cells, including using antibodies specifically targeted to the malignant cells but not injurious to the stem cells. The effect of purging in the long-term success of autologous transplantation is still unresolved, however.

The Transplant Procedure

Conditioning

Patients with a hematologic malignancy receiving an allogeneic transplant are treated initially with a conditioning regimen. This treatment has two functions:

1. To inactivate the patient's immune system and minimize the chance that the stem cell graft will be rejected and

2. To intensively treat the residual malignant cells so as to make a recurrence of the malignancy less likely.

Conditioning regimens are modified depending on the disease being treated. Although programs vary at different transplant centers, generally two regimens are used for treatment. Either several drugs are given together, such as cyclophosphamide (Cytoxan), busulfan (Myleran), cytarabine (Cytosar), melphalan (Alkeran), or etoposide (VePesid, VP-16), or chemotherapy is given along with total body irradiation. Radiation is administered in several smaller daily doses.

This technique is referred to as fractionation of the dose. Fractionation minimizes side effects such as lung injury, nausea, and vomiting. Side effects of conditioning treatment may include:

- Nausea and vomiting
- Diarrhea
- Ulcers in mouth
- Bleeding into urine from bladder
- Hair loss
- Loss of blood cell formation
- Pneumonitis (pneumonia)
- Occlusions of veins in liver
- Congestive heart failure
- Premature menopause*
- Sterility*
- Growth retardation*
- Cataracts*

*These effects are more likely to occur if total body irradiation is required for conditioning.

The drugs and radiation are given during the week before transplant. The precise duration and sequence of administration depends on the specific conditioning regimen. The days prior to the transplant are labeled minus 6, minus 5, etc., with the transplant (stem cell infusion) on day zero. The period after the transplant starts with day 1, day 2, and so forth, thereafter.

Nonmyeloablative Transplantation

This procedure is a technique that uses low rather than very high doses of either radiation or chemotherapy to condition the recipient of an allogeneic stem cell transplant. It may be advantageous for older patients, those with slowly progressive diseases, and those with nonmalignant inherited (e.g., sickle cell disease) or acquired diseases (severe immune diseases). Potent immune therapy can suppress the recipient's T lymphocytes so as to avoid rejection of the donor stem cells in order to insure that over time the latter will take up residence and dominate in the recipient's marrow. The immune cells made from the donor's stem cells attack and suppress the residual leukemia or lymphoma cells in the recipient. Thus, this technique relies on an immune suppression of the patient's hematopoietic malignancy over a more protracted period of time for success.

Infusion of Stem Cells

The cell suspension, derived from marrow or blood and containing the stem cells of the donor, is collected in a plastic blood transfusion bag. Similar to a blood transfusion, the cell suspension is infused through the patient's vein. Special filters are used to remove bone fragments, fatty particles, and large clusters of cells from the cell suspension before it enters the bloodstream if marrow is infused. Infusion of the cell suspension usually requires several hours; patients are checked frequently for signs of fever, chills, hives, a fall in blood pressure, or shortness of breath. Patients often experience no side effects from the infusion. Occasionally side effects occur, but these can be treated and the infusion completed. In patients receiving frozen-thawed stem cell suspensions, reactions may occur from the cryopreservative.

The Immediate Post-Transplant Period

By the second or third day after the transplant, the effects of the intensive conditioning regimen and the decrease in marrow function begin to have their effects. The patient is kept in a protected environment to minimize contact with infectious agents.

Two to five weeks after the transplant, the engraftment of donated cells becomes apparent by the appearance of normal white cells in the blood of the patient. Red cells and platelets are transfused periodically until marrow function is restored by the transplanted stem cells. The patient is monitored carefully by physical examinations, blood chemistries, imaging studies, and other tests to be sure major organs such as the heart, lung, kidneys, and liver are functioning normally. Periods of intravenous feeding, called hyperalimentation, may be needed in some patients to insure adequate nutritional intake in spite of poor appetite and diarrhea.

Special Problems

Most patients undergoing allogeneic transplantation for leukemia, lymphoma, or myeloma require blood cell replacement, nutritional support, and special drugs to treat graft versus host disease. The drug dosages are carefully adjusted, depending on the severity of the graft versus host reaction and whether the donor is related or unrelated.

343

The conditioning treatment prior to transplant can impair any system that is dependent on replacement by stem cells. In particular, the gastrointestinal tract, the skin, and hair follicles are very sensitive to cytotoxic drugs and radiation therapy. Ulcers and dysfunction of the gastrointestinal tract are frequent. Mouth sores, nausea, diarrhea, intestinal cramps, and rectal or anal ulceration may be troublesome. Rashes may develop. Hair loss is inevitable.

The lungs are particularly sensitive to the conditioning regimen, especially total body irradiation superimposed on prior chemotherapy. A reaction called interstitial pneumonitis (pneumonia) can occur. This lung change is caused by a tissue reaction and does not mean that an infection is present. However, it can be very severe and prevent the efficient exchange of oxygen in the lungs.

Leaky blood vessels can result from the accumulated injury of chemotherapy and radiotherapy. Chemicals released from the immune reactions that occur after transplant also contribute to this effect by damaging vessel walls. Fluid escapes from the circulation and causes edema or water-logging of tissues. In the lung, fluid accumulation can cause congestion and poor exchange of oxygen and shortness of breath.

The blood vessels that lead into and pass through the liver are prone to blockage after transplantation. This serious side effect is called veno-occlusive disease (or VOD) because the veins are plugged. This effect results from toxic changes in the liver from chemotherapy and radiotherapy. The changes cause injury to the liver, which is reflected in jaundice (yellowing of the skin and eyes), and accumulation of fluid in the abdomen and elsewhere. Sometimes toxins normally removed by the liver can accumulate, leading to mental confusion and sleepiness.

Infections

Intensive treatment is usually required to suppress immune function and kill tumor cells prior to transplant. The resulting suppression of white cells that normally prevent or combat infections leads to a very high risk of infection. Infections by bacteria, fungi, viruses, or other parasites are very likely. These organisms are present most often on the skin and in the mouth or the lower bowel. They are also found in uncooked food (salads, fresh fruits, and vegetables) and in the air.

When blood cell and immune cell levels are normal and when the skin and lining of the mouth and bowel are intact, the body easily fends off such microbes. These normal defenses are lost in transplant patients. For this reason, antibiotics and other antimicrobial drugs are sometimes administered to patients in anticipation of the nearly inevitable development of infection. The drugs are usually continued until the white cells reappear in the blood in sufficient numbers to make infections unlikely. The term *opportunistic microbes* is applied to infectious agents that rarely cause infection unless severe immunodeficiency is present. A few such organisms are varieties of Candida, Aspergillus, Pneumocystis, or Toxoplasma.

Many precautions are taken to minimize the risk of infection. Measures to combat infection include the use of a single room with filtered air, limiting contact with visitors, use of masks, and meticulous hand washing by staff and visitors who enter the patient's room. Indwelling catheter sites must be kept clean. Uncooked fruits and vegetables, which carry surface bacteria or fungi, are prohibited. Unfortunately, several of these measures isolate the patient for the month or more that it takes for the donor stem cells to begin forming enough blood and immune cells to replenish the body's immune system.

Graft Versus Host Disease

Graft versus host disease may be seen soon after the transplanted cells begin to appear in the recipient. This reaction occurs in many patients. It varies from barely perceptible to life-threatening and is most severe in older patients. With each advancing decade of age, the reaction occurs more frequently and severely.

An individual's immune cells recognize cells that are not genetically identical. The graft versus host reaction results when the donor's immune cells, especially the T lymphocytes, sense that the host cells are different from themselves. In the case of stem cell transplantation, the donor cells carefully measure the cells of the recipient's tissue for signs that they are different and attack them if they find significant variations. The differences may involve cell surface proteins that are not measured by HLA typing, or there may be subtle differences in HLA type that permit transplantation but not without engendering the reaction. With the exception of identical twins, some incompatibility will exist even though HLA testing indicates sufficient similarity to permit a transplant to be successful. This difference is particularly evident if the donor and recipient are of the opposite sex. The severity of graft versus host disease depends on the type and degree of differences between patient and donor.

Acute graft versus host disease starts in the first 90 days after transplantation. The first signs are usually a rash and burning and redness of the skin that occur on the patient's palms or soles. The rash, along with the burning and redness, may spread to the patient's trunk and eventually develop over the entire body. Blistering can occur, and the exposed surface of the skin may flake off. Nausea, vomiting, abdominal cramps, and loss of appetite are signs of graft versus host disease in the gastrointestinal tract. Diarrhea is frequent. Jaundice and pain in the abdomen indicate that graft versus host disease has injured the liver, which also may be swollen. Acute graft versus host disease may be mild, moderate, or severe. It may be life-threatening if the manifestations are difficult to control.

Chronic graft versus host disease usually occurs after the third month post-transplant and may not develop for a year or more after the transplant. As is the case with the acute reaction, older patients are more likely to develop chronic graft versus host disease. It is more likely to occur in patients who previously have had acute graft versus host disease.

Most patients experience skin problems. A rash and itching may occur first. The skin may become scaly. If the reaction is severe, patches of skin may be lost. Patients' skin color may deepen and the texture becomes very hard. The skin may heal by scarring, and the motion of nearby joints, such as the fingers, may be restricted. Hair loss may accompany the skin injury.

The inside of the mouth and the esophagus (a tube that extends from the mouth to the stomach) may become excessively dry and damaged. Ulcers can result. The tendency to drying may lead to loss of tear formation and dryness of the vagina and other surfaces. The lungs also may suffer from the drying and scarring effects of the attack by the donor immune cells. Liver injury may result in failure of liver function and the flow of bile, which may not be overt but can be detected by blood chemical measurements. In severe cases, the bile may back up into the blood and cause jaundice. The chronic graft versus host reaction can be mild with later improvement, or more severe, persistent, and incapacitating.

Several drugs are used to prevent or minimize graft versus host disease. These drugs include methotrexate, glucocorticoid hormones (steroids), cyclosporine, and tacrolimus. Another technique used to reduce the severity and incidence of graft versus host disease is called T lymphocyte depletion. Since T lymphocytes are the primary effector cells in graft versus host disease, the donor's marrow can be depleted of T cells in an effort to minimize the immune attack.

Leaving the Hospital

Some transplant centers perform autologous transplantation on an outpatient basis. Some patients may have a portion of either an autologous or allogeneic transplant performed on an outpatient basis.

By three to five weeks post-transplant, most patients have recovered sufficiently to leave the hospital. A patient is discharged when the bone marrow is producing a sufficient number of healthy red blood cells, white blood cells, and platelets, and there are no treatment complications. There is variability from patient to patient in their recovery of blood cell counts and the severity of other associated complications, especially graft versus host disease.

When blood cells return, a sense of well being begins to return. Mouth sores and diarrhea lessen or disappear. Appetite may improve. Before leaving the hospital, it is important that patients are able to eat and drink to get sufficient fluid and nourishment. The absence of fever, vomiting, and diarrhea are also important considerations. Before discharge, both the physician and patient should feel comfortable that there are no remaining needs that require very close surveillance or hospital-based resources.

Aftercare

In general, recovery from autologous transplantation is more rapid. Some of the difficulties and restrictions described are applicable principally to allogeneic transplantation.

After being discharged from the hospital, the patient continues recovery at home. Patients and families are instructed in the continuing care needed at home. They learn what signs, such as fever, pain, diarrhea, and others, should prompt rapid contact with the physicians responsible for care. Home visits by nurses or physicians and patient visits to the ambulatory care center permit appropriate follow-up and adjustment of activities and medications, in most cases. These visits may be frequent at first. After several months, if all is going as anticipated, the indwelling venous catheters can be removed and the frequency of patient visits can be decreased.

It takes six to 12 months (or somewhat longer) to recover nearly normal blood cell levels and immune cell function. During this time the patient should avoid contact with crowds, such as at shopping centers, religious services, parties, and concerts, to reduce the risk of infection. Patients also may be advised to avoid contact with children who have had recent immunization with live viruses. The immunity that the patient had from previous vaccinations may be decreased and reimmunization with vaccines made from inactivated organisms may be useful.

If the patient was treated with total body radiation during conditioning, the lenses of the eyes would have become irradiated and there is the possibility that cataracts may develop prematurely. Irradiation of the gonads leads to sterility in men and premature menopause in women. In the former case, hormone replacement is usually not necessary. In women so treated, estrogen and progesterone replacement therapy is invariably needed indefinitely. Children may have a slowed growth rate and may require growth hormone treatment and replacement of other hormones. In very young patients, puberty may be delayed and hormonal therapy required. Radiation may decrease thyroid function and require that thyroid hormone be administered orally. The severity of chronic graft versus host disease has a major impact on the long-term course. If this immune reaction is present, the patient is susceptible to troublesome infections.

Social and Emotional Aspects

Transplantation for leukemia, lymphoma, or myeloma is a daunting personal challenge. How the challenge will be met depends on different individuals' ability to endure the risks and hardships involved. The patient is faced with the risk of disease recurrence or progression and death if transplantation is not chosen or a possibility of an earlier death, severe side effects, or recurrence of the disease if transplantation is chosen. These challenges are counterbalanced by the hope of recovery and cure and the likelihood that new and better methods may make success more probable and the side effects less disabling.

The decision to undertake transplantation often is made under intense pressure, usually because of a medical crisis. Also, there are the mixed emotions created by whether or not a donor will be found and what is in store should one be found. If the transplant center is not nearby, the patient and family are placed under additional strains and are detached from support systems in their home community. The loss of autonomy, the isolation, the separation from work, school, friends, colleagues, and outside interests have to be endured.

There is disruption of family relationships as well. Children may worry about the outcome of a parent's illness and the separation from father or mother. Parents suffer the uncertainty of the outcome of a child's treatment and the strain put on siblings and other family members and friends. The cost of the procedure and relocation of family, if necessary, is usually in the range of several hundred thousand dollars. Although much of this cost may be recovered from insurance, some will not.

The challenges of a long hospital stay, much of this in isolation, loss of well-being, and many potential, very uncomfortable, painful or disfiguring side effects add up to a very trying experience. Patients require grit and the hope that better days are ahead. Even with great personal strength, the support of loved ones, nurses, physicians, and others is vitally important. Family can be the key to sustaining and supporting the patient through the ordeal. Several other techniques can be brought to bear on supporting the patient as he or she recovers strength and well-being and begins a return toward normal activities. For many patients, perhaps most, the experience is psychologically challenging and will result in changes in self-image and interpersonal relationships. For many, however, a successful outcome and a return to vitality and their school, job, or other roles and relationships is very satisfying to patient, family, and healthcare providers.

The Leukemia & Lymphoma Society would like to acknowledge Marshall A. Lichtman, MD, Executive Vice President, Research and Medical Programs, who contributed the material presented in this section.

Additional Information

The Leukemia & Lymphoma Society
1311 Mamaroneck Ave.
White Plains, NY 10605
Toll-Free: 800-955-4572
Tel: 914-949-5213
Fax: 914-949-6691
Website: www.leukemia-lymphoma.org

There are programs to help ease the emotional and economic strain created by leukemia, lymphoma or myeloma. The Leukemia & Lymphoma Society offers patients financial assistance and also provides the opportunity to join a support group or talk with a successfully treated patient with the same diagnosis.

Section 28.2.

Umbilical Cord Blood Stem Cell Transplantation

This section includes "Cord Blood Stem Cell Transplantation," updated September 15, 2000 © The Leukemia & Lymphoma Society, additional information available at www.leukemia-lymphoma.org, reprinted with permission; and "New Approaches in Umbilical Cord Blood Transplantation for Adult Patients," updated March 27, 2002 © University of Minnesota Cancer Center, reprinted with permission.

Cord Blood Stem Cell Transplantation

What Is Stem Cell Transplantation?

Stem cell transplantation is an accepted form of treatment for patients who require very high-dose chemotherapy or radiation therapy to treat their disease, usually a cancer. This treatment results in severe injury to blood cells formed in the marrow. In order to restore the patient's ability to make blood and immune cells, stem cells from a compatible donor can be administered. Stem cell transplantation is used to treat selected patients with leukemia or lymphoma, as well as some other severe inherited or acquired disorders of the marrow or the immune system.

Bone marrow is used for such transplants because it contains undifferentiated cells, called stem cells. Stem cells are very immature cells that can develop into any of the three types of blood cells (red cells, white cells, or platelets). Blood also contains stem cells, but in such small numbers that the cells cannot be counted or identified in ordinary blood tests. Nevertheless, with new procedures, stem cells can be induced to leave the marrow and enter the blood from which they are collected (harvested) for administration to patients who require stem cell transplantation. Stem cells are also present in umbilical cord and placental blood which can be collected after a baby is born.

Stem cell transplantation (marrow, blood, or cord blood) may be autologous (using the patient's own stem cells, which are collected

350

prior to high-dose chemotherapy) or allogeneic (using stem cells from a related or unrelated, matched donor).

What Is Cord Blood Stem Cell Transplantation?

Blood contained in the placenta and umbilical cord of newborn babies is emerging as a new source of stem cells. Cord blood contains significant numbers of stem cells and has advantages over bone marrow or adult blood stem cell transplantation for certain patients. Umbilical cord blood stem cell transplantation has transformed a waste product of the birth process into a life-saving resource.

What Disease May Be Treated with Cord Blood Stem Cell Transplantation?

The first cord blood stem cell transplant was performed in 1988 in Paris, France. The patient was a boy with Fanconi's syndrome (a rare and serious type of anemia) who is alive and healthy today. Since that first transplant, cord blood stem cell transplants have been successfully performed on patients (mostly children) with severe aplastic anemia, Gunther's disease, Hunter syndrome, Hurler syndrome, acute lymphocytic leukemia (ALL), acute myelogenous leukemia (AML), myelodysplasia, chronic myelogenous leukemia (CML), juvenile chronic myelogenous leukemia (JCML), neuroblastoma, non-Hodgkin's lymphoma, thalassemia, Wiskott-Aldrich syndrome, and X-linked lympho-proliferative syndrome. By September 2000, more than 800 cord blood stem cell transplants have been performed worldwide. Approximately 75% of these have been done with unrelated donors.

How Is Cord Blood Collected, Stored, and Used for Transplantation?

The most commonly used procedure for collecting cord blood is relatively simple. Immediately after a baby is delivered, the umbilical cord is clamped. The baby is then removed from the area and the placenta is placed in a sterile supporting structure with the umbilical cord hanging through the support. The cord is then cleansed with povidone-iodine (Betadine) and alcohol, and a needle is inserted into the umbilical vein. Blood is drawn through the needle into a standard blood collection bag containing nutrients and a solution to keep the blood from clotting (anticoagulant solution). Blood is then collected by gravity drainage, yielding an average 75 milliliters (mL) of blood.

A second method involves collecting the cord blood after delivery of the child, while the placenta is still in the mother. Theoretically, this method may be advantageous by beginning the collection earlier (before the blood has a chance to clot), and by using the contractions of the uterus to enhance blood collection. However, the technique is more intrusive, with the potential to interfere with the mother's care after delivery.

After collection, the bag of cord blood is immediately transported to a facility for testing and preservation. Testing procedures include tissue typing (a process called HLA-typing) to facilitate matching to potential recipients, as well as testing for infectious agents such as the AIDS virus, cytomegalovirus, and hepatitis viruses. The blood is then frozen and held in liquid nitrogen at very low temperature for future use. One can remove the red cells from the cord blood after collection to reduce the volume of material stored to minimize problems with incompatible red cell administration at the time of administration to the recipient.

At the time of transplant, the cord blood unit is thawed and infused through a vein into the patient.

What Facilities Are Used for the Collection of Cord Blood?

Facilities that collect and store this product are called cord blood banks. It is necessary to distinguish between cord blood banks designed to provide blood from unrelated donors (allogeneic use) from for-profit facilities that offer storage of cord blood in the event it is needed by the donor infant or family member at a later time (autologous use).

Public (not-for-profit) cord blood banks do not charge parents for donating cord blood. Private banks, however, offer cord blood preservation and storage (on a for-profit basis) for the potential use of the donor at a later time, if a condition develops that would benefit from transplantation.

Does One Type Have Advantages Over Another?

Theoretically, allogeneic stem cell transplants may be more successful for patients with certain cancers because of a lower risk of disease relapse than is the case with autologous transplants. However, this is unproven and varies with different disease states.

What Are the Benefits of Cord Blood Stem Cell Transplantation?

Potential advantages of cord blood stem cell transplantation over bone marrow transplants include:

- large potential donor pool;
- rapid availability, since the cord blood has been prescreened and tested;
- greater racial diversity can be attained in the banks by focusing collection efforts on hospitals where children of underrepresented ethnic backgrounds are born;
- no risk or discomfort for the donor;
- rare contamination by viruses; and
- lower risk of graft-versus-host disease (where the donor's cells attack the patient's organs and tissues), even for recipients with a less-than-perfect tissue match.

What Are the Potential Disadvantages of Cord Blood Stem Cell Transplantation?

Cord blood stem cell transplantation is a new, experimental procedure, compared with other sources of stem cells. It is possible that genetic or congenital diseases (those that are present at the time of birth) carried by stem cells, although not immediately apparent, may be transmitted to patients receiving allogeneic cord blood stem cell transplantation. Follow-up procedures to track this possibility would require creating a long-term link between the medical facility caring for the recipient and the donor center and the donor. This procedure has raised concerns about privacy. One solution, which is used by some centers, is to obtain from potential donors complete and detailed questionnaires, prior to cord blood collection. These questionnaires have particular emphasis on individual and family histories of disease, as well as a detailed sexual history. If responses to the questionnaire generate medical concern, the unit is not collected. This technique is similar to that used to screen blood donors.

Another area of uncertainty relates to the requirements for predicting long-term success using stem cells from cord blood. For example, the minimum number of cells required is based on the recipient's weight, age, and disease status. Cord blood might contain too few stem cells for the recipient's size.

Cord blood stem cells take hold more slowly than stem cells from marrow or adult blood. Until engraftment occurs, patients are at risk of developing life-threatening infections. So far, however, the incidence of fatal infections in patients receiving cord blood stem cell transplant does not appear to be higher than that seen in other types of stem cell transplantation.

A fourth concern is the potential for contamination of the cord blood with blood from the mother. The mother's blood cells are mature (not stem cells) and they are not of the same HLA type as the cord blood cells. These maternal cells (lymphocytes) could cause severe and even fatal graft-versus-host disease in the transplant recipient.

Finally, the length of time in which cord blood can be stored without losing its effectiveness is not known. Cord blood samples have been preserved and then successfully transplanted for as long as 5 years, thus far. Autologous bone marrow stored longer than 2 years has been successfully transplanted in 94% to 97% of patients. In one of these cases, the marrow had been stored for 11 years. It is not known whether these findings will be true of cord blood as well, but this information is critical to the success of cord blood storage efforts. The supply of cord blood is potentially so great that banks could replenish older samples, circumventing this issue.

What Recommendations Can Parents and Patients Follow?

- Healthy parents with healthy children, or couples expecting their first child, can donate their child's cord blood to banks and research programs, if their hospital is actively engaged in public cord blood banking or university-based research programs.

- Parents who have a child or family member with cancer, immune deficiencies, or genetic disease that may benefit from transplantation should discuss with their physicians the potential for cord blood collection and transplantation that is directed for use in a specific recipient.

- Selected cord blood banks monitor donor infants up to 2 years after donation. If the cord blood unit has not yet been shipped or used, parents can withdraw their permission to transplant the unit to an unrelated recipient.

- Well before delivery, parents considering private collection should contact their health insurance carrier to find out whether cord blood collection and storage are covered benefits.

- Parents who do not have another child or family member in need of a stem cell transplant must consider the cost associated with private cord blood banking, given the low likelihood that the blood will be used. Companies currently charge approximately $1000 to $3000 for collection and storage, with or without an additional yearly storage fee.

- To minimize the risk to mothers and newborn infants, normal procedures related to delivery should not be altered in order to collect cord blood.

- Because cord blood collection and transplantation are investigational, they should only be done at centers with experience in the transplantation of unrelated sources of stem cells.

- Parents and patients should discuss any questions and concerns with health care professionals who understand cord blood banking and stem cell transplantation.

References

1. Kline RM, Bertolone SJ. Umbilical cord blood transplantation: providing a donor for everyone needing a bone marrow transplant? *South Med J* 1998; 91(9):821-828.

2. Rubinstein P and others. Outcomes among 562 recipients of placental blood transplants from unrelated donors. *New England Journal of Medicine* 339: 1565, 1998.

3. Smith FO, Kurtzberg J, Karson al. Umbilical cord blood collection, storage, and transplantation: issues and recommendations for parents and patients (unpublished paper).

New Approaches in Umbilical Cord Blood Transplantation for Adult Patients

The University of Minnesota, under the leadership of Dr. Juliet Barker, Assistant Professor in the Department of Medicine and Cancer Center member, is currently investigating a number of new transplant approaches using umbilical cord blood in adults. Umbilical cord blood offers several advantages over bone marrow for use in adults, most notably:

- Faster availability of unrelated donor umbilical cord blood as compared with bone marrow. This is important for patients who require urgent transplant.

- The tissue type match between the patient and the umbilical cord blood donor does not have to be perfect (i.e. 1-2 HLA mismatch may be tolerated). Therefore, umbilical cord blood offers the potential to extend the opportunity of transplantation to those patients who cannot find a matched unrelated bone marrow donor.

- Reduced incidence and severity of graft-versus-host disease. This has clearly been demonstrated in children and may also be true for adult patients.

However, there are some unique problems to be overcome in the transplantation of adults using umbilical cord blood. We know that the number of stem cells in cord blood (i.e. the cell dose) has a very important impact on survival after transplant. For larger teenagers and adults, a single cord blood unit may not contain enough stem cells to perform the transplant safely. Therefore, we are currently investigating transplantation of two closely matched cord blood units or double umbilical cord blood transplant as a way to increase the number of cord blood stem cells transplanted. The first clinical trial to investigate the feasibility, safety and efficacy of mixing two closely matured umbilical cord blood (UCB) units is underway. Early results are encouraging in that:

- There has been no harmful side effects, and

- We have demonstrated engraftment of both UCB units in some patients.

In addition to speeding recovery of white cells, it is possible that double UCB transplantation in adults may decrease the risk of relapse such that there are two healthy immune systems capable of rejecting the leukemia or tumor cells. Furthermore, immune recovery could be benefited. It is important to note that the latter two attributes have been thus far only hypothetical and remain to be proven.

Second, we know that older adult patients, those that have relapsed after a prior transplant, those that have already had extensive therapy for their cancer, or those who have other illnesses or complications, will not be strong enough to undergo high dose chemotherapy and radiation. Therefore, we are investigating a less intense or non-myeloablative transplant protocol that still enables the growth of the umbilical cord blood cells in the body. These transplants are designed to be less toxic and are effective by means of an immunological effect of the umbilical cord blood cells attacking cancer cells known as the graft-versus-malignancy effect.

The first clinical trial to investigate the feasibility, safety, and efficacy of umbilical cord blood after non-myeloablative preparative regimen is underway. Early results are encouraging in that:

- Engraftment of UCB has been seen in most patients
- Toxicity of this regimen is less than conventional transplants

Future directions at the University of Minnesota include:

- Improvement in homing and ex vivo expansion
- Expansion of T cells from UCB to augment anti-leukemia effect

Additional Information

Blood and Bone Marrow Transplant Newsletter
2900 Skokie Valley Road
Suite B
Highland Park, IL 60035
Toll Free: 888-597-7674
Tel: 847-433-3313
Website: www.bmtnews.org
E-mail: help@bmtinfonet.org

The Leukemia & Lymphoma Society of America
1311 Mamaroneck Avenue
White Plains, NY 10605
Toll-Free Information Resource Center: 800-955-4572
Tel: 914-949-5213
Fax: 914-949-6691
Website: www.leukemia-lymphoma.org

For cord blood collection sites, contact:

American Red Cross
431 18ᵗʰ Street, NW
Washington, DC 20006
Tel: 202-639-3520
Website: www.redcross.org

National Marrow Donor Program (NMDP)
3001 Broadway Street Northeast
Suite 500
Minneapolis, MN 55413-1753
Toll Free: 800-627-7692
Tel: 612-627-5800
Website: www.marrow.org

Section 28.3

Transplant Outcome by Disease

This section includes "Disease and Transplant Outcome Data," from the National Marrow Donor Program at http://www.marrow.org © 2003 by the National Marrow Donor Program. Reprinted with permission. "Factors Leading to Improved Transplant Outcomes," from the National Marrow Donor Program at http://www.marrow.org © 2003 by the National Marrow Donor Program. Reprinted with permission. Also, "Cancer Patients Overestimate Transplant Success Rate," by Janet Haley Dubow, February 28, 2001 © Dana Farber Cancer Institute, reprinted with permission.

Disease and Transplant Outcome Data

National Marrow Donor Program (NMDP)-Facilitated Transplant Outcomes

When the NMDP was founded in 1987, unrelated donor bone marrow transplantation was an investigational therapy with uncertain benefits. Since then, morbidity and mortality have decreased and the indications for stem cell transplantation have increased. Unrelated donor stem cell transplantation is now an appropriate first course of treatment for some patients. For some diseases and disease stages, outcome of transplantation using an unrelated donor is nearly equivalent to transplantation using a comparably matched related donor.

Since its inception, the NMDP has collected data on unrelated donor transplants facilitated through its Network. The tables that follow illustrate outcomes by disease.

Table 28.1. NMDP Transplant Outcomes for Acute Leukemias

Disease	# of Transplants	Kaplan-Meier 5-Year Survival*
AML 1st complete remission (CR)	302	32% ± 7%
AML 2nd CR	398	29% ± 5%
AML 3rd or greater CR or relapse	920	11% ± 2%
ALL 1st CR	223	34% ± 8%
ALL 2nd CR	244	27% ± 7%
ALL 3rd or greater CR	83	18% ± 9%
ALL relapse or primary induction failure	340	7% ± 3%

June 2001, *with 95% Confidence Interval

Table 28.2. NMDP Transplant Outcomes for Non-Leukemias

Disease	# of Transplants	Kaplan-Meier 5 Year Survival*
Severe Aplastic Anemia	381	40% ± 5%
Myelodysplastic & Related Syndromes	895	28% ± 3%
Non-Hodgkin's Lymphoma	490	20% ± 5%
Other Non-Malignant Diseases	657	44% ± 4%

June 2001, *with 95% Confidence Interval

Table 28.3. NMDP Transplant Outcomes for Chronic Myelogenous Leukemia

Disease	# of Transplants	Kaplan-Meier 5-Year Survival*
CML 1st chronic phase (CP)	1,896	43% ± 3%
CML 2nd CP & accelerated phase	753	22% ± 3%
CML blast phase	165	10% ± 5%

June 2001, *with 95% Confidence Interval

Factors Leading to Improved Transplant Outcomes

The decision to undertake an unrelated donor stem cell transplant is complex and involves many factors. The NMDP collects and analyzes comprehensive baseline and follow-up data on all NMDP blood stem cell recipients. Analyses of these data identify factors that can improve a patient's likelihood of a successful transplant.

HLA Match Quality

It is important that the human leukocyte antigens (HLA) of a donor or cord blood unit match the patient as closely as possible. The more closely they match, the less likely the patient will have complications such as graft failure or graft-versus-host disease (GVHD), which can occur after the new stem cells engraft. The NMDP requires HLA-A and B typing at the intermediate resolution level and HLA-DRB1 typing at the high resolution level. The donor and the recipient must be matched for 5 of 6 or 6 of 6 antigens. Some transplant centers will consider additional HLA antigens in donor selection. Advancing technology and clinical research have resulted in continued refinement of HLA match criteria; there is not yet an established standard within the transplant community.

Patient Factors

NMDP analyses of stem cell transplant recipient data show that, in general, the following patient-specific factors lead to more favorable transplant outcomes:

- Transplant performed during a stable disease period
- Transplant performed on younger patients
- Transplant performed during an earlier disease phase
- Cytomegalovirus (CMV) sero-negative recipient

NMDP analyses also show that impaired organ function increases the risk of toxicity of the transplant conditioning regimen, so patients with impaired organ function should be evaluated carefully to ensure their suitability for transplant.

Donor Factors

Donor-specific factors are also considered when selecting a donor. NMDP Transplant Centers often prefer:

- Younger donors (better transplant outcomes)

- Larger donors (can provide larger volume of marrow or stem cells)

- CMV sero-negative donors (to prevent CMV transmission when the patient is CMV sero-negative)

- Male donors or female donors who have never been pregnant (to avoid transplanting cells that may have been alloimmunized to HLA antigens by prior pregnancies)

NMDP outcome studies, however, have shown that the only donor factor influencing patient survival is donor age.

NMDP-Facilitated Transplant Outcomes

When the NMDP was founded in 1987, unrelated donor bone marrow transplantation was an investigational therapy with uncertain benefits. Since then, morbidity and mortality have decreased and the indications for stem cell transplantation have increased. Unrelated donor stem cell transplantation is now an appropriate first course of treatment for some patients. For some diseases and disease stages, outcome of transplantation using an unrelated donor is nearly equivalent to transplantation using a comparably matched related donor.

Since its inception, the NMDP has collected data on unrelated donor transplants facilitated through its Network.

Cancer Patients Overestimate Transplant Success Rate

Patients with leukemia, lymphoma and other cancers who choose to undergo bone marrow transplantation often overestimate the success rate of the procedure, according to a study published in the February 21, 2001 issue of the *Journal of the American Medical* Association (JAMA).

Researchers at Dana-Farber Cancer Institute led by Stephanie J. Lee, MD, MPH, measured the survival expectations of 313 patients and their physicians prior to bone marrow or stem cell transplantation and then compared those expectations with actual outcomes. Some 72% of their patients were considered lower risk because they either had early stage disease or were given their own bone marrow or blood back as part of the transplant. These patients correctly estimated that they had a low risk of death from the procedure.

However, patients with advanced leukemia, lymphoma, or other cancers undergoing more risky types of transplant procedures experienced treatment-related death rates more than twice what they estimated. Their physicians provided more accurate estimates, but they too tended to underestimate mortality.

"Stem cell transplantation offers the potential of life extension or cure for otherwise fatal diseases, but there is always a risk of cancer relapse or treatment-related death after the transplant." says Lee. "We do not know the reasons for discrepancies between patient expectations, physician expectations, and reality, but it is easy to imagine that as prognosis worsens, both patients and physicians may avoid dwelling on discouraging statistics and focus instead on the possibility of cure."

Researchers also measured patient and physician expectations for cure. Each of the four patient risk groups studied anticipated very high cure rates regardless of the type of transplant or stage of disease. In reality, those with the highest risk of death and relapse (8% of patients in the study) had only a 10% chance of being alive and free of their disease 2 years following transplantation.

"These are emotionally difficult situations for both patients and physicians," said Lee. "If all patients asked for explicit prognostic information, discussions would be more straightforward. When patients don't ask these questions or don't seem to want to know the answers, I think physicians struggle with the balance between informing patients about treatment risks and maintaining hope. "We do not know if patients undergoing bone marrow transplantation, particularly those who have no other options for cure, would be helped or harmed if forced to acknowledge grim statistics."

Researchers note they do not know how prognostic information was communicated or what process led to the formation of patient expectations because they did not observe doctor-patient interactions. However, they believe that these research findings have important implications for physicians and patients.

"Discrepancies between doctor and patient expectations are certainly not new," says Jane Weeks, MD, senior author of the study and director of the Center for Outcomes and Policy Research at Dana-Farber. "However, this study emphasizes the need for physicians to ask patients what they expect from treatment options, especially when high risks are involved. "Even if this discussion doesn't change their desire to undergo transplantation, it may help patients and their families better prepare themselves for the challenges ahead."

Dana-Farber Cancer Institute is a principal teaching affiliate of the Harvard Medical School and is among the leading cancer research and care centers in the United States. It is a founding member of the Dana-Farber/Harvard Cancer Center (DF/HCC), a designated comprehensive cancer center by the National Cancer Institute.

Section 28.4

Donation of Marrow, Peripheral Blood Stem Cells, and Umbilical Cord Blood

"Steps of Marrow and PBSC Donation," from the National Marrow Donor Program at http://www.marrow.org. © 2003 by the National Marrow Donor Program. Reprinted with permission. Also, "Umbilical Cord Blood Donation, Basic," from the National Marrow Donor Program at http://www.marrow.org © 2003 by the National Marrow Donor Program. Reprinted with permission.

Steps of Marrow and Peripheral Blood Stem Cell (PBSC) Donation

Each year, thousands of people develop diseases treatable with marrow or blood stem cell transplants. The National Marrow Donor Program (NMDP) has been a leader in unrelated bone marrow transplantation for more than 10 years. Now, the role of peripheral blood stem cell (PBSC) donation as an alternative to bone marrow donation for unrelated transplants is being evaluated under a research protocol accepted by the U.S. Food and Drug Administration. The following is what you can expect if you volunteer to donate stem cells through the NMDP.

1. The first step is to join the NMDP Registry. NMDP representatives inform you about marrow and peripheral blood stem cell (PBSC) donation processes. You complete a brief health questionnaire, sign a form consenting to have your tissue type listed on the Registry, and provide a small blood sample to determine your tissue type. Once listed on the Registry, your tissue type will be compared to the tissue types of thousands of patients around the world who need transplants.

2. If you are identified as a potential match for a patient, NMDP Donor Center representatives will ask for another blood sample to see whether you match well enough to be an actual donor for the patient. If you are indeed a match, you will receive further education about marrow and PBSC donation processes and which is the preferred process for this patient.

3. To prepare for either donation procedure, you will attend an information session about the donation process and potential side effects of the procedure. You will have a physical exam to determine your health status and to discover if there are any special risks to you with either donation procedure. The health requirements are the same for marrow and PBSC donation.

4. You decide whether or not you will donate. After being fully informed about the donor experience, you, with the support of your friends and loved ones, make the decision whether or not to become a donor.

Marrow

5. The marrow collection process is a surgical procedure lasting approximately one to two hours. The procedure occurs in a hospital operating room while you receive regional or general anesthesia. Part of your marrow is removed from the back of your pelvic bone using sterile needles and syringes.

6. You should recover quickly from the procedure. Most donors have some bone pain and aches for several days or a few weeks. Your marrow naturally replenishes itself within four to six weeks.

Peripheral Blood Stem Cell (PBSC)

5. For a PBSC donation, you will receive injections of Filgrastim for four or five consecutive days. Filgrastim is a drug that increases the number of stem cells released from your marrow into your blood stream so they can be collected through an apheresis procedure.

6. During apheresis, which is done at a blood center or hospital, your blood is removed through a sterile needle placed in a

vein in one arm and passed through an apheresis machine that separates out the stem cells. The remaining blood, minus the stem cells, is returned to you through a sterile needle in your other arm. The number of stem cells required by the recipient will determine if the procedure needs to be repeated the following day.

7. Apheresis donors commonly experience bone and muscle pain, headache, and fatigue prior to the donation procedure as a result of receiving Filgrastim. These effects diminish over one to two days after the last dose of Filgrastim is given.

After you donate stem cells, your NMDP Donor Center coordinator will call you to follow up on your experience. Your coordinator will continue to call you regularly until you are able to resume normal activity, and annually for long-term follow up.

Umbilical Cord Blood Donation, Basic

The blood in the umbilical cord and placenta is unique because it contains large numbers of blood stem cells. The blood stem cells from cord blood are being studied under research protocols as a new method for treating patients with life-threatening diseases. Blood stem cells to treat these patients can come from donated bone marrow or peripheral (circulating) blood or cord blood. Although some patients have a family member who can donate blood stem cells, nearly 75% of patients will not find a matching donor in their family. Cord blood donations can give more patients hope of finding a match.

Cord Blood Donation Process

When a mother decides to donate her child's umbilical cord blood:

1. She looks for a cord blood bank in her community. (Because cord blood banking is relatively new, many communities do not have a cord blood bank.)

2. The cord blood bank asks the mother to complete a consent form and health history questionnaire and give a small blood sample. The cord blood is collected after the baby's birth.

3. Doctors search the NMDP Registry of donors and cord blood units to find a match for their patients who need a transplant.

If selected, the cord blood unit is transplanted to a matching patient.

Umbilical Cord Blood Collection

Collecting cord blood poses no health risk to the mother or infant donor. The cord blood is collected after delivery and would normally be discarded. The cord blood is stored only with the mother's signed consent, and no collection is made if there are any complications during delivery.

After the baby's birth, the umbilical cord is clamped, breaking the link between the baby and the placenta. Trained staff drain the blood from the umbilical cord and placenta. Methods vary somewhat at different hospitals. The blood is usually collected using a needle to draw the blood into a blood bag. The collection usually takes ten minutes or less.

Amount Collected

On average, about three to five fluid ounces are collected from the umbilical cord. If the amount is too small, there will not be enough stem cells to be used for transplantation and the cord blood unit (CBU) will not be stored. CBUs that do not meet the criteria for transplant may be used by researchers in the search for new and more effective medical uses for cord blood stem cells.

CBU Storage

The collected cord blood is taken to a laboratory where it is tested and processed.

1. It is tested for signs of infection or other possible problems.

2. It is tested for the HLA type, which is listed on the NMDP Registry and used to match the CBU with patients who need a transplant.

3. Often, the red blood cells and plasma, which are not needed for transplants, are removed so the CBU takes less storage space.

If the CBU meets eligibility standards, it is then stored in a plastic or vinyl bag in a liquid nitrogen freezer. It can be stored for a long time. Studies have shown good cell recovery after up to ten years of storage (*Clin Exp Immunol* 1997; 107, Suppl 1). Studies are ongoing to determine the storage life of CBUs.

Process of Consent

The cord blood bank always gets the mother's written permission before banking the cord blood. The mother is also asked to provide a blood sample for infectious disease testing and to fill out health history forms. All information that would identify the mother or infant donor is kept confidential at the cord blood bank. The mother will be informed if tests performed on a sample of her blood or the umbilical cord blood show information that may be important for her or her baby to know for health purposes.

Section 28.5.

Search Process for Human Leukocyte Antigen (HLA) Match

"Physician FAQs," from the National Marrow Donor Program at http://www.marrow.org © 2003 by the National Marrow Donor Program. Reprinted with permission.

What is a preliminary search?

The preliminary search report tabulates and summarizes the volunteer donors who are potentially HLA identical with the patient, as well as those who are, at most, one antigen mismatched. The purpose of the preliminary search is to provide a first look, a "snapshot" of potential volunteer donors in the NMDP's Registry who meet the HLA matching criteria on the day the search is conducted.

Who can submit a preliminary search request?

Any licensed physician can submit a preliminary search of the NMDP Registry. The search is submitted to the NMDP Office of Patient

Advocacy, which can be contacted through the NMDP Coordinating Center at 888-999-6743. Required information includes the patient's HLA typing for HLA-A, B and DR. In addition, the NMDP requires the patient's name, address, telephone number, and date of diagnosis.

How does a formal search differ from a preliminary search?

The purpose of the formal search is to identify the best stem cell donor for the patient. This search involves additional HLA typing of the potential donor and the proposed recipient. If a marrow or peripheral blood stem cell donor is selected, his or her health is assessed through a physical examination and other health testing. Only an NMDP Transplant Center manages formal searches.

How long are preliminary search results kept on file?

Preliminary search results are kept on the NMDP computer system for 45 days. If you wish to continue the process, an NMDP-approved Transplant Center must request a formal search. If more than 45 days has passed, a new preliminary search must first be requested by the transplant physician to see which potential stem cell donors are currently available.

Should I always HLA type the patient's family before submitting an unrelated donor search?

Ideally, family typing should include the patient, all full-blooded siblings, and the patient's parents. The results should be reviewed by a knowledgeable HLA expert to ensure consistency in the results. Unless HLA typing results are carefully reviewed, potential donors within the patient's family may be overlooked.

What about HLA typing the patient's extended family?

HLA typing the extended family (aunts, uncles, cousins, etc.) could, in unique situations, identify a suitable donor. When given the patient's HLA typing, the NMDP can provide assistance about the usefulness of extended family typing. If you need assistance, the NMDP Search Coordinating Unit has HLA experts available to consult. You can reach the Search Coordinating Unit at 800-526-7809.

What alternatives are there if the preliminary search shows no fully matched potential volunteer donors?

NMDP histocompatibility experts can suggest strategies for finding a fully matched volunteer donor from among the partially matched volunteers identified by a preliminary search. These strategies include:

- Repeat tissue typing to ensure that the initial typing used was the most specific.

- Identifying and retyping volunteer donors who may have HLA types that were possibly mis-assigned.

- Identifying and retyping donors whose HLA type was determined at a broad level of specificity.

- Consulting antigen tables to identify low frequency antigens, then re-testing volunteer donors.

- Running the search with alternate HLA phenotypes, which may identify suitable donors that may have been missed in the preliminary search.

These alternate strategies may require consultation with an expert in HLA and histocompatibility. If you wish to speak with an NMDP histocompatibility expert, contact the NMDP Office of Patient Advocacy at 888-999-6743.

Approximately how long does a formal search take?

The median time from formal search to transplant is four months. The NMDP recommends starting the search process early in the course of investigating treatment options.

What steps should I take if my patient has inadequate insurance to cover transplantation?

Contact the NMDP's Office of Patient Advocacy. Concerns about inadequate financial resources should not prevent referral for transplantation evaluation. NMDP Transplant Centers are frequently able to help establish adequate coverage. The NMDP's Office of Patient Advocacy also works closely with insurers to explore coverage options.

Chapter 29

Gleevec™
Newest Treatment for CML

What Is Gleevec™?

Gleevec™, also known as STI571, is a new drug that the Food and Drug Administration approved December 20, 2002 for accelerated approval for initial treatment of newly diagnosed Philadelphia chromosome-positive (Ph+) chronic myelogenous leukemia (CML), a cancer of white blood cells. It was designed in the laboratory to target an abnormal version of a normal cellular protein, present in nearly all CML patients. The abnormal protein is much more active than the normal version and is probably the cause of the disease. By blocking the abnormal protein, called bcr-abl, Gleevec™ kills the leukemia cells.

Why Is Gleevec™ Different from Most Chemotherapy Drugs?

Gleevec™ represents a new class of cancer drugs and a new way of thinking about cancer. These molecularly targeted drugs are different

This chapter begins with excerpts from "Questions and Answers: Gleevec™," National Cancer Institute (NCI), May 10, 2001; "Gleevec™ Confirmed as More Effective Than Conventional Treatment for CML," National Cancer Institute (NCI), 3/13/2003. Also included are "Practical Issues in the Use of Gleevec™," November 12, 2001 © Healthology, Inc., reprinted with permission; and "Resistance to Gleevec™: How Common Is It?" December 8, 2001 © Healthology, Inc., reprinted with permission.

because they target abnormal proteins that are fundamental to the cancer itself. Most current cancer therapies lack specificity, killing both cancer and normal cells. This is one reason why many people who undergo chemotherapy experience unwanted side effects from their medications. But Gleevec™ and other drugs in the development are designed to zero in on specific cancer-causing molecules, eliminating cancer cells while avoiding serious damage to other, non-cancerous cells. In the case of Gleevec™, the drug is targeted at the bcr-abl protein in CML cells. (Gleevec™ also affects other messenger systems in a cell which may contribute to its toxicity.)

Gleevec™ Confirmed as More Effective Than Convention Therapy for CML

The molecularly targeted drug Gleevec™ delayed progression of disease for longer, produced milder side effects, and resulted in a significantly better response than conventional therapy in patients with previously untreated chronic myelogenous leukemia (CML), researchers reported in the March 13, 2003, issue of the *New England Journal of Medicine*.

At 18 months of follow-up, however, the researchers found no evidence that treatment with Gleevec™ lengthens patients lives: 97 percent of patients treated with Gleevec™ (imatinib, formerly known as STI571) survived, compared with 95 percent of those who got conventional therapy.

Early results of this study were considered so significant that they were released ahead of schedule at the American Society of Clinical Oncology annual meeting in May 2002. At that time, patients had been followed for an average of six to eight months.

Randomized Study

The study—known as the *International Randomized Study of Interferon and STI571*—involved 1,106 patients in 16 countries. Patients were randomly assigned to receive either Gleevec™ or conventional therapy with interferon and low-dose cytarabine. The research team was led by Stephen G. O'Brien, MD, of the University of Newcastle in the United Kingdom.

At 18 months of follow-up, 92 percent of patients on Gleevec™ had no progression of disease, compared with 73.5 percent of patients on conventional therapy. Eighty-five percent of patients on Gleevec™ had a major cytogenetic response (a significant reduction in the number of cancerous cells), compared with 22 percent of patients on conventional therapy.

Crossover Permitted

Patients were permitted to cross over to the other treatment group if they stopped responding to therapy or had intolerable side effects. Seventy-nine patients (14 percent) in the Gleevec™ group either stopped treatment or crossed over, whereas 493 patients (89 percent) on conventional therapy did so.

The high rate of crossover to Gleevec™ from conventional therapy made it impossible to detect whether Gleevec™ had a beneficial effect on patients' survival, say the authors. The study will continue for at least five years. Longer-term results may provide a clearer picture of Gleevec's™ impact on survival.

Transplant: Curative but Risky

Some CML patients may continue to opt for the only treatment known to cure the disease—a bone marrow transplant. However, the risk of death or serious side effects from transplantation increases with age. Many patients are not young or healthy enough to tolerate transplantation or do not have a suitable marrow donor. An editorial accompanying the study report says Gleevec™ "now seems to be the initial treatment of choice for patients with CML who do not have a suitable bone marrow donor or who are not candidates for transplantation."

Gleevec™ was approved by the U.S. Food and Drug Administration in May 2001 to treat CML in patients for whom interferon had failed.

Gleevec™ Turns Off Protein Signal

The drug targets an abnormal version of a normal cellular protein that is present in nearly all CML patients. The abnormal protein called bcr-abl, is much more active than the normal version and is probably the cause of the disease. By blocking the abnormal protein, Gleevec™ kills the leukemic cells. It is the first approved drug that directly turns off the signal of a protein known to cause a cancer. Unlike other drugs used in cancer treatment, Gleevec™ does not kill normal cells in addition to cancer cells.

CML is a disease in which too many white blood cells are made in the bone marrow, the spongy tissue inside large bones. Most of the

4,500 Americans diagnosed with CML each year are middle-aged or older, although the cancer can occur in children. In the first stages of CML, most people do not have any symptoms of cancer, and the disease progresses slowly.

Practical Issues in the Use of Gleevec™

This section presents a November 12, 2001 radio discussion hosted by Shawne Duperon, with participants Charles Schiffer, MD, Karmanos Cancer Institute, Detroit, Michigan; and Mike Benninger, patient.

How Long Have You Been Using Gleevec™, and What Are Some of the Practical Issues That You've Encountered?

Charles Schiffer, MD: "I've been using it for a couple of years. It's a relatively simple drug to use. It's oral. It comes in 100 mg dosages. The dose for patients in chronic phase is 400 mg/day taken all at once. The dose for patients with more advanced disease is 600 mg/day, again, taken all at once. Patients can take it in the morning or the evening, whenever they choose, and generally we recommend that it be taken with meals."

Transitioning to Gleevec™ When Using Other Drugs

Charles Schiffer, MD: "Usually, patients when they're newly diagnosed, are treated initially with hydroxyurea to bring the white count down. In fact, Gleevec™ works extremely rapidly, so it's possible to immediately transfer from hydroxyurea to Gleevec™ without any problems. The transition from interferon to Gleevec™ is also pretty straightforward. In general, we stop the interferon and begin Gleevec™ a few days later."

Has Gleevec™ Been Easy to Take?

Mike Benninger, patient: "Yes, it has. The transition was extremely easy. I experienced some side effects initially, such as leg cramps, muscle cramps, but those went away with absolutely no additional medication. My liver counts went up to the point where I was taken off the drug for a period of two weeks. This was approximately two months into the treatment, but after that I was put back on it, and my liver counts have returned to virtually normal. My blood counts across the board are very close to that of a normal person."

How Long Should a Patient Be on Gleevec™?

Charles Schiffer, MD: "At the moment, all people who are having terrific responses, such as Mike, are staying on the drug perhaps indefinitely. Again, with more follow-up, we'll be able to answer that question somewhat better."

What Is Cytogenetic Response?

Charles Schiffer, MD: "Cytogenetics refers to the way of looking at the abnormal chromosome in this disease, which is called the Philadelphia chromosome, so called because it was discovered in Philadelphia in the late 1960s. There's pretty good evidence that if you have a treatment that will reduce or eliminate the Philadelphia chromosome that this will turn into long-term benefit for patients. So you're looking at therapies or you're trying to identify therapies that will do so. In patients treated with Gleevec™ in chronic phase, at least half, and probably appreciably more, will have these major reductions in the Philadelphia chromosome, and in some they will have apparent elimination of the Philadelphia chromosome. What we don't know yet is how long these responses will last, but some of them have now lasted at least a couple of years."

What about Patients That Want to Switch from Using More Traditional Therapies, like Interferon? How Do You Recommend They Do That?

Charles Schiffer, MD: "The decision to switch from interferon can sometimes be a difficult one. If a patient is having no response to interferon or intolerable side effects from the interferon, then that's a no-brainer, and the switch is very, very simple. You stop the interferon and you start the Gleevec™ a few days later. The more difficult decision is, there are patients who are having major benefit from interferon, and that they've had major reductions in the Philadelphia chromosome. We know from many years' experience that these patients can do well for many, many years as a consequence of their favorable effect from the interferon, and it's still an open question as to whether they should be switched to Gleevec™. Some choose to be switched because the side effect profile favors Gleevec™. Others say, 'No, I'm going to take my ride on interferon, and then I'm going to take my ride on STI, and hope that they're going to add up to a very long benefit for me.'"

375

Tips for Anybody Who's Going to Be Taking Gleevec™

Mike Benninger, patient: "First of all, when you're put on the drug initially, you may experience side effects that you find very inconvenient. In my case, most of those side effects have passed, and they passed without me taking additional medication, although it was available to me. Just be patient. Wait it out. You will acclimate to the drug over a period of time. Another thing is that I found taking the drug in the morning had a very profound effect on me. I was very fatigued, [it] took many hours out of my day. By switching to the evening, I basically sleep off those initial effects, and although I still experience fatigue, it's certainly not at the level that I was experiencing before."

Future Use of Gleevec™

Charles Schiffer, MD: "I think we are going to see it used in combination, particularly for advanced disease, and quite possibly for early stage disease, as well. Obviously, in a few years, we'll know more about the duration of these effects and how long it should be continued. We'll probably learn more about dosage effects and whether a higher dosage might be useful in some patients. We'll know a heck of a lot more about why the drug doesn't work in some people, mechanisms of resistance, and we might be able to get around that by different scheduling, different combinations, et cetera."

"This has been one of the most exciting things that has certainly happened to me personally in medicine, and I've been doing clinical trials in leukemia for almost 30 years. Usually when you do a clinical trial, you treat hundreds and hundreds of patients, and if you're lucky, five years later you see a small difference between the two groups. Here you went down to clinic and you saw the benefit under your very nose every single day. This is obviously something that we hope is going to happen with other targeted therapies and in other tumors, and it's really not a fantasy. The fruits of the molecular biology revolution are producing a remarkable increase in our understanding of different tumors, and also the production of lots of compounds like this. So I'd stay tuned."

Resistance to Gleevec™: How Common Is It?

This section includes information given in an interview hosted by Brett Scott. Charles L. Sawyers, MD, UCLA Jonsson Cancer Center, Los Angeles, CA, and Nicholas Donato, PhD., M.D. Anderson Cancer Center, reported about Gleevec™ resistance presented at the American Society of Hematology annual meeting December 2001.

Since approval of Gleevec™ for the treatment of CML in 2000, the drug has shown impressive results. But as with many cancer medications, researchers are concerned about patients developing a resistance to the drug.

Dr. Charles Sawyers: "Resistance to Gleevec™ occurs fairly commonly in patients who have the advanced stages of chronic myeloid leukemia, and by advanced, I mean blast crisis. The drug is actually very effective in controlling the disease, but it only is controlled for a couple of months or a year in most of those patients. So when they relapse, that's what's called resistance."

In patients with blast crisis, it happens in probably 60%-70% of the patients. So it's a big problem at that stage of the disease. The resistance is actually very rare in patients who have the earlier stage of the disease, the chronic phase."

What Are Some of the Ways Resistance to Gleevec™ Develops?

Nicholas Donato, PhD: "It turns out that the target is somewhat elusive. Even though it's well-defined, it can go through many alterations that provide it with an escape hatch, if you will. So STI-571 actually works by penetrating into the cell, and interacting with its individual target. But there are some mechanisms that allow that target to be changed."

"Some of the ways that we've seen—along with Dr. Sawyer—is that some mutations arise within the gene itself that prevent the drug from actually interacting with the target in a sufficient way to provide sufficient inhibition of the target and therefore under those conditions, you have very limited anti-tumor responsiveness. We've also seen that the target itself can become secondary to some other target. So that even though the target is still expressed, it may be expressed at such a low level that it really doesn't play much of a role in the progression of the disease. So therefore, even though the drug is still inhibiting the target, there are some other factors that are present within the cell that provide the oncogenic influence to provide the tumor to keep going and going."

Are Certain Patients at Higher Risk for Developing Resistance to Gleevec™?

Charles Sawyers, MD: "Definitely. Patients who are in advanced-stage accelerated phase or blast crisis are the ones at risk. We don't yet know for sure if patients in chronic phase are not at risk, and it's a research question at this point."

What Are Some of the Possible Solutions to the Resistance Problem?

Nicholas Donato, PhD: "We've found that there are a couple of different ways of approaching it. We've found that every one of the patients that we've screened that had developed resistance to STI continues to respond to conventional chemotherapy. So there is a possibility that you can combine conventional chemotherapy with STI to elicit a better or a more long-standing antitumor response with STI."

"Based on our studies, we can also define some other molecular targets that arise when patients become resistant to STI. So we're working with other companies as well as other individuals within our institution to try to determine ways of interacting with those individual molecules that come up that we think propagate the resistance phenomena. And, using a combination approach with STI and perhaps another inhibitor that will inhibit the secondary target would certainly benefit the patients and perhaps overcome resistance."

Charles Sawyers, MD: "One solution to the resistance problem might be to increase the dose of the Gleevec™. The idea would be that some mutations might be overcome by higher doses. But I think it's also pretty clear that some cases are not going to respond to the higher doses, and in those cases we need to combine Gleevec™ with other treatments."

What Is the Future Direction of Research in This Area? What Additional Questions Need to Be Answered?

Nicholas Donato, PhD: I think what really needs to be known is what's going on besides the individual target that's being affected by this individual agent. Keep in mind that this drug actually has a very, very narrow spectrum of activity, and that is, in fact, part of the reason that it's so effective and also part of the reason that it's so nontoxic."

"Patients do very well on this drug. They don't typically develop nasty side effects that are commonly occurring with standard chemotherapeutic agents. So it's of big benefit to the patient to actually seek out the individual target that's expressed in the tumor and inhibit that target and therefore have an antitumor effect."

"But I think what is much more pressing is to understand what other targets may exist in these cells, because it seems as if, when we look at the resistance phenomena, we find that the individual target varies. It can either vary by mutations, it can vary by changes in its level of expression, or it can vary by changes that are provided by other signals that are engaged within the cell. So the research in this area should be focused on and will be focused on understanding what the new targets are that are arising in patients that become resistant to the drug, and therefore hit those targets as well as the individual target that is affected by STI."

Should Resistance Be a Major Concern for Patients?

Charles Sawyers, MD: "Patients who are in the chronic phase of CML should not be worried about resistance. Less than 10% of patients, after two years of follow-up, show any signs of resistance. So it's definitely not a big issue there. But I think patients with blast crisis or accelerated phase definitely have a high risk of resistance, and I think they should be talking with their physicians about enrolling in clinical trials in which Gleevec™ is studied in combination with other drugs like chemotherapy or other signal transduction inhibitors."

Chapter 30

Targeting Treatment in AML

According to Professor Cheryl Willman of the University of New Mexico, it will become increasingly possible to customize therapy for individual patients with acute myelogenous leukemia (AML). In order for targeted therapy to become a reality for most patients, the biologic and genetic characteristics of a patient's leukemia cells as well as those of the patient's noncancerous cells need to be assessed in order to determine which individual patient should receive which specific treatment. About a third of patients with AML have one of three gene mutations: translocation involving 15 and 17, translocation involving chromosome 8 and 21, and abnormalities of chromosome 16. The remaining patients have a wide variety of acquired genetic changes that represent different molecular targets.

In some cases common pathways may permit patients with different specific gene abnormalities to be treated with a single drug. Consequently, one area being examined is the transcriptional regulation of human gene expression. Many mutations in AML cells are the result of encoded proteins that are involved in the process of transcription.

It is through this pathway that a DNA strand is copied into a complementary RNA strand. Dr. Willman suggests that one step, chromatin remodeling, might be considered the target for new agents because dysregulated chromatin remodeling could result in the creation of a mutated leukemia cell.

Another aspect of the transcription process is DNA methylation, making it a potential target for therapy. DNA methyltransferase is the enzyme that transfers a methyl group to DNA. Because increased DNA methyltransferase activity is a hallmark of most cancers, inhibiting DNA methyltransferase activity appears to be a logical goal of targeted therapy.

In order to determine which patients would benefit from treatment with methylation-altering agents, Dr. Willman and collaborators from the M.D. Anderson Cancer Center looked at 14 genes known to be under- or over-methylated in AML cells. Their data strongly suggest that in the future patients can receive agents that either promote methylation or diminish methylation, depending on the individual patient's methylation status.

Another application of molecular analysis of patients with leukemia is the use of very sensitive techniques to measure residual leukemia that is not detectable by blood cell counts or marrow examination using a microscope, the standard tools of diagnosis. Using specific assays to measure minimal tumor burden, these investigators also determined which of 800 APL patients with acute promyelocytic leukemia in remission would be most likely to relapse by quantifying the amount of leukemia cells detectable by ultrasensitive methods. In the future, strategies to monitor disease burden will be implemented earlier in the design of clinical trials in order to monitor the efficacy of new therapies.

Dr. Willman and colleagues are also analyzing gene expression patterns of 30,000 genes in AML patients with the same genotype but different clinical outcomes. Their long-term goal is to identify genetic patterns that forecast the response to a specific therapy and predict in advance which therapy would be better for a specific patient.

The relationship of leukemia cells to the supporting structure of marrow plays an important role in the expression of leukemia. The ability of AML cells to adhere to bone marrow endothelium, for example, a process that must occur in order for the disease to progress, might also attract future targeted therapy. Because several conditions must be in place in order to effect successful cell adherence, Dr. Willman points to the marrow macroenvironment as an area ripe for the development of novel therapeutic targets.

This report highlights several advances in our knowledge of leukemia biology investigation that might hold promise as sites for future targeted therapies in AML.

Source: *Leukemia,* vol. 15, no. 4 April 2001.

New Gene-Targeted Therapy Promises Improved Cure Rates for Deadly Type of Leukemia

Researchers at the Johns Hopkins Oncology Center have developed a new gene-based therapy that they hope will transform one of the most lethal types of adult leukemia to one of the most treatable. The test-tube findings, related to the treatment of acute myeloid leukemia (AML), also the most common form of adult leukemia, were reported in the August 1, 2001, issue of *Blood.*

AML is characterized by the uncontrolled growth of myeloid cells of the blood and bone marrow, which eventually crowds out and destroys normal blood cells. Normally, FLT3 is involved in the growth and maturation of healthy blood cells. In AML patients with FLT3 mutations, the cells acquire an abnormally altered FLT3 gene that promotes the uncontrolled growth. Existing therapies using chemotherapy cure the disease in fewer than 10 percent of patients who have a mutation of the FLT3 gene. But, researchers say a new treatment that targets and blocks the abnormal action of mutant FLT3 has the potential to dramatically improve the cure rate for these patients. Still, Donald Small, MD, Ph.D., associate professor of oncology and director of the research, cautions that the Hopkins studies are preliminary, and the safety and effectiveness of the therapy have yet to be confirmed in animal and human clinical trials.

Specifically, researchers have identified a compound that targets the signaling ability of mutant FLT3 (pronounced: flit three) genes. These mutations occur in and account for up to 40 percent of AML cases and are associated with a more aggressive, less curable form of the disease. Mutant FLT3 genes signal leukemia cells to grow and prevent the cells from dying. The new treatment specifically inhibits this activity, blocking the signal for growth and inducing leukemia cells to die.

In their study, the Hopkins investigators used the drug AG1295 to interfere with abnormal FLT3 signaling. "By blocking the action of the altered FLT3 protein, we can render it powerless. It's as if the mutation no longer exists. This is really proof of concept that a FLT3 inhibitor can kill human leukemia cells," says, Small, the first to clone the human FLT3 gene*.

The investigators tested AG1295 on clusters of human leukemia cells called blasts obtained from 23 AML patients. The compound caused many of the leukemia cells to die, with the most significant activity occurring in the blasts of patients with FLT3 mutations.

"This is the payoff of more than a decade of laboratory research to pinpoint the genetic alterations associated with this type of leukemia. Now, as hoped, we have evidence that the very abnormalities that cause the disease to progress may provide part of the cure," says Small.

The first human trials at Johns Hopkins of a FLT3 inhibitor are currently in planning.

AML strikes more than 10,000 adults and children in the U.S. annually making it the most common form of adult leukemia and the second most common childhood leukemia.

In addition to Small, other participants in this study include Mark Levis, Kam-Fai Tse, B. Douglas Smith, and Elizabeth Garrett. This work was supported by grants from the National Cancer Institute, Leukemia and Lymphoma Society, Children's Cancer Foundation, Alexander and Margaret Stewart Trust, and the National Institutes of Health.

*Small, D., Levenstein, M., Kim, E.K., Carow, C., Amin, S., Rockwell, P., Witte, L., Burrow, C., Ratajczak, M., Gewirtz, A.M., and Civin, C.I. STK-1, the human homolog of Flk-2/Flt-3, is selectively expressed in CD34+ human bone marrow cells and is involved in the proliferation of early progenitor/stem cells. *Proc. Natl. Acad. Sci.* 91: 459-463, 1994.

Reference: "A FLT3 Tyrosine Kinase Inhibitor is Selectively Cytotoxic to AML Blasts Harboring FLT3/ITD Mutations." *Blood* vol. 98, no. 3, August 1, 2001.

Treatment Outcome for t(8;21) AML Defined by White Blood Cell Index

According to a 2002 article published in the journal *Blood*, the white blood cell index (white blood cell count multiplied by the percentage of immature white blood cells called marrow blasts) appears to be the most accurate indicator of treatment outcomes in patients with t(8;21) acute myeloid leukemia.

Acute myeloid leukemia (AML) is a cancer of the bone marrow and blood characterized by the rapid uncontrolled abnormal growth of immature white blood cells known as myelocytes. The disease is more common in adults than in children, with the average age at diagnosis being over 65 years. Treatment for AML consists of remission induction, which is initial therapy utilized to induce a remission (disappearance of cancer), followed by consolidation therapy, which is therapy used during a complete remission to kill any cancer cells that may have remained following previous therapy.

A genetic abnormality referred to as the 8;21 translocation (t(8;21))occurs in approximately 8% of patients with AML. Clinically, t(8;21) AML has been associated with a high rate of complete remission and favorable outcomes as compared with other AML subsets, except in pediatric patients. Intensive consolidation therapy during complete remission has consistently resulted in survivals in excess of 50%. However, up to 50% of patients with t(8;21) AML will ultimately relapse and die of their disease. Very little is known about the disease characteristics of patients with t(8;21) AML and possible variables that may be associated with differing responses to treatment.

Researchers from the French AML Intergroup recently analyzed disease characteristics of 161 patients with t(8;21) AML. Patients were treated with either an allogeneic stem cell transplant or intensive chemotherapy as consolidation therapy. Of the patients in this study, 150 had achieved a complete remission. These researchers found that the white blood cell (WBC) index was the disease characteristic that best determined outcomes of these patients. Cancer-free survival and overall survival were estimated to be 52% and 59%, respectively, for the entire group. Disease-free survival was approximately 75% for 31 patients with a low WBC index, 55% for 89 patients with an intermediate index and 35% for 30 patients with a high index. Consolidation treatment with an allogeneic stem cell transplantation did not appear to result in a better outcome than intensive chemotherapy, even in high-risk patients from the high WBC index group. It appeared that the relatively worse outcome for children with t(8;21) AML was explained by a higher frequency of patients with a high WBC index compared to adults.

These authors concluded that the WBC index was the only variable associated with prognostic significance in regards to the duration of complete remission and overall survival in patients with t(8;21) AML. Although there was a relatively small number of patients receiving stem cell transplants, these results appear to indicate that allogeneic stem cell transplants as consolidation therapy may not provide a survival advantage over intensive chemotherapy in patients with t(8;21) AML. However, it is important that patients speak with their physician regarding the risks and benefits of all treatment options.

Reference: Nguyen S, Leblanc T, Fenaux P, et al. A white blood cell index as the main prognostic factor in t(8;21) acute myeloid leukemia (AML): A survey of 161 cases from the French AML Intergroup. *Blood.* 2002;99:3517-3523.

Chapter 31

What's New in Adult Acute Leukemia Research and Treatment?

Genetics of Leukemia

Research on the causes, diagnosis, and treatment of acute leukemia is being done at many world-renowned cancer research centers. Scientists are making progress in understanding how changes in a person's DNA can cause normal bone marrow cells to develop into leukemia. A greater understanding of the genes (regions of the DNA) involved in certain translocations that often occur in acute leukemia is providing insight into why these cells become abnormal. These cells may grow too rapidly, live too long, and fail to develop into mature cells that fail to function normally. As this information unfolds, it may be used in developing gene therapy. This approach replaces the abnormal DNA of cancer cells with normal DNA in order to restore normal control of cell growth.

Detection of Minimal Residual Disease

Progress in understanding DNA changes in acute leukemia has already provided an improved and highly sensitive test for detecting leukemia cells after treatment, even when so few are present that they cannot be found by routine bone marrow tests. Tests such as the polymerase chain reaction (PCR) can identify acute leukemia cells based on their gene translocations or rearrangements. This test can find one leukemic cell among a million normal cells. A PCR test can be useful in determining how completely the chemotherapy has destroyed the acute leukemia cells, and whether a relapse is likely.

Clinical Trials of Chemotherapy

Studies are currently in progress to find the most effective combination of chemotherapy drugs while still avoiding unnecessary side effects. New drugs are continually being developed and tested. Studies are underway to determine whether patients with certain unfavorable prognostic features benefit from more intensive chemotherapy. One factor limiting the effectiveness of chemotherapy is that leukemia cells become resistant. Ways to prevent or reverse resistance by using other drugs along with chemotherapy are being studied.

Stem Cell Transplantation

Studies continue to refine this procedure to increase effectiveness, reduce complications, and determine which patients are likely to be helped by this treatment.

Arsenic for Acute Promyelocytic Leukemia

A new drug, arsenic trioxide, has been developed which is also effective in this disease. Studies are now in progress to learn how to combine this with the other treatments to make them more effective.

A New Drug for Chronic Myelocytic Leukemia (CML)

This drug, which is a pill, appears to be effective for all patients with CML. It is also effective in some patients whose CML has changed into AML. The drug Gleevec™ was called STI571. It is too early to know how long this drug will work, but it has almost no side effects and can be combined with other treatments. Studies of this drug combined with other treatments are planned.

Monoclonal Antibodies

These proteins are manufactured in the laboratory and designed to attach to acute leukemia cells. Radioactive chemicals or cell poisons are attached to the antibodies. When the monoclonal antibodies are injected into the person with leukemia, they attach to the leukemia cells and the radioactivity or the cell poison kills the cells. Mylotarg, a monoclonal antibody with a cell poison attached, has recently been approved for use in older adults with acute myelocytic leukemia who might not be able to tolerate the side effects of chemotherapy. But it will still cause very low blood counts because it, like chemotherapy, will kill normal blood-forming cells. Studies are in progress to see how it might best be used.

Chapter 32

Azacytidine for Patients with Pre-Leukemia

Myelodysplastic syndrome (MDS), sometimes referred to as pre-leukemia or smoldering leukemia, is a group of diseases characterized by failure of the bone marrow to produce enough normal blood cells. In about one-third of patients, the disease transforms into acute leukemia. In high-risk MDS, the bone marrow contains too many immature blood cells known as blasts. Patients with high-risk MDS survive for an average of six to 12 months. Standard treatment for MDS consists of blood transfusions and antibiotics (supportive care). Anti-leukemia chemotherapy, hormonal therapy, and other treatments have been tested and generally found to be ineffective against MDS. Now two papers published in the May 15, 2002, issue of the *Journal of Clinical Oncology* suggest that the drug azacytidine may improve survival and quality of life for patients with MDS, compared to supportive care.

The two papers both report on a clinical trial in which 191 patients with MDS were randomly assigned to receive either supportive care plus azacytidine or supportive care alone. The trial was not blinded, so patients (and their doctors) knew which treatment group they were in. Patients assigned to supportive care alone could switch to azacytidine after four months if their condition got worse. The multicenter trial was conducted by the Cancer and Leukemia Group B, a cooperative group sponsored by the National Cancer Institute.

"Azacytidine May Improve Survival, Quality of Life for Patients with Pre-Leukemia," National Cancer Institute (NCI), 7/1/2002.

Patients' quality of life was assessed through telephone interviews conducted at the time they entered the study and after 7 weeks, 15 weeks, and 6 months of treatment. Patients were asked to rate their symptoms, physical functioning, fatigue, social and emotional functioning, depression, and anxiety.

Seven percent of patients treated with azacytidine experienced a complete response (disappearance of most abnormal cells from the bone marrow), 16 percent experienced a partial response (disappearance of at least half of the abnormal cells from the bone marrow), and 37 percent experienced an improvement (higher blood cell counts and reduced need for blood transfusions).

By contrast, just 5 percent of patients who received supportive care alone experienced an improvement and none had a partial or complete response. Death or transformation to acute leukemia occurred in 15 percent of patients treated with azacytidine and in 38 percent of those in the supportive care group.

During the study, 49 patients who were randomly assigned to receive supportive care alone—53 percent of all patients in that group—switched to azacytidine therapy because their condition got worse.

Patients taking azacytidine survived for an average of 20 months compared with 14 months for patients who received only supportive care. However, the number of patients enrolled in the study was too small for this difference in survival to be statistically significant. In other words, the difference could be the result of chance rather than an effect of the drug.

Over time, patients receiving azacytidine reported experiencing better mood and physical functioning—less fatigue, shortness of breath, and psychological distress—than patients who were treated with supportive care alone. Patients who switched to azacytidine reported feeling better and having less fatigue and shortness of breath after the switch.

The results of this trial should be interpreted with caution, writes Hagop M. Kantarian, MD of the University of Texas M.D. Anderson Cancer Center in Houston in an accompanying editorial. Assessments of quality of life might have been influenced by the fact that both patients and doctors knew whether a patient was receiving azacytidine or not, he notes. Secondly, supportive care might have been delivered differently at different study sites.

Chapter 33

Using the Immune System to Treat Leukemia

Can the body's own immune system be enlisted to fight leukemia, lymphoma, and myeloma?

Immunotherapy is treatment that boosts the body's own immune system to fight disease or lessen its side effects. Immunotherapy can be used with standard treatments for leukemia, lymphoma, Hodgkin's disease, and myeloma. In many cases, immunotherapy is still considered experimental and is given only through clinical trials—studies designed to see if a treatment is safe and effective. To participate in clinical trials, you must meet the eligibility criteria and agree to follow study guidelines.

Is immunotherapy the same as biological therapy?

Yes. Because this form of treatment relies on the living body and seeks to change or enhance the body's response to disease, it is also known as biological therapy, biotherapy, or biological response modifier therapy.

What is a biological response modifier?

The substances used in immunotherapy or biological therapy are called biological response modifiers. Originally available only in the

"Immunotherapy," Fact Sheet, © 2000 The Leukemia & Lymphoma Society, find additional information at www.leukemia-lymphoma.org, reprinted with permission.

small quantities produced by the body itself, biological response modifiers can now be manufactured in large quantities in laboratories.

Are there different types of biological response modifiers?

Yes. Biological response modifiers include interferons, monoclonal antibodies, colony-stimulating factors, and cancer vaccines. While research on biological response modifiers is still continuing, they may prove to work best when used in combination with each other and/or with chemotherapy and radiation to treat leukemia, lymphoma, and myeloma.

The major challenge in immunotherapy is to get the immune system to mount a specific immune response to cancer cells. Some of the newest cancer therapy, based on molecular science, aims to individualize treatments for each patient.

How do biological response modifiers work against cancer?

The immune system, which works to defend the body against disease and infection, may recognize the difference between healthy cells and cells which become abnormal and lead to leukemia, lymphoma, and myeloma. Biological response modifiers may aid the immune system in a number of ways.

Among their possible roles, biological response modifiers may be used to:

- Enhance the immune system to fight the uncontrolled growth of cells that occurs with leukemia, lymphoma, and myeloma.

- Eliminate, regulate, or suppress conditions that permit uncontrolled cell growth.

- Make cancer cells more vulnerable to destruction by the immune system.

- Change the growth patterns of cancer cells so that they are more like normal cells.

- Block or reverse the process that changes a normal or pre-cancerous cell into a cancerous cell.

- Enhance the body's ability to repair normal cells damaged by other forms of treatment for leukemia, lymphoma, and myeloma, such as chemotherapy and radiation.

- Prevent a cancer cell from spreading to other parts of the body.

What are cytokines?

Cytokines are powerful substances that control important cell processes, such as cell growth, activation migration, and aging. Cytokines are types of biological response modifiers.

How can cytokines help in the treatment of blood cancers?

Cytokines that stimulate the production of blood cells can be used to restore blood counts depleted by treatments or to boost blood counts in patients with inadequate blood cell production. Cytokines that stimulate the production of red blood cells, white blood cells, or platelets have been approved by the Food and Drug Administration or are undergoing clinical trials that may lead to such approval.

What are interferons?

Interferons are types of cytokines that occur naturally in the body. As with other types of biological response modifiers, interferons can now be produced in the laboratory.

How are interferons used to fight blood cancers?

Research has shown that interferons can improve the body's immune response against cancer cells and may work directly on cancer cells by inhibiting their growth or getting them to behave more normally. Alpha interferon was the first biological response modifier approved by the Food and Drug Administration for treating cancer, including chronic myelogenous leukemia and hairy cell leukemia.

For patients with chronic myelogenous leukemia who are not eligible for bone marrow transplantation, alpha interferon offers a most effective treatment. It also has better results than chemotherapy in delaying the rate at which chronic myelogenous leukemia progresses and extending survival time for the patient.

Alpha interferon can be used to treat Hairy Cell Leukemia for patients who do not respond to chemotherapy with cladribine (2-chlorodeoxyadenosine or 2-CdA) or pentostatin (Deoxycoformycin or Nipent).

Alpha interferon may also be used to treat multiple myeloma, non-Hodgkin's lymphoma, and cutaneous T-cell lymphoma.

What are monoclonal antibodies?

Monoclonal antibodies are mass produced antibodies that can be targeted to specific cells. Injecting cancer cells into mice makes their immune systems produce antibodies against these cancer cells. The cells making these monoclonal antibodies are then removed from the mice and fused with a laboratory grown "immortal" cell to create a hybrid cell or hybridoma that can indefinitely produce large quantities of monoclonal antibodies. Antibodies work against cancer and other diseases by latching onto or binding with specific antigens, substances the body recognizes as foreign, similar to the way a key fits a lock.

How do monoclonal antibodies work against leukemia and lymphoma?

Because they can target specific cells, monoclonal antibodies by themselves—so-called naked antibodies—have been used to identify and diagnose some forms of cancer. Monoclonal antibodies could also be clothed with radioactive isotopes or chemotherapy drugs to target and kill cancer cells. The antibodies can then be injected into patients in the hope that the antibodies would latch on to the antigen on the surface of the cancer cells and destroy the cells.

The first monoclonal antibody to be approved by the Food and Drug Administration for the treatment of lymphoma is called Rituxan. In early studies, about one-half of patients who had not responded to chemotherapy experienced shrinkage of their lymphoma tumors when treated with Rituxan. It is expected that therapy using monoclonal antibodies will become an important part of lymphoma treatment in the next several years.

Other monoclonal antibody treatments are being tested against a number of cancers, including leukemia and lymphoma. In clinical trials, anti-CD20 monoclonal antibody has produced good response rates in patients with relapsed low-grade or follicular non-Hodgkin's lymphoma. Monoclonal antibodies directed against B cell lymphoma have also yielded impressive results in clinical trials.

What are colony-stimulating factors?

Colony-stimulating factors (CSFs), also know as hematopoietic growth factors, are a class of cytokines that play an important role in the growth and survival of blood cells. CSFs also encourage bone marrow cells to divide and develop into specialized white blood cells, platelets, and red blood cells. Three hematopoietic growth factors have been approved by the Food and Drug Administration: granulocyte colony-stimulating factor (G-CSF, filgrastim), granulocyte-macrophage colony-stimulating factor (GM-CSF, sargramostim), and erythropoietin (EPO). Others are being developed.

How do colony-stimulating factors work?

Colony-stimulating factors act by stimulating the young blood cells in the marrow to make new white blood cells more effectively. This effect can help to restore white cell counts more rapidly after intensive chemotherapy, lessening the risk of infection.

Used in elderly patients with acute myelogenous leukemia following chemotherapy, CSFs can reduce recovery time and life-threatening infections. CSFs may also shorten the recovery time after bone marrow transplantation, which is now standard treatment for selected patients with leukemia, lymphoma, and myeloma. Short-term use of CSFs may also be helpful to myelodysplastic syndrome patients with severely reduced levels of neutrophils (a type of white blood cell) and recurrent infections. Myelodysplastic syndromes are a group of blood disorders that often progress to acute leukemia.

Can vaccines help prevent cancer?

Researchers are working on vaccines that could help the body reject tumors or prevent cancer from recurring. Vaccines could also be used in combination with biological response modifiers. Lymphomas are among the cancers being targeted by vaccines.

What are the side effects of biological response modifiers?

Although biological response modifiers originated as natural treatments, they do have side effects. As with other cancer treatments, these side effects can vary widely. Major side effects are listed:

- Biological response modifiers given by injection can cause rashes or swelling at the injection site.

- Interferons, can cause flu-like symptoms, including fever, chills, tiredness, and digestive problems, and can affect blood pressure.

- Monoclonal antibodies may cause allergic reactions.

- Cancer vaccines could cause fever and muscle aches.

How can I find out if immunotherapy treatments might be suitable for me?

If you are interested in immunotherapy, talk it over with your doctor. Get a clear picture of your current health status and if the treatments you are currently receiving are working. If immunotherapy might be right for you, your doctor can refer you to a clinical trial, help you enroll, and follow your progress.

Everyone has the right to apply to a clinical trial, but must meet eligibility criteria. Clinical trials are designed to answer specific research questions. The eligibility criteria ensure that the questions will be answered and that trial results are reliable. These criteria also help protect you—there must be at least a good chance that you will be helped by the treatment being tested in the clinical trial.

In addition to talking to your doctor, you can also find out more about promising new treatments by contacting the resources listed.

Additional Information

The Leukemia & Lymphoma Society of America
1311 Mamaroneck Avenue
White Plains, NY 10605
Toll-Free: 800-955-4572
Tel: 914-949-5213
Fax: 914-949-6691
Website: www.leukemia-lymphoma.org

Cancer Information Service
National Cancer Institute
6166 Executive Blvd., MSC 8322
Suite 3036A
Bethesda, MD 20892-8322
Toll-Free: 800-4-CANCER (800-422-6237)
Website: www.cancer.gov

American Cancer Society (ACS)
P.O. Box 102454
Atlanta, GA 30368-2454
Toll-Free: 800-ACS-2345 (800-227-2345)
Website: www.cancer.org

References

1. *Biological Therapies: Using the Immune System to Treat Cancer,* Cancer Fax from the National Cancer Institute, current as of 3/01/99.

2. *Cancer Facts: Questions and Answers About Gene Therapy*, National Cancer Institute, reviewed 1993.

3. *Cancer Management: A Multidisciplinary Approach* (second edition). Richard Pazdur, MD, et al (editors). PRR, Inc., Huntington, NY, 1998.

4. Cancer Trailblazer Follows the Genetic Fingerprints, *New York Times*, April 13, 1999.

5. *Chronic Myelogenous Leukemia*, Cancer Fax from the National Cancer Institute, current as of 3/01/99.

6. *Hairy Cell Leukemia*, The Leukemia & Lymphoma Society, 9/99

7. T-Cell Based Immunotherapy For Cancer: A Virtual Reality? CA-*A Cancer Journal for Clinicians*, 1999;49:74-100.

8. *1998 Cancer Facts and Figures*, American Cancer Society, 1998.

9. *1999 Facts*, The Leukemia & Lymphoma Society, 1999.

Chapter 34

Complementary and Alternative Therapies for Leukemia

Standard medical treatment for leukemia, lymphoma, Hodgkin's disease, or myeloma usually involves either chemotherapy, radiation therapy, or both. This treatment has been proven through scientific studies to be effective against these cancers and safe for the patient. There is no evidence that anything but current medically approved standard therapy can stem the progression of or cure these cancers. Therefore, standard therapy should not be replaced by any unproven remedy.

Although standard treatment has greatly improved survival for individuals with these cancers, the side effects can be difficult. Some persons will wish to seek out other remedies or techniques, sometimes called complementary and alternative therapies, in addition to the treatment prescribed by their doctor. The information provided here is meant to assist persons who have leukemia, lymphoma, Hodgkin's disease, or myeloma—diseases which are referred to from this point as blood-related cancers.

Many complementary therapies—from vitamins and herbal therapies to massage and acupuncture—work well for persons with blood-related cancers, helping to relieve the side effects of the radiation and chemotherapy involved in the standard medical treatment of cancer. However, because many complementary and alternative therapies

401

have not yet been studied, it is not known which are potentially helpful, which potentially harmful. For this reason, it is important to speak with your doctor about any complementary or alternative therapies you are currently using or considering. Asking about your concerns—such as which therapies are likely to be helpful, which therapies might have no effect or might be harmful, or where to find reliable information—will help you to make informed treatment decisions that are right for you.

Is There a Difference Between Complementary and Alternative Therapies?

Although many people use the term alternative therapies to include both complementary and alternative therapies, these two types of treatment have important differences. Complementary therapies are those that are used in combination with, or in addition to, the standard medical treatment prescribed by your doctor. Complementary therapies are usually used to relieve symptoms, alleviate pain or the side effects of standard cancer treatment, and to improve overall physical, emotional, and spiritual well-being. Alternative therapies are promoted for use instead of the standard cancer treatment prescribed by your doctor. Any therapy promoted for use instead of the standard medical treatment to fight cancer is considered alternative.[1,2]

What Is the Difference Between These Treatments and Those Prescribed by My Doctor?

Until recently, complementary and alternative therapies were not offered by medical doctors or hospitals and were not taught in medical schools. All the standard treatments (also called mainstream, conventional, or proven treatments) prescribed by your doctor to fight blood-related cancers have been well studied, and the drugs used in your treatment have been approved by the Food and Drug Administration (FDA). To receive approval from the FDA, a treatment must undergo a thorough series of investigations, called clinical trials. In these clinical trials, researchers determine whether the treatment works against the cancer (or treatment side effects) and whether it is safe for your use. The researchers also determine the side effects, any dangerous reactions that might occur if the treatment is combined with certain other drugs, and the dose of the drug that will work best against the cancer and still be safe for your use. The standard treatment prescribed by your doctor has been approved by the FDA to be effective against blood-related cancers and, importantly, its side effects and possible interactions with other drugs are known.

FDA approval is required for drugs to be prescribed for a particular condition or illness. Complementary and alternative therapies such as vitamins or herbal medicines are not considered drugs, but foods. Although there are FDA regulations for these diet products, thorough studies have not been conducted for many of these therapies, leaving their effectiveness and safety unknown.[3,4,5] Fortunately, science has responded to the public's growing interest in and use of these products. Scientific studies of numerous complementary and alternative therapies are underway, and others are being planned by the National Institutes of Health and other organizations.

Do Complementary and Alternative Therapies Work? Are They Safe?

Complementary Therapies

Many complementary therapies work well to relieve pain, alleviate the side effects of radiation therapy and chemotherapy, and enhance overall health and well-being. It is possible that some complementary therapies may interfere with or have a dangerous reaction with your medical treatment. For this reason, it is important to consult your doctor about any therapies you are considering or using. Your doctor can advise you about which therapies might be helpful and which are potentially harmful.

However, since research on these therapies is limited, little is known about how these therapies might affect adults. Less is known about their impact on children. Because children are still developing and growing, some therapies that are safe and helpful in adults could be harmful to children. One example is that of cranio-sacral therapy, a manual method of healing that involves manipulation of the head, neck, and spine. Because young children's bones are still forming, this therapy could be hazardous to very young children.[6] If you are considering a complementary therapy for your child with a blood-related cancer, be sure to consult your child's doctor before beginning any new treatment.

Alternative Therapies

Alternative therapies have not been tested and approved by the FDA for effectiveness against cancer or for safety. There are no alternative therapies that have been proven to kill cancer cells or stop the malignant process. Like complementary therapies, all the potential side effects and hazards of these therapies are not known, but the biggest danger of alternative therapies is the requirement to forego the standard medical treatment for cancer. The use of alternative therapies may cost persons with cancer their best opportunity for survival.

What Types of Complementary and Alternative Therapies Are Available?

Complementary and alternative therapies are available for treatment of physical, psychological, and spiritual needs. The National Center for Complementary and Alternative Medicine lists seven categories of complementary and alternative therapies—alternative systems of medical practice; diet, nutrition, and lifestyle changes; mind/body control; bioelectromagnetic applications; pharmacologic and biologic treatments; manual healing; and herbal medicine—with each category consisting of a large number of remedies or techniques.[7]

The National Center for Complementary and Alternative Medicine, American Cancer Society, and University of Texas Center for Alternative Medicine provide detailed descriptions of these and more therapies. They describe information on how each therapy works, whether it works, and whether it is safe or potentially harmful. In addition, the American Institute for Cancer Research Nutrition Hotline provides information to help you determine the best diet for you in achieving optimal health and well-being.

Are There Complementary and Alternative Therapies Specifically for Persons with Leukemia and Related Cancers?

At this time, many complementary and alternative cancer therapies are not marketed to persons with specific cancers. Certain advocates of alternative therapies claim their treatments work to cure or slow all types of cancer. Some complementary therapies are said to the relieve nausea, fatigue, and other common side effects of chemotherapy and radiation. Persons with leukemia, lymphoma, and related cancers may benefit from the use of helpful complementary therapies. Also of particular interest might be those therapies that are promoted to boost the immune system or build the blood. The following is a select list of therapies—some potentially helpful, some potentially harmful—which claim to relieve treatment side effects or stimulate the immune system.

Potentially Promising Results

Acupuncture

Developed in China more than 2000 years ago, this is a complementary therapy that has been studied thoroughly. Acupuncture is a technique which involves the placing of needles into the skin at certain points, called meridians. This therapy has been proven effective as a complementary therapy against general muscle pain and the nausea and vomiting of chemotherapy.[8]

Coenzyme Q10 (CoQ10)

CoQ10, an antioxidant and potential immune stimulator, is sold in capsule form and is being studied in persons with leukemia, non-Hodgkin's lymphoma, and other cancers. Some results indicate that this therapy may be useful as a complementary therapy, enhancing the immune system and providing protection against the harmful effects of radiation and/or some chemotherapy drugs on healthy tissues. On occasion, individuals taking this supplement have experienced mild side effects such as headache, heartburn, fatigue, diarrhea, and rash. CoQ10 is being studied to further determine whether it is beneficial, whether it is safe, and for whom.[9]

Polysaccharide K, or PSK

This mushroom-derived treatment is used in Japan, usually in combination with surgery, chemotherapy, and/or radiation to treat some cancers. In addition, one U.S. company sells PSK extract as a tea to various clinics. Some studies have shown this treatment to have immune-enhancing qualities, and it remains under study for possible anticancer activity. Some individuals have experienced gastrointestinal upset while on this treatment.[10]

Unknown or Potentially Harmful Effects

Camphor, or 714-X

This treatment, taken by injection, drops, or nebulizer, is said by some to bolster the body's immune system, thereby curing cancer and other diseases. Those who promote 714-X claim that it arms the immune system by interfering with cancer cells' protection against the immune system, regaining balance, and killing the cancer cells. While there are no major risks reported, no clinical studies have been performed with 714-X. Therefore, there is no evidence to support the use of 714-X for the treatment of leukemia or any other cancer and its safety has not been established.[11]

Green Tea

Green tea is used widely, and is said by some to enhance the immune system. However, this tea has been studied mainly for its ability to prevent cancer, not to treat cancer. Ten studies have shown a protective effect against developing cancer, while two studies have shown the opposite effect. Some laboratory studies show that green tea may slow tumor growth. However, it is not known whether this is true in humans, and it is not known whether this is the case for different types of cancers. Mild insomnia has been experienced by some persons taking green tea.[12]

Hoxsey

Purported to be an immune-boosting remedy, this herbal formula was developed in the early 1900s to treat cancer and is now offered in Tijuana. The formula, which may be used on the skin or taken as a liquid, consists of agents such as bloodroot, arsenic sulfide, sulfur, licorice, red clover, burdock root, barberry, cascara, and other herbs. Advocates of this treatment say that it strengthens the immune system and causes cancer cells to die. Side effects, such as diarrhea, nausea and vomiting—and some more serious conditions—have been observed with the ingredients used in the Hoxsey treatment.[13]

Vitamin Megadoses

Taking vitamins as dietary supplements may be helpful to promote health in some persons with cancer; however, large overdoses of these same vitamins can be harmful. In the 1970s, some began recommending high doses of vitamin C (10 grams or more daily) to prevent and cure cancer. However, studies showed that these vitamin megadoses had no benefit in comfort and survival, and may cause diarrhea, renal stones, iron overload, and gastrointestinal discomfort. Other vitamin overdoses that might cause harmful effects include vitamin A (25,000 IU or more daily), which may cause severe liver disease and vitamin B6 (more than 100 mg daily), which may cause balance difficulties or nerve injury.[4, 14]

Will My Insurance Pay for Complementary and Alternative Therapies?

More and more, insurance policies are covering the costs of certain complementary and alternative therapies. Several insurers have developed major medical plans that include select complementary and alternative therapies as part of their regular plans. Other insurance companies are developing plans to cover complementary and alternative therapies specifically. For detailed information about insurance coverage, consult your insurance provider and your healthcare providers.[15]

How Do I Talk to My Doctor about Complementary and Alternative Therapies?

Because of possible side effects and dangerous interactions of some complementary and alternative therapies, it is important that you consult your doctor about any therapies you are considering or using. Likewise, if you are considering foregoing standard treatment for an alternative therapy, please discuss your options with your doctor. Together, you and your doctor can determine which therapies will be the most effective and safe for you.

In the past, some patients have had difficulty talking with their doctors about complementary and alternative therapies. They felt that their doctors believed only in standard medical treatment and were not willing to consider the benefits of some complementary and alternative medicine. Fortunately, this is changing.

The potential benefits and risks of complementary and alternative therapies are now being taught in many medical schools, and select complementary therapies are being offered at hospitals and cancer clinics. In addition, cancer healthcare professionals are eagerly awaiting the results of ongoing studies of such therapies.

The following questions are examples of how you might ask your doctor about complementary and alternative therapies:

- "I was on the Internet recently and came across some information that said acupuncture might be helpful in relieving the nausea after chemo. Is that something that might be helpful for me?"

- "A friend said that using echinacea really helped her to feel less fatigued. Do you think that is something I should try?"

- "With my recent diagnosis and difficult treatments, I am feeling discouraged lately. Do you have any suggestions to help me get through this?"

You might also consider bringing any materials that you find from the Internet,[16] from a friend, or from various cancer organizations for your doctor's review. Your doctor can then address your questions, keep a record of which therapies you are using, and avoid any harmful interactions. Your doctor may also refer you to a nurse or social worker who can help you further.

Additional Information

American Cancer Society
P.O. Box 102454
Atlanta, GA 30368-2454
Toll-Free: 800-227-2345
Website: www.cancer.org

ACS provides Fact Sheets on specific complementary and alternative therapies, how to speak with your doctor, and how to choose a reliable provider.

American Institute for Cancer Research Nutrition Hotline
1759 R Street NW
Washington, DC 20009
Toll-Free: 800-843-8114
Tel: 202-328-7744
Fax: 202-328-7226
Website: www.aicr.org
E-mail: aicrweb@aicr.org

AICRN provides information on different nutritional regimens and potential health benefits.

Food and Drug Administration
5600 Fishers Lane
Rockville, MD 20857-0001
Toll Free: 888-463-6332
Website: www.fda.gov

The FDA provides a number of articles on dietary supplements, discussions of specific products with potentially serious side effects, and warnings about specific products.

National Cancer Institute
6166 Executive Blvd., MSC 8322
Suite 3036A
Bethesda, MD 20892-8322
Toll-Free: 800-422-6237
Toll-Free TTY: 800-332-8615
Website: www.cancer.gov

The NCI provides information on clinical trials and Fact Sheets on complementary and alternative therapies.

National Center for Complementary and Alternative Medicine
P.O. Box 7923
Gaithersburg, MD 20898
Toll Free: 888-644-6226
TTY: 866-464-3615
Fax: 866-464-3616
Website: http://nccam.nih.gov
E-mail: info@nccam.nih.gov

NCCAM provides Fact Sheets on specific complementary and alternative therapies and ongoing studies; its clearinghouse provides information and publications on various topics, including how to discuss the topic with your doctor and how to find a practitioner in your area.

Oncolink
University of Pennsylvania Cancer Center
3400 Spruce Street
2 Donner
Philadelphia, PA 19104-4283
Fax: 215-349-5445
Website: www.oncolink.upenn.edu

Oncolink provides information and video segments on specific complementary and alternative therapies, how to discuss the topic with your doctor, how to choose a reliable provider.

Reuters Health
45 West 36th Street, 12th Floor
New York, NY 10036
Tel: 212-273-1700
Website: www.reutershealth.com
E-mail: support@reutershealth.com

Reuters Health provides the latest news in medical advances, including those related to complementary and alternative therapies.

University of Texas M.D. Anderson Cancer Center
1515 Holcombe Blvd.
Houston, TX 77030
Toll Free: 800-392-1611
Tel: 713-792-6161
Website: www.mdanderson.org/departments/cimer

UT Center for Alternative Medicine Research provides extensive information on specific complementary and alternative therapies, with detailed scientific summaries of study results.

Quackwatch
P.O. Box 1747
Allentown, PA 18105
Tel: 610-437-1795
Website: www.quackwatch.org
E-mail: sbinfo@quackwatch.com

Quackwatch provides information on claims of complementary and alternative therapies that are unproven, proven to be ineffective, or proven to be unsafe.

Glossary

Acupuncture. Well studied Chinese therapy that uses placement of needles to relieve various symptoms including the nausea and vomiting associated with chemotherapy.

Alternative Therapy. Treatments or techniques that are used instead of standard medical treatment to fight cancer. Also called unproven, unconventional, or unorthodox treatments.

Bioelectromagnetic Application. Type of complementary or alternative treatment, such as electrostimulation, as categorized by the National Cancer Institute.

Chemotherapy. Treatment with drugs, often prescribed by the doctor as part of standard medical treatment, to fight cancer cells.

Complementary Therapy. Treatments or techniques that are used in addition to the standard treatment prescribed by the doctor. Also called unproven, unconventional, unorthodox, or integrated treatments.

Craniosacral Therapy. Type of complementary or alternative therapy which involves massage or manipulation of the head, neck, and spine.

Herbal Medicine. Type of complementary or alternative treatment, involving use of herbs, as categorized by the National Cancer Institute.

Immune System. The body's defense system against disease or infection.

Manual Healing. Type of complementary or alternative treatment, such as massage, as categorized by the National Cancer Institute.

Mind/Body Control. Type of complementary or alternative treatment, such as biofeedback or meditation, as categorized by the National Cancer Institute.

Pharmacologic and Biologic Treatment. Type of complementary or alternative treatment, such as the use of antioxidizing agents or metabolic therapy, as categorized by the National Cancer Institute.

Radiation Therapy. Treatment with radiation, often prescribed by the doctor as part of standard medical, to fight cancer cells.

Side Effect. Symptoms or discomfort that can be caused by certain standard medical treatments for cancer as well as by some complementary and alternative therapies.

Standard Medical Treatment. Treatment prescribed by the doctor to fight cancer cells. Drugs and techniques, such as those used in chemotherapy and radiation therapy have been studied and proven safe and effective. Also called proven, conventional, or mainstream medicine.

References

1. *Q and A about Complementary and Alternative Medicine in Cancer Treatment*. National Cancer Institute online 3/2/99.

2. Cassileth BR. Resources for Alternative and Complementary Cancer Therapies. *Cancer Practice* 1998; 6(5): 299-301.

3. *Overview of Dietary Supplements.* US Food and Drug Administration online 3/2/99.

4. *Supplements Associated with Illnesses and Injuries.* US Food and Drug Administration online 3/2/99.

5. Jensen CB. Clinical Trials of Herbal and Pharmaceutical products: A comparison. *Alternative & Complementary Therapies* 1998; 4(1): 30-35.

6. *Craniosacral Therapy.* American Cancer society online 3/2/99.

7. *Classification of alternative Medicine Practices.* National Center for complementary & Alternative Medicine online 3/2/99.

8. *Acupuncture.* American Cancer Society online 3/2/99.

9. *Coenzyme Q10 Summary.* University of Texas Center for Alternative Medicine online 2/3/99.

10. *Coriolus Versicolor.* University of Texas Center for Alternative Medicine online 3/2/99.

11. *714X Summary.* University of Texas Center for Alternative Medicine online 3/2/099.

12. *Green Tea Summary.* University of Texas Center for Alternative Medicine online 3/2/99.

13. *Hoxsey.* University of Texas Center for Alternative Medicine online 3/2/99.

14. Metz J. OncoTip: *Megadose Vitamin C.* www.oncolink.upenn.edu/support/tips/tip25.html. October 18, 1999.

15. Sapight BM. Managed Care Update. *Alternative & Complementary Therapies* 1998; 4(1): 5-7.

16. Compilation of home pages mentioned in this Fact Sheet.

Chapter 35

Access to Investigational Drugs

What is an investigational drug?

An investigational drug is one that is under study but does not yet have permission from the Food and Drug Administration (FDA) to be legally marketed and sold in the United States.

FDA approval is the final step in the process of drug development. The first step in the process is for the new drug to be tested in the laboratory. If the results are promising, the drug company or sponsor must apply for FDA approval to test the drug in people. This is called an Investigational New Drug (IND) Application. Once the IND is approved, clinical trials can begin. Clinical trials are research studies to determine the safety and measure the effectiveness of the drug in people. Once clinical trials are completed, the sponsor submits the study results in a New Drug Application (NDA) or Biologics License Application (BLA) to the FDA. This application is carefully reviewed and, if the drug is found to be reasonably safe and effective, it is approved.

How do patients get investigational drugs?

By far, the most common way that patients get investigational drugs is by participating in a clinical trial sponsored under an IND. A patient's doctor may suggest participation in a clinical trial as

"Access to Investigational Drugs: Questions and Answers," Fact Sheet 7.42, National Cancer Institute (NCI), reviewed 05/04/2001.

one treatment option. Or a patient or family member can ask the doctor about clinical trials or new drugs available for cancer treatment.

Another way of learning about new drugs being tested in clinical trials is through the National Cancer Institute's (NCI) PDQ® database. This database contains information on a large number of ongoing studies. Individuals can search this database on their own at http://cancer.gov/clinical_trials or they can call the NCI's Cancer Information Service at 800-4-CANCER (800-422-6237). Information specialists can search the database and provide a list of trials for individuals to share with their doctor.

Are there other ways to get investigational drugs?

Less common ways that patients can receive investigational drugs are through an expanded access protocol or by a mechanism known as a special or compassionate exception.

Expanded Access

Expanded access protocols are available for a limited number of investigational drugs that have been well studied and are awaiting final FDA approval for marketing. Expanded access allows a wider group of people to be treated with the drug. The purpose of an expanded access program is to make investigational drugs that have significant activity against specific cancers available to patients before the FDA approval process has been completed.

The drug company or IND sponsor must apply to the FDA to make the drug available through an expanded access program. There must be enough evidence from studies already completed to show that the drug may be effective to treat a specific type of cancer and that it does not have unreasonable risks. The FDA generally approves expanded access only if there are no other satisfactory treatments available for the disease.

Special Exception / Compassionate Exemption

Patients who do not meet the eligibility criteria for a clinical trial of an investigational drug may be eligible to receive the drug under a mechanism known as a special exception or a compassionate exemption to the policy of administering investigational drugs only in a clinical trial. The patient's doctor contacts the sponsor of the investigational agent and provides the patient's medical information and treatment history. Requests are evaluated on a case-by-case basis. The FDA must approve each request to provide the drug outside a clinical trial. There should be reasonable expectation that the drug will prolong survival or improve quality of life.

These are some questions that are considered when determining if a patient may be a candidate to receive an investigational drug as a special exception:

- Is the patient ineligible for a clinical trial?

- Have standard therapies been exhausted?

- Is there objective evidence that the investigational agent is active in the disease for which the request is being made?

- Can the drug potentially benefit the patient?

- What is the risk to the patient?

In some cases, even patients who qualify for treatment with an investigational drug on a compassionate basis might not be able to obtain it if the drug is in limited quantity and high demand.

Are all investigational drugs available through an expanded access or special exception mechanism?

No. The drug company or sponsor decides whether to provide an investigational drug outside the clinical trial setting. Availability may be limited in part by drug supply, patient demand, or other factors.

What is the NCI's role in providing access to investigational drugs?

The NCI acts as the sponsor for many, but not all, investigational drugs. When acting as sponsor, the NCI provides the investigational drug to the physicians who are participating in clinical trials of the drug. A physician who wishes to treat a patient with the investigational drug as a special exception must request the drug from the NCI. The request must include the patient's age, sex, diagnosis, date of diagnosis, previous cancer therapy, current clinical status, intended dose and schedule of the requested drug, any proposed concomitant cancer drugs or other therapies, and pertinent laboratory data. These requests are reviewed on a case-by-case basis.

Who can provide access to investigational drugs being developed by pharmaceutical companies?

In the case of investigational drugs sponsored by a drug company, the drug company in collaboration with the FDA provides access to the drug. The process is similar to that described.

A request to treat a patient with an investigational drug outside a clinical trial must be made to the drug company and to the FDA. The request to the FDA is sent as general correspondence to the appropriate reviewing division where the IND application is filed. The drug company can provide the name of the appropriate reviewing division. (FDA reviewing divisions are prohibited from divulging proprietary information such as whether a sponsor has filed an IND or the status of an IND.)

Are there specific criteria used to determine whether patients can receive an investigational drug outside the clinical trial setting?

Generally, patients must meet the following criteria to be considered for treatment with an investigational drug outside the clinical trial setting:

- They have undergone standard treatment that has not been successful.

- They are ineligible for any ongoing clinical trials.

- They have a cancer diagnosis for which an investigational drug has demonstrated activity and is being studied in ongoing Phase 2 or Phase 3 protocols

The potential benefits of receiving the drug should outweigh the risks involved.

What should patients do if they are interested in receiving an investigational drug through a special exception or expanded access mechanism?

Patients interested in gaining access to investigational drugs should talk to their physician about available options. Physicians can make requests for special exceptions by contacting the study sponsor. Physicians will be required to follow strict guidelines, including gaining approval from their Institutional Review Board and obtaining informed consent from the patient. Informed consent is a process that includes a document to be signed by the patient which outlines the known risks and benefits of the treatment, as well as the rights and responsibilities of the patient.

What are the costs involved in receiving an investigational drug?

In general, the drug is provided free of charge. However, there may be other costs associated with the treatment. Patients should check with their insurer about coverage of these costs prior to beginning treatment.

What are some of the potential drawbacks to receiving an investigational drug?

There are some potential drawbacks to receiving an investigational drug. It is not known whether an investigational drug is better than standard therapy for treating a disease, and a patient who is receiving an investigational drug may not receive any benefit from it. Side effects (both long-term and short-term) from the drug may not be fully understood, especially if the drug is in early phases of testing. Finally, a patient's health insurance company may not pay expenses associated with receiving the investigational drug.

How can patients find out more information about a specific investigational drug?

Patients can find out more about a specific drug by contacting the drug company that is developing the drug. Information may also be available from the Cancer Information Service at 800-4-CANCER (800-422-6237).

Additional Information

National Cancer Institute
Cancer Information Service
6166 Executive Blvd., MSC 8322
Suite 3036A
Bethesda, MD 20892-8322

Toll-Free: 800-4-CANCER (800-422-6237)
Toll-Free TTY: 800-332-8615
Fax: 800-624-2511
Website: www.cancer.gov
E-mail: cancermail@cips.nci.nih.gov (use the word "help in the body of the message to obtain a contents list)

NCI's website has a feature titled *Understanding the Approval Process for New Cancer Drugs: Summary*, available at http://cancer.gov/clinical_trials/doc_header.aspx?viewid=d94cbfac-e478-4704-9052-d8e8a3372b56

NCI's Cancer Therapy Evaluation Program (CTEP) has a website titled *Developing Cancer Therapies* available at http://ctep.cancer.gov.

U.S. Food and Drug Administration (FDA)

5600 Fishers Lane
Rockville, MD 20857-0001
Toll-Free: 888-463-6332
Website: www.fda.gov

FDA Center for Drug Evaluation and Research website has *Oncology Tools*, which contains a variety of information related to cancer including a section on access to unapproved drugs. That address is www.fda.gov/cder/cancer/index.htm.

Part Five

Life during and after Treatment for Leukemia

Chapter 36

Cancer Survivor's Treatment Record

Editor's Note: This chapter may be copied for your personal use, or may be used as a guide for your medical record keeping.

Taking Care of Yourself for Life

This chapter helps you keep track of your medical history with:

- A summary of your cancer treatment

- Guidelines for health monitoring that may reduce your chances of medical problems in the future.

- Suggestions for additional resources for information and assistance.

Your Name: _____

Medical Record Number:_____

General Health History Information

1. Name of disease you had: _____

2. Date of diagnosis (month/year): _____

3. Date all treatment was completed (month/year): _____

4. Date of any relapses: _____

5. Place of treatment (institution, address, and phone number):

    _____

6. The doctor and/or nurse practitioner most responsible for your care (names and telephone number):

    _____

Treatment Information

Chemotherapy

List for each treatment:

- Drug Name:_____
- Total Dose:_____
- How given: IV, by mouth, intrathecally?: _____

    _____

Surgery

- Date: _____
- Type of Surgery: _____
- Surgeon's Name: _____

Radiation Therapy

- Date: _____
- Area Treated: _____
- Total Dose: _____

Place of treatment:

Institution: _____

Address: _____

Telephone number: _____

Your radiation therapy was supervised by Dr. _____

Bone Marrow Transplantation

Date and types of BMT(s):

- Month/Year/Type _____
- Month/Year/Type _____

BMT Chemotherapy

List for each treatment:

- Drug Name: _____
- Total Dose: _____
- How given: IV, by mouth, intrathecally?: _____

BMT Radiation Therapy

- Date: _____
- Area Treated: _____
- Total Dose: _____

Place of treatment:

Institution: _____

Address: _____

Telephone number: _____

Doctor responsible for your BMT was Dr. _____

Disease/Treatment Complications

These problems were complications you had during treatment (other than fever and low blood counts):

- Date: _____
- Complication: _____
- Date: _____
- Complication: _____
- Date: _____
- Complication: _____

Your Medical Follow-Up

These are special instructions for monitoring your health in the future, based on the treatment you received:

- Treatment: _____
- Organs at Risk: _____
- Tests: _____

- Treatment: _____
- Organs at Risk: _____
- Tests: _____

Things to Do for Your Health

You have an important responsibility for your health. Today more people are cured of cancer than ever before. You can help yourself and anyone who gives you medical care by:

- Knowing about your disease and its treatment.
- Having checkups once a year, with a physical examination, blood count, urinalysis, and recommended tests.
- Staying in touch with the medical center or clinic where you were originally treated for cancer, at least once a year.
- Learning the 10 steps to a healthier life and a reduced adult cancer risk suggest by the American Cancer Society.
- Making use of available resources for information and support.
- Keeping a copy of all your test results (MRI, CT scan, etc.) so they are available if needed for comparison.

Resources

American Cancer Society
P.O. Box 102454
Atlanta, GA 30329
Toll-Free: 800-227-2345
Website: www.cancer.org

The Association of Cancer Online Resources, Inc., (ACOR)
173 Duane Street, Suite 3A
New York, NY 10013-3334
Website: www.acor.org

   Offers a wide range of electronic discussion groups that provide information and support to patients, caregivers, and families.

Canadian Cancer Society
565 W. 10ᵗʰ Ave.
Vancouver, BC V5Z 4J4
Toll-Free: 888-939-3333
Tel: 604-872-4400
Website: www.bc.cancer.ca
E-mail: inquiries@bc.cancer.ca

Cancervive
11636 Chayote Street
Los Angeles, CA 90049
Toll-Free: 800-4-To-Cure (800-486-2873)
Tel: 310-203-9232
Fax: 310-471-4618
Website: www.cancervive.org
E-mail: cancervivr@aol.com

Candlelighters Childhood Cancer Foundation
P.O. Box 498
Kensington, MD 20895-0498
Toll-Free: 800-366-2223
Tel: 301-962-3520
Fax: 301-962-3521
Website: www.candlelighters.org
E-mail: info@candlelighters.org

National Cancer Institute
NCI Public Inquiries Office
6166 Executive Blvd. MSC 8322
Suite 3036A
Bethesda, MD 20892-8322
Toll-Free: 800-4-CANCER (800-422-6237)
Toll-Free TTY: 800-332-8615
Website: www.cancer.gov

The National Coalition for Cancer Survivorship
1010 Wayne Ave, Suite 770
Silver Spring, MD 20910
Toll-Free: 877-622-7937
Tel: 301-650-9127
Fax: 301-565-9670
Website: www.canceradvocacy.org
E-mail: info@canceradvocacy.org

Patient-Centered Guides
1005 Gravenstein Highway North
Sebastopol, CA 95472
Toll-Free: 800-998-9938
Tel: 707-829-0515
Fax: 707-829-0104
Website: www.patientcenters.com
E-mail: patientguides@oreilly.com

Other Resources in Your Area

Record other resources:_____

This Summary of Your Disease and Treatment Was Prepared By

Name: _____

Date: _____

Keep this copy for your records. Make copies as needed for your doctors or nurses. Determine and record whom you should contact where you were treated whenever your medical condition or address changes, or if you have questions about your follow-up.

Chapter 37

Nutrition in Cancer Care

Nutrition Implications of Cancer Therapies

The nutritional status of someone diagnosed with cancer entering the treatment process varies from patient to patient. Not everyone begins therapy with anorexia, weight loss, and other symptoms of nutritional problems. For patients who do, however, anticancer therapies can complicate the treatment and expected recovery. Many individuals also present with pre-existing comorbid diseases and illnesses that further complicate their treatment. Surgery, chemotherapy, and radiation can have a direct (or mechanical) and/or an indirect (or metabolic) negative effect on nutritional status. The success of the anticancer therapy will be influenced by a patient's ability to tolerate therapy, which will, in turn, be affected by nutritional status preceding treatment. The treating clinician should assess baseline nutritional status and be aware of the possible implications of the various therapies. Patients receiving aggressive cancer therapies typically need aggressive nutrition management.

Chemotherapy

In 2000, more than 90 different chemotherapy agents were approved for use. These agents are divided into several functional categories.

Excerpted from PDQ® Cancer Information Summary, National Cancer Institute; Bethesda, MD, "Nutrition in Cancer Care (PDQ®): Supportive Care," updated 02/2003, available at: http://cancer.gov, accessed 03/31/2003.

Chemotherapy agents can be used in combination or as single agents, depending on the disease type and health condition of the individual.[4]

Unlike surgery and radiation therapy, cancer chemotherapy is a systemic treatment (not a localized treatment) that affects the whole body (not just a specific part).[5] Consequently, there are potentially more side effects with chemotherapy than with surgery and radiation therapy. The most commonly experienced nutrition-related side effects are anorexia, taste changes, early satiety, nausea, vomiting, mucositis/esophagitis, diarrhea, and constipation. Because side effects of chemotherapy, as well as the cancer itself, can greatly affect nutritional status, healthcare providers need to anticipate, and educate the patient about possible problems[5] in an effort to prevent malnutrition and weight loss. Malnutrition and weight loss can affect a patient's ability to regain health and acceptable blood counts between chemotherapy cycles; this can directly affect the ability to stay on treatment schedules, which is important in achieving a successful outcome.

Nutrition support or high-calorie/high-protein liquid supplements may be used in an effort to maintain adequate calorie and nutrient intake. Special formulas are available for people with secondary medical conditions such as hyperglycemia or compromised renal function.

Radiation Therapy

Nutritional support during radiation therapy is vital. The effect of radiation therapy on healthy tissue in the treatment field can produce changes in normal physiologic function that may ultimately diminish a patient's nutrition status by interfering with ingestion, digestion, or absorption of nutrients. Medications such as pilocarpine (Salagen) may be useful in treating the xerostomia (dry mouth) that accompanies radiation therapy. This medicine may reduce the need for artificial saliva agents or other oral comfort agents such as hard candy or sugarless gum.

The side effects of radiation therapy depend on the area irradiated, total dose, fractionation, duration, and volume irradiated. Most side effects are acute, begin around the second or third week of treatment, and diminish 2 or 3 weeks after radiation therapy is completed. Some side effects can be chronic and continue or occur after treatment has been completed.[6]

Individuals receiving radiation therapy to any part of the gastrointestinal tract are more susceptible to nutrition-related side effects. Patients most at risk for developing nutrition-related side effects are those whose cancers involve the aerodigestive tract, including the head and neck, lungs, esophagus, cervix, uterus, colon, rectum, and pancreas. Patients who are receiving radiation therapy to the head and neck region may present to radiation therapy with pre-existing malnutrition secondary to an inability to ingest foods because of the disease itself or any surgery to treat the disease. Many of these patients have a history of high alcohol intake, which also places them at a higher nutritional risk. These individuals are generally at the greatest risk for developing significant nutrition problems and severe weight loss.[7]

Nutrition intervention is based on symptom management. Patients who maintain good nutrition are more likely to tolerate the side effects of treatment. Adequate calories and protein can help maintain patient strength and prevent body tissues from further catabolism. Individuals who do not consume adequate calories and protein use stored nutrients as an energy source, which leads to protein wasting and further weight loss.

Some of the more common nutrition-related side effects caused by irradiation to the head and neck include taste alterations or aversions, odynophagia (pain produced by swallowing), xerostomia, thick saliva, mucositis, and/or dysphasia. Thoracic irradiation may be associated with esophagitis, dysphasia, or esophageal reflux. Diarrhea, nausea, vomiting, enteritis, and malabsorption of nutrients are possible side effects of pelvic or abdominal radiation.[8]

Many patients who are undergoing radiation therapy will benefit from nutritional supplements between meals.[9] Aggressive nutritional support is indicated when oral intake alone fails to maintain an individual's weight. Tube feedings are used more frequently than parenteral nutrition, primarily to preserve gastrointestinal function. Tube feedings are usually well tolerated, pose less risk to the patient than parenteral feedings, and are more cost effective. Numerous studies demonstrate the benefit of enteral feedings initiated at the onset of treatment, specifically treatment to head and neck regions, before significant weight loss has occurred.[10,11]

Many nutrition-related side effects result from radiation therapy. Quality of life and nutritional intake can be improved by managing these side effects through appropriate medical nutritional therapy and dietary modifications.

Immunotherapy

Monoclonal antibodies, used to block cancer-cell receptors for growth-stimulating factors, may cause a cascade of symptoms; however, the symptoms most likely to impact nutritional status are fever, nausea, vomiting, and diarrhea.[1] Interferon (a nonspecific immunotherapy) has had the noted nutrition-related side effects of anorexia, nausea, vomiting, and fatigue.[1] Interleukin-2, approved by the Food and Drug Administration (FDA) for the single-agent treatment of metastatic renal cell cancer, can also cause symptoms such as fatigue, nausea, vomiting, or diarrhea [1,12] Response to interleukin-2 treatment varies; some patients gain weight, and some require nutrition support.[12] Most patients taking interleukin however, gain weight. Finally, granulocyte-macrophage colony-stimulating factor (GM-CSF), a very common therapy used to increase the production of white blood cells, may also cause fever, nausea, vomiting, and diarrhea.[1]

If ignored, these symptoms can cause gradual or drastic weight loss (depending on the severity of the symptoms), which may lead to malnutrition. Malnutrition can complicate the expected healing and recovery process.

Hemopoietic and Peripheral Blood Stem Cell Transplantation

Hemopoietic and stem cell transplant patients have special nutritional requirements.[13] Before their transplant, patients receive high-dose chemotherapy and may also be treated with total-body irradiation (TBI).[14] These treatments, in addition to medications used during transplantation, frequently result in nutritional side effects, which may affect the ability to consume an adequate diet. The goal of nutrition support should be the maintenance of nutrition status and protein stores. In addition, transplant patients are at very high risk for neutropenia, an abnormally small number of neutrophils in the blood, that makes them susceptible to multiple infections.[15,16]

To reduce the risk of infections related to stem cell transplantation, most healthcare setting guidelines recommend only cooked and processed foods and restrict raw vegetables and fresh fruits that could cause a food-related infection. Specific dietary restrictions and their duration depend on the type of transplant and the cancer site. In addition to specific dietary restrictions, food safety guidelines should be reviewed and stressed with all transplant patients.

The chemotherapy regimen and complications associated with the transplant may result in numerous problems that adversely affect nutritional intake and status.[17] During the transplant process, patients may experience nutrition-related side effects such as taste changes, oral dryness, thick saliva, mouth and throat sores, nausea and vomiting, diarrhea, constipation, lack of appetite/weight loss, and weight gain. Often during the first few weeks post-transplant, patients are fed intravenously to ensure they receive sufficient calories, protein, vitamins, minerals, and fluids.[18]

Many patients experience mouth and throat sores 2 to 4 weeks after transplantation. Mucositis is the general term that refers to the erythema, swelling, and ulceration of the intraoral soft-tissue structures and the oral and esophageal mucosa in response to the cytotoxic effect of radiation therapy and high-dose chemotherapy. Mouth and throat sores can make eating and swallowing difficult. TBI may also cause dryness of the mouth, temporarily alter the taste of food, and/ or cause thick saliva to form in the mouth and throat. Nausea and vomiting are common problems experienced by transplant patients. Nausea and vomiting may be caused by TBI, chemotherapy, and some medications. TBI, chemotherapy, infection, depression, and fatigue can cause a decrease in appetite and weight loss. Lack of appetite may continue to be a problem long after discharge from the hospital. Patients may also experience gastrointestinal problems such as diarrhea and constipation that could be caused by TBI, chemotherapy, gastrointestinal graft-versus-host disease (GVHD), infection, and some medications.[19,20]

References

1. American Cancer Society Web Site. Atlanta, GA: American Cancer Society, 2003 Available online. Last accessed February 5, 2003.

2. McGuire M: Nutritional care of surgical oncology patients. *Semin Oncol Nurs* 16 (2): 128-34, 2000.

3. Allison G, Dixon D, Eldridge B, et al.: Nutrition implications of surgical oncology. In: McCallum PD, Polisena CG, eds.: *The Clinical Guide to Oncology Nutrition*. Chicago, IL: The American Dietetic Association, 2000, pp 79-89.

4. Eldridge B: Chemotherapy and nutrition implications. In: McCallum PD, Polisena CG, eds.: *The Clinical Guide to Oncology Nutrition*. Chicago, IL: The American Dietetic Association, 2000, pp 61-9.

5. Fishman M, Mrozek-Orlowski M, eds.: *Cancer Chemotherapy Guidelines and Recommendations for Practice*. 2nd ed. Pittsburgh, PA: Oncology Nursing Press, 1999.

6. Donaldson SS: Nutritional consequences of radiotherapy. *Cancer Res* 37 (7 Pt 2): 2407-13, 1977.

7. Chencharick JD, Mossman KL: Nutritional consequences of the radiotherapy of head and neck cancer. *Cancer* 51 (5): 811-5, 1983.

8. Polisena CG: Nutrition concerns with the radiation therapy patient. In: McCallum PD, Polisena CG, eds.: *The Clinical Guide to Oncology Nutrition*. Chicago, IL: The American Dietetic Association, 2000, pp 70-8.

9. McCarthy D, Weihofen D: The effect of nutritional supplements on food intake in patients undergoing radiotherapy. *Oncol Nurs Forum* 26 (5): 897-900, 1999.

10. Tyldesley S, Sheehan F, Munk P, et al.: The use of radiologically placed gastrostomy tubes in head and neck cancer patients receiving radiotherapy. *Int J Radiat Oncol Biol Phys* 36 (5): 1205-9, 1996.

11. Heymsfield SB, Greenwood T, Roongpisuthipong C: Dietetics and enteral nutrition: past, present, and future. *J Am Diet Assoc* 85 (6): 667-8, 1985.

12. Samlowski WE, Wiebke G, McMurry M, et al.: Effects of total parental nutrition (TPN) during high-dose interleukin-2 treatment for metastatic cancer. *J Immunother* 21 (1): 65-74, 1998.

13. Charuhas PM: Bone marrow transplantation. In: Skipper A, eds.: *Dietitian's Handbook of Enteral and Parenteral Nutrition*. 2nd ed. Gaithersburg, MD: Aspen Publishers, 1998, pp 273-94.

14. Johns A: Overview of bone marrow and stem cell transplantation. *J Intraven Nurs* 21 (6): 356-60, 1998 Nov-Dec.

15. Ninin E, Milpied N, Moreau P, et al.: Longitudinal study of bacterial, viral, and fungal infections in adult recipients of bone marrow transplants. *Clin Infect Dis* 33 (1): 41-7, 2001.

16. Jantunen E, Ruutu P, Piilonen A, et al.: Treatment and outcome of invasive Aspergillus infections in allogeneic BMT recipients. *Bone Marrow Transplant* 26 (7): 759-62, 2000.

17. Roberts SR: Bone marrow and peripheral blood stem cell transplantation. In: Lysen LK, eds.: *Quick Reference to Clinical*

Dietetics. Gaithersburg, MD: Aspen Publishers, Inc., 1997, pp 162-68.

18. Weisdorf SA, Schwarzenberg SJ: Nutritional support of bone marrow transplantation recipients. In: Forman SJ, Blume KG, Thomas ED, eds.: *Bone Marrow Transplantation.* Boston, MA: Blackwell Scientific Publications, 1994, pp 327-36.

19. Charuhas PM: Medical nutrition therapy in bone marrow transplantation. In: McCallum PD, Polisena CG, eds.: *The Clinical Guide to Oncology Nutrition*. Chicago, IL: The American Dietetic Association, 2000, pp 90-8.

20. Shapiro TW, Davison DB, Rust DM, eds.: *A Clinical Guide to Stem Cell and Bone Marrow Transplantation*. Boston, MA: Jones and Bartlett Publishers, 1997.

Nutrition Therapy

Nutrition Screening and Assessment

Nutrition in cancer care embodies prevention of disease, treatment, cure, or supportive palliation. Caution should be exercised when considering alternative or unproven nutritional therapies during all phases of cancer treatment and supportive palliation, as these diets may prove harmful. Patient nutritional status plays an integral role in determining not only risk of developing cancer, but also risk of therapy-related toxicity and medical outcomes. Whether the goal of cancer treatment is cure or palliation, early detection of nutritional problems and prompt intervention are essential.

The original principles of nutrition care for people diagnosed with cancer developed in 1979[1] are still very relevant today. Proactive nutritional care can prevent or reduce the complications typically associated with treatment of cancer.[1]

Screening and nutrition assessment should be interdisciplinary; the healthcare team (e.g., physicians, nurses, registered dietitians, social workers, psychologists) should all be involved in nutritional management throughout the continuum of cancer care.[5]

A number of screening and assessment tools are currently available for use in nutritional assessment. Examples of these tools include the Prognostic Nutrition Index,[6,7] delayed hypersensitivity skin testing, institution-specific guidelines, and anthropometrics. Each of these tools can help in identify the person at nutritional risk; unfortunately, the values obtained using such tools can be altered by the hydration status and the immune compromise frequently found in individuals diagnosed with cancer. In addition, each of these objective measures can carry a cost in terms of laboratory or practitioner time.

Another example of a screening and assessment procedure is the Patient-Generated Subjective Global Assessment (PG-SGA). Based on earlier work on a protocol called Subjective Global Assessment (SGA),[8] the PG-SGA is an easy-to-use and inexpensive approach to identifying individuals at nutritional risk and to triaging for subsequent medical nutritional therapy in a variety of clinical settings.[9] The individual and/or caretaker complete sections on weight history, food intake, symptoms, and function. A member of the healthcare team evaluates weight loss, disease, and metabolic stress and performs a nutrition-related physical examination. A score is generated from the information collected. The need for nutrition intervention is determined according to the score.

Bioelectrical impedance analysis (BIA) is also used to assess nutritional status, as determined by body composition.[10] The BIA measures electrical resistance based on lean body mass and body fat composition. Single BIA measures show body cell mass, extracellular tissue, and fat as a percent of ideal, while sequential measurements can be used to show body composition changes over time. Because of cost and accessibility, use of BIA is currently limited and often unavailable to most ambulatory settings.

Because nutritional status can quickly become compromised from illness and decreased dietary intake, and because nutritional well-being plays an important role in treatment and recovery from cancer, early screening and intervention, as well as close monitoring and evaluation throughout all phases of cancer treatment and recovery are imperative in the pursuit of health and for the individual with cancer.

Goals of Nutrition Therapy

Optimal nutrition status is an important goal in the management of individuals diagnosed with cancer. While nutrition therapy recommendations may vary throughout the continuum of care, maintenance of adequate intake is important. Therefore, a waiver from most dietary restrictions observed during religious holidays is granted for those undergoing active treatment. Individuals with cancer are encouraged to speak to their religious leader regarding this matter before a holiday. Whether patients are undergoing active therapy, recovering from cancer therapy, or in remission and striving to avoid cancer recurrence, the benefit of optimal caloric and nutrient intake is well documented.[11-13]

The goals of nutrition therapy are to:

- Prevent or reverse nutrient deficiencies.
- Preserve lean body mass.
- Help patients better tolerate treatments.
- Minimize nutrition-related side effects and complications.
- Maintain strength and energy.
- Protect immune function, decreasing the risk of infection.
- Aid in recovery and healing.
- Maximize quality of life.

Patients with advanced cancer can receive nutrition support even when nutrition therapy can do little for weight gain.[14,15] Such support may help:

- Lessen side effects.
- Reduce risk of infection (if given enterally).
- Reduce asthenia.
- Improve well-being.

In individuals with advanced cancer, the goal of nutrition therapy should not be weight gain or reversal of malnutrition, but rather comfort and symptom relief.[16]

Nutrition continues to play an integral role for individuals whose cancer has been cured or who are in remission.[17] A healthy diet helps prevent or control comorbidities such as heart disease, diabetes, and hypertension. With as many as 35% of cancer deaths being nutrition related, following a healthful nutrition program might help prevent another malignancy from developing.

Nutritional Suggestions for Symptom Management

Optimal nutrition can improve the clinical course, outcome, or quality of life of patients undergoing treatment for cancer.[25] Each cancer patient should consult with a registered dietitian or physician to formulate a plan for nutrition and to begin meal planning. Oral nutrition, or eating by mouth, is the preferred method of feeding, whenever possible. Appetite stimulants may be used to enhance the enjoyment of foods and to facilitate weight gain in the presence of significant anorexia.[26]

Recommendations during treatment may focus on eating high-energy, protein, and micronutrient foods to help maintain nutrition status. This may be especially true for individuals with early satiety, anorexia, and alteration in taste, xerostomia, mucositis, nausea, or diarrhea. Under most of these circumstances, eating frequently and including high-energy and protein snacks may help overall intake.[27]

Anorexia

Loss of appetite or poor appetite is one of the most common problems that occur with cancer and its treatment. Anorexia is a complex problem involving abnormalities in protein, carbohydrate, and fat metabolism.[28] The cause of anorexia may be multifactorial. Treatment modality, the cancer itself, and psychosocial factors may all play a role in appetite.[28] Eating frequent meals and snacks that are easy to prepare may be helpful. Liquid supplements may improve total energy intake and body function [29] and may work well when eating solids is difficult. Other liquids that contain energy may also help, such as juices, soups, milk, shakes, and fruit smoothies. Eating in a calm, comfortable environment and regular exercise may also improve appetite.[28]

Suggestions for Appetite Improvement [30-32]

- Plan a daily menu in advance.

- Eat small, frequent, high-calorie meals (every 2 hours).

- Arrange for help in preparing meals.

- Add extra protein and calories to food.

- Prepare and store small portions of favorite foods.

- Consume one-third of daily protein and calorie requirements at breakfast.

- Snack between meals.

- Seek foods that appeal to the sense of smell.

- Be creative with desserts.

- Experiment with different foods.

- Perform frequent mouth care to relieve symptoms and decrease aftertastes.

What Types of Foods Are Usually Recommended?

- Cheese and crackers
- Muffins
- Puddings
- Nutritional supplements
- Milkshakes
- Yogurt
- Ice cream
- Powdered milk added to foods such as pudding, milkshakes, or any recipe using milk
- Finger foods (handy for snacking) such as deviled eggs, cream cheese or peanut butter on crackers or celery, or deviled ham on crackers

Taste Alterations

Alterations in taste can be related to treatment, dental problems, or medications. Simply changing the types of foods eaten, as well as adding additional spices or flavorings to foods may help. Citrus may be tolerated well if no mouth sores or mucositis is present. Rinsing the mouth before eating may help improve the taste of food.[28]

While undergoing cancer therapy, patients may experience taste changes or develop sudden dislikes for certain foods. Their sense of taste may return partially or completely, but it may be a year after therapy ends before their sense of taste is normal again. A randomized clinical trial found that zinc sulfate during treatment may be helpful in expediting the return of taste after head and neck irradiation.[33]

Suggestions for Helping Cancer Patients Manage Taste Changes

- Eat small, frequent meals and healthy snacks.
- Be flexible. Eat meals when hungry rather than at set mealtimes.
- Use plastic utensils if foods taste metallic.

- Try favorite foods.

- Plan to eat with family and friends.

- Have others prepare the meal.

- Try new foods when feeling best.

- Substitute poultry, fish, eggs, and cheese for red meat.

- A vegetarian or Chinese cookbook can provide useful nonmeat, high-protein recipes.

- Use sugar-free lemon drops, gum, or mints when experiencing a metallic or bitter taste in the mouth.

- Add spices and sauces to foods.

- Eat meat with something sweet, such as cranberry sauce, jelly, or applesauce.

Xerostomia

Xerostomia (dry mouth) is most commonly caused by radiation therapy that is directed at the head and neck.[31] A number of medications may also induce xerostomia. Dry mouth may affect speech, taste sensation, ability to swallow, and use of oral prostheses. There is also an increased risk of cavities and periodontal disease because less saliva is produced to cleanse the teeth and gums. A primary method of coping with xerostomia is to drink plenty of liquids (25-30 mL/kg) per day and eat moist foods with extra sauces, gravies, butter, or margarine.[27,32,34] In addition, hard candy, frozen desserts such as frozen grapes, chewing gum, flavored ice pops, and ice chips may be helpful.[28] Oral care is very important to help prevent infections. Irradiation to the head and neck of a patient who has permanent dry mouth symptoms may result in reduced intake of energy, iron, zinc, selenium, and other key nutrients.[35] Special efforts should be made to help tailor meals and snacks for individuals with xerostomia.

Suggestions for Lessening or Alleviating Dry Mouth[32]

- Perform oral hygiene at least four times per day (after each meal and before bedtime).

- Brush and rinse dentures after each meal.

- Keep water handy at all times to moisten the mouth.

- Avoid liquids and foods with high sugar content.

- Avoid rinses containing alcohol.
- Consume very sweet or tart foods and beverages, which may stimulate saliva.
- Drink fruit nectar instead of juice.
- Use a straw to drink liquids.

Mucositis/Stomatitis

Stomatitis, or a sore mouth, can occur when cells inside the mouth, which grow and divide rapidly, are damaged by treatment such as bone marrow transplantation, chemotherapy, and radiation therapy. These treatments may also affect rapidly dividing cells in the bone marrow, which may make patients more susceptible to infection and bleeding in their mouth. By carefully choosing foods and by taking good care of their mouths, patients can usually make eating easier.[36-38] Individuals who have mucositis, mouth sores, or tender gums, should eat foods that are soft, easy to chew and swallow, and nonirritating.[28] Some conditions may require processing foods in a blender. Irritants may include acidic, spicy, salty, and coarse-textured foods. A recent pilot study found that oral glutamine swishes might be helpful in reducing the duration and severity of mucositis.[39] Glutamine may also reduce the duration and severity of stomatitis during cytotoxic chemotherapy.[39,40]

Suggestions for Helping People with Cancer Manage Stomatitis

- Eat soft foods that are easy to chew and swallow, including bananas and other soft fruits; applesauce; peach, pear, and apricot nectars; watermelon; cottage cheese; mashed potatoes; macaroni and cheese; custards; puddings; gelatin; milkshakes; scrambled eggs; oatmeal or other cooked cereals; pureed or mashed vegetables such as peas and carrots; and pureed meats.

- Avoid foods that irritate the mouth, including citrus fruit or juices such as oranges, grapefruit, or tangerines; spicy or salty foods; rough, coarse, or dry foods, including raw vegetables, granola, toast, and crackers.

- Cook foods until soft and tender.

- Cut foods into small pieces.

- Use a straw to drink liquids.

- Eat foods cold or at room temperature; hot and warm foods can irritate a tender mouth.

- Practice good mouth care, which is very important because of the absence of the antimicrobial effects of saliva.

- Increase the fluid content of foods by adding gravy, broth, or sauces.

- Supplement meals with high-calorie, high-protein drinks.

- Numb the mouth with ice chips or flavored ice pops.

Nausea

Nausea can affect the amount and types of food eaten during treatment. Eating before treatment is important, as well as finding foods that do not trigger nausea. Frequent triggers for nausea include spicy foods, greasy foods, or foods that have strong odors.[28] Once again, frequent eating, and slowly sipping on fluids throughout the day may help.

Additional Eating Suggestions[16]

- Eat dry foods such as crackers, breadsticks, or toast, throughout the day.

- Sit up or recline with a raised head for one hour after eating.

- Eat bland, soft, easy-to-digest foods rather than heavy meals.

- Avoid eating in a room that has cooking odors or is overly warm; keep the living space comfortable but well ventilated.

- Rinse out the mouth before and after eating.

- Suck on hard candies such as peppermints or lemon drops if the mouth has a bad taste.

Diarrhea

Radiation, chemotherapy, gastrointestinal surgery, or emotional distress can result in diarrhea. Avoiding hyponatremia, hypokalemia, and dehydration during episodes of diarrhea, requires the intake of additional oral fluids and electrolytes. Broth, soups, sports drinks, bananas, and canned fruits may be helpful for the replenishment of electrolytes. Diarrhea may worsen with greasy foods, hot or cold liquids, or caffeine.[28] In the presence of radiation enteritis, fibrous foods—especially dried beans and cruciferous vegetables—may contribute to frequent stools.[41] Meal planning should be individualized to meet nutritional needs and tolerances. Oral glutamine may also help prevent intestinal toxicity from fluorouracil.[42]

Additional Suggestions[16]

- Drink plenty of fluids through the day; room temperature may be better tolerated.
- Limit milk to 2 cups or eliminate milk and milk products until the source of the problem is determined.
- Limit gas-forming foods and beverages such as soda, cruciferous vegetables, legumes and lentils, and chewing gum.
- Limit the use of sugar-free candies or gum made with sugar alcohol (sorbitol).
- Drink at least one cup of liquid after each loose bowel movement.

Neutropenia

People with cancer may have a low white blood cell count for a variety of reasons, some of which include radiation therapy, chemotherapy, or the cancer itself. Patients who have a low white blood cell count are at an increased risk for developing an infection.[43]

Suggestions for Helping People Prevent Infections Related to Neutropenia

- Check expiration dates on food and do not buy or use if the food is out of date.
- Do not buy or use food in cans that are swollen, dented, or damaged.
- Thaw foods in the refrigerator or microwave—never thaw foods at room temperature.
- Cook foods immediately after thawing.
- Refrigerate all leftovers within 2 hours of cooking and eat them within 24 hours.
- Keep hot foods hot and cold foods cold.
- Avoid old, moldy, or damaged fruits and vegetables.
- Avoid tofu in open bins or containers.

- Cook all meat, poultry, and fish thoroughly; avoid raw eggs or raw fish.

- Buy individually packaged foods, which are better than larger portions that result in leftovers.

- Use caution when eating out—avoid salad bars and buffets.

- Limit exposure to large groups of people and people who have infections.

- Wash hands frequently to prevent the spread of bacteria.

Hydration and Dehydration

Adequate hydration is critically important for health maintenance. There are several common scenarios found in cancer treatment that may lead to altered hydration status and electrolyte imbalance. Hydration status can become compromised with prolonged disease or treatment-related diarrhea and/or episodes of nausea and vomiting.[44] Acute and chronic pain can also adversely affect the appetite; hence, the desire to eat and drink. Fatigue, an all too common complaint of people with cancer, can be one of the first signs of dehydration.[45]

Suggestions to Promote Adequate Hydration[28,46,47]

- Drink 8 to 12 cups of liquids a day; take a water bottle whenever leaving home. It is important to drink even if not thirsty, as the thirst sensation is not a good indicator of fluid needs.

- Add food to the diet that contains a significant portion of fluid, such as soup, flavored ice pops, flavored ices, and gelatins.

- Limit consumption of caffeine-containing products, including colas and other caffeine-containing sodas, coffee, and tea (both hot and cold); these foods may not be as nourishing as noncaffeinated beverages.

- Drink most liquids after and/or between meals to increase overall consumption of both liquids and solids.

- Use antiemetics for relief from nausea and vomiting; antiemetic use can be very helpful and may prevent hospital admissions from dehydration. The classes of available antiemetics include anticholinergics, phenothiazines, antihistamines, butyrophenones, benzamides, and serotonin receptor antagonists. Of note, all of these antiemetics have side effects, which many would consider less problematic than nausea and vomiting.

Constipation

Constipation is defined as fewer than 3 bowel movements per week.[48] It is a very common problem among individuals with cancer and may result from lack of adequate fluids or dehydration; lack of fiber in the diet; physical inactivity or immobility; anticancer therapies such as chemotherapy; and medications used in the treatment of side effects of anticancer therapy such as antiemetics and opioids.[48,49] In addition, commonly used pharmacologic agents such as minerals (calcium, iron), nonsteroidal anti-inflammatory drugs, and antihypertensives can cause constipation.[48]

An effective bowel regimen should be in place before the problem of constipation occurs. Preventive measures should be common practice, and special attention should be paid to the possibility of constipation as a side effect of certain therapies.

Suggestions for Avoiding Constipation[46,48]

- Eat more fiber-containing foods on a regular basis. The recommended fiber intake is 25 to 35 grams per day. Fiber should be gradually added to the diet, and adequate fluids must be consumed at the same time.

- Drink 8 to 10 cups of fluid each day; beverages such as water, prune juice and warm juices, decaffeinated teas, and lemonade can be particularly helpful.

- Take walks and exercise regularly (proper foot wear is important).

If prevention does not work and constipation is a problem, the application of a three-pronged approach for treatment is suggested: diet (fiber and fluids), physical activity, and over-the-counter or prescription medication. The use of biofeedback or surgery may also be considered.[50]

Additional Suggestions [12,46,48,50,51]

- Continue to eat high-fiber foods and drink adequate fluids. Try adding wheat bran to the diet; begin with 2 heaping tablespoons each day for 3 days, then increase by 1 tablespoon each day until constipation is relieved. Do Not Exceed 6 Tablespoons per day.

443

- Maintain physical activity.

- Include over-the-counter treatments if necessary. This refers to bulk-forming products (e.g., psyllium, methylcellulose (Citrucel), psyllium hydrophilic mucilloid (Metamucil, Fiberall), calcium polycarbophil (FiberCon, Fiber-Lax); stimulants [e.g., bisacodyl (Dulcolax) tablets or suppositories, glycerin suppositories, and calcium salts of sennosides (Senokot)]; stool softeners (e.g., docusate sodium (Colace), docusate calcium (Surfak and Dialose); and osmotics (e.g., milk of magnesia, lactulose, and magnesium sulfate/epsom salts); cottonseed and aerosol enemas can also help relieve the problem. Lubricants such as mineral oil would be included in this group but are not recommended because of the potential for binding and preventing absorption of essential nutrients.

References

1. Shils ME: Principles of nutritional therapy. *Cancer* 43 (5 Suppl): 2093-102, 1979.

2. Langstein HN, Norton JA: Mechanisms of cancer cachexia. *Hematol Oncol Clin North Am* 5 (1): 103-23, 1991.

3. Dewys WD, Begg C, Lavin PT, et al.: Prognostic effect of weight loss prior to chemotherapy in cancer patients. Eastern Cooperative Oncology Group. *Am J Med* 69 (4): 491-7, 1980.

4. Ottery FD, Kasenic S, DeBolt S, et al.: *Volunteer network accrues >1900 patients in 6 months to validate standardized nutritional triage.* [Abstract] Proceedings of the American Society of Clinical Oncology 17: A-282, 73a, 1998.

5. Eldridge B, Rock CL, McCallum PD: Nutrition and the patient with cancer. In: Coulston AM, Rock CL, Monsen ER, eds.: *Nutrition in the Prevention and Treatment of Disease.* San Diego, CA: Academic Press, 2001, pp 397-412.

6. Dempsey DT, Mullen JL: Prognostic value of nutritional indices. *JPEN J Parenter Enteral Nutr* 11 (5 Suppl): 109S-114S, 1987 Sep-Oct.

7. Dempsey DT, Mullen JL, Buzby GP: The link between nutritional status and clinical outcome: can nutritional intervention modify it? *Am J Clin Nutr* 47 (2 Suppl): 352-6, 1988.

8. Ottery FD: Rethinking nutritional support of the cancer patient: the new field of nutritional oncology. *Semin Oncol* 21 (6): 770-8, 1994.

9. McMahon K, Decker G, Ottery FD: Integrating proactive nutritional assessment in clinical practices to prevent complications and cost. *Semin Oncol* 25 (2 Suppl 6): 20-7, 1998.

10. Lukaski HC: Requirements for clinical use of bioelectrical impedance analysis (BIA). *Ann N Y Acad Sci* 873:72-6, 1999.

11. Bloch AS: *Nutrition Management of the Cancer Patient*. Rockville, MD: Aspen Publishers, 1990.

12. McCallum PD, Polisena CG, eds.: *The Clinical Guide to Oncology Nutrition*. Chicago, IL: The American Dietetic Association, 2000.

13. Rivlin RS, Shils ME, Sherlock P: Nutrition and cancer. *Am J Med* 75 (5): 843-54, 1983.

14. Zeman FJ: Nutrition and cancer. In: Zeman FJ: *Clinical Nutrition and Dietetics*. 2nd ed., New York, NY: Macmillan Pub. Co., 1991, pp 571-98.

15. Albrecht JT, Canada TW: Cachexia and anorexia in malignancy. *Hematol Oncol Clin North Am* 10 (4): 791-800, 1996.

16. American Cancer Society: *Nutrition for the Person with Cancer: a Guide for Patients and Families*. Atlanta, GA: American Cancer Society, Inc., 2000.

17. Brown J, Byers T, Thompson K, et al.: American Cancer Society Workgroup on Nutrition and Physical Activity for Cancer Survivors: Nutrition during and after cancer treatment: a guide for informed choices by cancer survivors. *CA Cancer J Clin* 51 (3): 153-87; quiz 189-92, 2001 May-Jun.

18. Wong PW, Enriquez A, Barrera R: Nutritional support in critically ill patients with cancer. *Crit Care Clin* 17 (3): 743-67, 2001.

19. Piazza-Barnett R, Matarese LE: Enteral nutrition in adult medical/surgical oncology. In: McCallum PD, Polisena CG, eds.: *The Clinical Guide to Oncology Nutrition*. Chicago, IL: The American Dietetic Association, 2000, pp 106-18.

20. DeChicco RS, Steiger E: Parenteral nutrition in medical/surgical oncology. In: McCallum PD, Polisena CG, eds.: *The Clinical Guide to Oncology Nutrition*. Chicago, Il.: The American Dietetic Association, 2000, pp 119-25.

21. Bozzetti F, Braga M, Gianotti L, et al.: Postoperative enteral versus parenteral nutrition in malnourished patients with gastrointestinal cancer: a randomised multicentre trial. *Lancet* 358 (9292): 1487-92, 2001.

22. Shils ME, Olson JA, Shike M, et al., eds.: *Modern Nutrition in Health and Disease*. 9th ed. Baltimore, MD: Williams & Wilkins, 1999.

23. Heys SD, Walker LG, Smith I, et al.: Enteral nutritional supplementation with key nutrients in patients with critical illness and cancer: a meta-analysis of randomized controlled clinical trials. *Ann Surg* 229 (4): 467-77, 1999.

24. Brennan MF, Pisters PW, Posner M, et al.: A prospective randomized trial of total parenteral nutrition after major pancreatic resection for malignancy. *Ann Surg* 220 (4): 436-41; discussion 441-4, 1994.

25. Rivadeneira DE, Evoy D, Fahey TJ, et al.: Nutritional support of the cancer patient. *CA Cancer J Clin* 48 (2): 69-80, 1998 Mar-Apr.

26. Seligman PA, Fink R, Massey-Seligman EJ: Approach to the seriously ill or terminal cancer patient who has a poor appetite. *Semin Oncol* 25 (2 Suppl 6): 33-4, 1998.

27. Zeman FJ: *Clinical Nutrition and Dietetics*. 2nd ed., New York, NY: Macmillan Pub. Co., 1991.

28. National Cancer Institute: *Eating Hints for Cancer Patients: Before, During & After Treatment*. Bethesda, MD: National Cancer Institute, 1998. Publication No. 98-2079. Also available online. Last accessed January 10, 2003.

29. Stratton RJ: Summary of a systematic review on oral nutritional supplement use in the community. *Proc Nutr Soc* 59 (3): 469-76, 2000.

30. Tait NS: Anorexia-cachexia syndrome. In: Yarbo CH, Frogge MH, Goodman M, eds.: *Cancer Symptom Management*. 2nd ed. Sudbury, MA: Jones and Bartlett Publishers, 1999, pp 183-97.

31. Ottery FD: Supportive nutrition to prevent cachexia and improve quality of life. *Semin Oncol* 22 (2 Suppl 3): 98-111, 1995.

32. Farmer G: *Pass the Calories, Please! A Cookbook and Problem-Solving Guide for People Who Need To Eat More.* Chicago, IL: The American Dietetic Association, 1994.

33. Ripamonti C, Zecca E, Brunelli C, et al.: A randomized, controlled clinical trial to evaluate the effects of zinc sulfate on cancer patients with taste alterations caused by head and neck irradiation. *Cancer* 82 (10): 1938-45, 1998.

34. Ship JA, Fischer DJ: The relationship between dehydration and parotid salivary gland function in young and older healthy adults. *J Gerontol A Biol Sci Med Sci* 52 (5): M310-9, 1997.

35. Backstrom I, Funegard U, Andersson I, et al.: Dietary intake in head and neck irradiated patients with permanent dry mouth symptoms. *Eur J Cancer B Oral Oncol* 31B (4): 253-7, 1995.

36. Miller SE: Oral and esophageal mucositis. In: Yasko JM, eds.: *Nursing Management of Symptoms Associated with Chemotherapy.* West Conshoshocken, PA: Meniscus Health Care Communications, 2001, pp 71-83.

37. da Fonseca MA: Management of mucositis in bone marrow transplant patients. *J Dent Hyg* 73 (1): 17-21, 1999 Winter.

38. Wardley AM, Jayson GC, Swindell R, et al.: Prospective evaluation of oral mucositis in patients receiving myeloablative conditioning regimens and haemopoietic progenitor rescue. *Br J Haematol* 110 (2): 292-9, 2000.

39. Huang EY, Leung SW, Wang CJ, et al.: Oral glutamine to alleviate radiation-induced oral mucositis: a pilot randomized trial. *Int J Radiat Oncol Biol Phys* 46 (3): 535-9, 2000.

40. Anderson PM, Schroeder G, Skubitz KM: Oral glutamine reduces the duration and severity of stomatitis after cytotoxic cancer chemotherapy. *Cancer* 83 (7): 1433-9, 1998.

41. Sekhon S: Chronic radiation enteritis: women's food tolerances after radiation treatment for gynecologic cancer. *J Am Diet Assoc* 100 (8): 941-3, 2000.

42. Bozzetti F, Biganzoli L, Gavazzi C, et al.: Glutamine supplementation in cancer patients receiving chemotherapy: a double-blind randomized study. *Nutrition* 13 (7-8): 748-51, 1997 Jul-Aug.

43. Bumpous JM, Snyderman CH: Nutritional considerations in patients with cancer of the head and neck. In: Myers EN, Suen JY, eds.: *Cancer of the Head and Neck*. 3rd ed. Philadelphia, PA: Saunders, 1996, pp 105-16.

44. Eremita D: Dolasetron for chemo nausea. *RN* 64 (3): 38-40, 2001.

45. Newton S, Smith LD: Cancer-related fatigue: how nurses can combat this most common symptom. *Am J Nurs* 101 (suppl): 31-4, 2001.

46. Weihofen DL, Marino C: *The Cancer Survival Cookbook: 200 Quick and Easy Recipes With Helpful Eating Hints*. Minneapolis, MN: Chronimed Publications, 1998.

47. Kovac AL: Prevention and treatment of postoperative nausea and vomiting. *Drugs* 59 (2): 213-43, 2000.

48. Vickery G: Basics of constipation. *Gastroenterol Nurs* 20 (4): 125-8, 1997 Jul-Aug.

49. Bernhard J, Maibach R, Thürlimann B, et al.: Swiss Group for Clinical Cancer Research: Patients' estimation of overall treatment burden: why not ask the obvious? *J Clin Oncol* 20 (1): 65-72, 2002.

50. Xing JH, Soffer EE: Adverse effects of laxatives. *Dis Colon Rectum* 44 (8): 1201-9, 2001.

51. Schiller LR: Review article: the therapy of constipation. *Aliment Pharmacol Ther* 15 (6): 749-63, 2001.

Additional Reading

Walker MS, Masino, K: Oncology Nutrition Patient Education Materials. The Oncology Nutrition Dietetic Practice Group of The American Dietetic Association, 1998.

Ghosh K, Carson L, and Cohen E: *Betty Crocker's Living with Cancer Cookbook: Easy Recipes and Tips through Treatment and Beyond*. New York, NY: Hungry Minds, 2002.

Nixon D: *The Cancer Recovery Eating Plan: The Right Foods to Fuel Your Recovery*. New York, NY: Random House, 1996.

American Cancer Society's *Healthy Eating Cookbook: A Celebration of Food, Friends, and Healthy Living*. 2nd ed. Atlanta, Ga: The American Cancer Society, 2001.

Weihofen, DL, Robbins J, Sullivan PA: *Easy-to-Swallow, Easy-to-Chew Cookbook: Over 1250 Tasty and Nutritious Recipes for People Who Have Difficulty Swallowing.*

Additional Information

American Botanical Council
6200 Manor Road
Austin, TX 78723
Toll-Free: 800-373-7105
Tel: 512-926-4900
Fax: 512-926-2345
Website: www.herbalgram.org
E-mail: abc@herbalgram.org

American Cancer Society
P.O. Box 102454
Atlanta, GA 30368-2454
Toll-Free: 800-227-2345
Website: www.cancer.org

American Dietetic Association
120 South Riverside Plaza
Suite 2000
Chicago, IL 60606-6995
Toll-Free: 800-877-1600
Tel: 312-899-0040
Website: www.eatright.org
E-mail: education@eatright.org

American Institute for Cancer Research
1759 R Street NW
Washington, DC 20009
Toll-Free: 800-843-8114
Tel: 202-328-7744
Fax: 202-328-7226
Website: www.aicr.org
E-mail: aicrweb@aicr.org

American Society of Clinical Oncology
1900 Duke Street
Suite 200
Alexandria, VA 22314
Tel: 703-299-1044
Fax: 703-299-1044
Website: www.asco.org
E-mail: asco@asco.org

American Society for Parenteral and Enteral Nutrition
8630 Fenton Street, Suite 412
Silver Spring, MD 20910
Tel: 301-587-6315
Fax: 301-587-2365
Website: www.nutritioncare.org
E-mail: aspen@nutr.org

Integrative Medicine
1029 Chestnut Street
Newton, MA 02464
Toll-Free: 877-426-6633
Tel: 617-641-2300
Fax: 617-641-2301
Website: www.onemedicine.com
E-mail:
customerservice@onemedicine.com

National Cancer Institute
6166 Executive Blvd. MSC 8322
Suite 3036A
Bethesda, MD 20892-8322
Toll-Free: 800-422-6237
Toll-Free TTY: 800-332-8615
Website: www.cancer.gov

National Center for Complementary and Alternative Medicine (NCCAM)
P.O. Box 7923
Gaithersburg, MD 20898
Toll-Free: 888-644-6226
Toll-Free TTY: 866-464-3615
Fax: 866-464-3616
Website: www.nccam.nih.gov
E-mail: info@nccam.nih.gov

Office of Dietary Supplements
National Institutes of Health
6100 Executive Blvd.
Room 3B01, MSC 7517
Bethesda, MD 20892-7517
Tel: 301-435-2920
Fax: 301-480-1845
Website: http://ods.od.nih.gov
E-mail: ods@nih.gov

Oncology Nursing Society
125 Enterprise Drive
RIDC Park West
Pittsburgh, PA 15275-1214
Toll-Free: 866-257-4667
Tel: 412-859-6100
Fax: 877-369-5497
Website: www.ons.org
E-mail: customer.service@ons.org

Chapter 38

Neutropenic Diet

After bone marrow/stem cell transplantation, it is important to avoid food-borne pathogens as one means of minimizing the risk of infection. For allogeneic transplant patients, avoid all milk and milk products—even those in the allowed category—until it is approved by your physician. Duke University Medical Center Adult Bone Marrow/ Stem Cell Transplant Program recommends that patients who have undergone allogeneic BMT/SCT follow neutropenic diet guidelines for at least 60 days post-transplant.

For autologous transplant patients, milk and milk products may be included as tolerated. They recommend that patients who have undergone autologous BMT/SCT follow neutropenic diet guidelines for at least 2 weeks, or until the ANC is > 500 for at least 3 days.

Safe Food Handling

- Keep foods at safe temperatures; cook hot foods to a minimum internal temperature of 165° F and keep cold foods below 40° F.

- Cook meats until well done—there should be no remaining pink. Red meats should be cooked to an internal temperature of 165° F and poultry to 180° F.

"What Is a Neutropenic Diet," Duke University Medical Center Adult Bone Marrow/Stem Cell Transplant Program. © 2002 Duke University Medical Center, reprinted with permission.

- Cook ground meats until well done—gray or brown with no pink remaining.

- Thaw meat, fish, or poultry in the refrigerator or microwave in a dish to catch drips. Use defrosted foods right away; do not re-freeze.

- Never leave perishable food out of the refrigerator for over two hours. Egg dishes and cream- and mayonnaise-based foods should not be left unrefrigerated for more than one hour.

- Divide large amounts into small, shallow containers for quick cooling in the refrigerator. Refrigerate only as much as can be eaten in 2 to 3 days; freeze the rest.

- Wash fruits and vegetables thoroughly under running water before peeling and cutting; cut away bruised areas.

- Wash tops of canned foods before opening. Wash can opener after each use with warm soapy water.

- During food preparation, do not taste the food with the same utensil used for stirring.

- **Never taste food that looks or smells strange!**

- Cook eggs until the whites are completely hard and the yokes begin to thicken. The yolk should no longer be runny but need not be hard.

Microwave Cooking

- Microwave cooking can leave cold spots in food where bacteria can survive. Rotate the dish a quarter turn once or twice during cooking if there is no turntable in the appliance.

- When heating leftovers, use a lid or vented plastic wrap for thorough heating; stir several times during reheating.

Grocery Shopping

- Check the *sell by* and *use by* dates.

- Check packaging date on fresh meats, poultry, and seafood. Check for off-odor and mold or insect contamination.

- Reject damaged, swollen, rusted, or deeply dented cans. Check that packaged and boxed foods are properly sealed.

Table 38.1. Specific Food Guidelines (*continued on next page*)

Food Groups	Allowed	Not Allowed
Dairy	All pasteurized, grade A milk and milk products	Unpasteurized or raw milk, cheese, yogurt, and other milk products
	Commercially-packaged cheese and cheese products made with pasteurized milk (i.e. mild and medium cheddar, mozzarella, parmesan, Swiss, etc.)	Cheeses from delicatessens
		Cheeses containing chili peppers or other uncooked vegetables
	Pasteurized yogurt	Cheese with molds (i.e. blue, Stilton, Roquefort, gorgonzola)
	Dry, refrigerated, and frozen pasteurized whipped topping	Sharp cheddar, brie, camembert, feta cheese, farmer's cheese
	Ice cream, frozen yogurt, sherbet, ice cream bars, homemade milkshakes	
	Commercial nutritional supplements and baby formulas, liquid and powdered	
Vegetables	All cooked frozen or canned vegetables	Raw vegetables, salads
		Caesar Salads with Caesar dressing
	All cooked herbs and spices (add at least 5 minutes before end of cooking)	Pepper
		Garnishes
		Uncooked herbs and spices
Fruits and Nuts	Canned and frozen fruit and fruit juices	Dried fruits
		Raw fruit; foods containing raw fruits
	Thick skinned fruits (oranges, bananas)	Unpasteurized fruit and vegetable juices
	Melons cut up and used immediately	
		Raw nuts
	Canned or bottled roasted nuts	
		Roasted nuts in the shell
	Nuts in baked products	
		Precut fresh fruits
	Commercially packaged peanut butter	

Table 38.1. Specific Food Guidelines (continued from page 453)

Food Groups	Allowed	Not Allowed
Bread, Grain, and Cereal Products	All breads, bagels, rolls, pancakes, sweet rolls, waffles, French toast	Raw grain products
	Potato chips, corn chips, tortilla chips, pretzels, popcorn	Bakery breads, cakes, donuts, muffins
	Cooked pasta, rice, and other grain	Potato/macaroni salad
	All cereals, cooked and ready-to-eat	
Entrees, Soups	All cooked entrees and soups	All miso products (i.e. miso soup)
Meat and Meat Substitutes	All well-cooked or canned meats (beef, pork, lamb, poultry, fish, shellfish, game, ham, bacon, sausage, hot dogs)	Raw or undercooked meat, poultry, fish, game, tofu
	Well-cooked eggs (white cooked firm with thickened yolk acceptable, i.e. hard boiled, over hard)	Meats and cold cuts from delicatessen
		Hard cured salami in natural wrap
	Pasteurized egg substitutes (i.e. Egg Beaters)	Cold smoked salmon, lox
		Pickled fish
	Commercially packaged salami, bologna, and other luncheon meats	Tempe (tempeh) products
	Canned and commercially-packaged hard smoked fish, refrigerated after opening	Sushi
		Raw oysters/clams
	Cooked tofu (which must be cut into 1" cubes or smaller and boiled a minimum of five minutes in water or broth before eating or using in recipes)	
Beverages	Tap water	Well water (unless tested yearly and found safe)
	Commercial bottled distilled and natural waters	Cold-brewed tea made with warm or cold water sun tea
	All canned, bottled, powdered beverages	Eggnog

(*Beverages continued on next page*)

Table 38.1. Specific Food Guidelines (*continued from page 454*)

Food Groups	Allowed	Not Allowed
Beverages (*continued*)	Instant and brewed coffee, tea; brewed tea made with boiling cold water	Fresh apple cider
		Homemade lemonade
	Brewed herbal teas using commercially-packaged tea bags	Spring water
	Commercial nutritional supplements, liquid and powdered	
Fats	Oil, shortening	Fresh salad dressings containing aged cheese (i.e. blue, Roquefort) or raw eggs, stored in refrigerated case
	Refrigerated lard, margarine, butter	
	Commercial shelf-stable mayonnaise and salad dressings (including cheese-based salad dressings, refrigerated after opening)	
Desserts	Refrigerated commercial and homemade cakes, pies, pastries, and pudding	Unrefrigerated cream-filled pastry products (not shelf-stable)
	Refrigerated cream-filled pastries	Cream or custard filled donuts
	Homemade and commercial cookies	
	Shelf-stable cream-filled cupcakes (i.e. Twinkies, Ding Dong), fruit pies (i.e. Pop tarts, Hostess fruit pies), and canned pudding	
Other	Salt, granulated sugar, brown sugar Jam, jelly, syrups (refrigerated after opening)	Raw or unpasteurized honey
	Commercially packaged (pasteurized) honey	Herbal and non-traditional (health food store) nutritional supplements, Chinese herbs
	Catsup, mustard, BBQ sauce, soy sauce, other condiments (refrigerated after opening)	Brewers yeast, if eaten uncooked
	Pickles, pickle relish, olives (refrigerated after opening)	

- Select unblemished fruits and vegetables.

- Avoid delicatessen foods.

- In the bakery, avoid unrefrigerated cream- and custard-containing desserts and pastries.

- Avoid foods from self-select, bulk containers.

- Avoid yogurt and ice cream products dispensed from soft-serve machines.

- Avoid tasting free food samples.

- Reject cracked, unrefrigerated eggs.

- Purchase frozen and refrigerated foods last, especially during the summer months.

- Store groceries promptly; never leave food in a hot car.

- Read labels for information about ingredients/cooking style.

Dining Out

- Eat early to avoid crowds.

- Select restaurants with a reputation for cleanliness.

- Check grades at restaurants; look for A with score in the 90s.

- Ask that food be prepared fresh in fast food establishments.

- Request single-serving condiment packages; avoid self-serve bulk condiment containers.

- Avoid high risk food sources: garnishes, salad bars, delicatessens, buffets and smorgasbords, potlucks, and sidewalk vendors.

Home Sanitation

- Have available liquid or bar hand soap for hand washing.

- Wash hands with soap and warm, running water before and after every step in food preparation.

- Wash hands before eating, especially when eating hand-held foods.

- Wash hands after using the rest room, handling garbage, and touching pets.

- Use paper towels for drying hands.

- Use separate cutting boards (plastic, glass, and wooden are acceptable) for cooked foods and raw foods.

- Wash cutting boards after each use in hot, soapy water or in the dishwasher. Boards are sanitized weekly using a solution of 1 part household bleach to 10 parts water.

- Keep appliances free of food particles.

- Check microwave oven, toaster, can openers, and blender and mixer blades. Blender blades and bottom should always be removed when washing the jar. Use bleach solution to sanitize these items.

- Keep counter and kitchen surfaces free of food particles.

- Replace dishcloths and dish towels daily.

- Replace sponges at least weekly.

- Sanitize dishcloths and sponges daily in a bleach solution.

- Do not store food under the sink. Do not store chemicals and cleaning solutions near food supplies.

- Use liquid dish soap when washing dishes and pans.

- Clean spills in refrigerator or freezer immediately; keep shelves and doors sanitized.

- Maintain refrigerator temperature between 34° F–40° F.

- Maintain freezer temperature to below 5° F.

- Store all food in covered containers after cooling. First, cool hot foods, uncovered, in the refrigerator; cover storage containers after cooling. Make sure that covers seal tightly.

- Discard eggs with cracked shells.

- Discard foods older than their *use by* expiration dates; discard all prepared foods after 72 hours (3 days).

- Discard entire food packages or containers with *any* mold present, including yogurt, cheese, cottage cheese, fruit, vegetables, jelly, and bread or pastry products.

- Discard freezer-burned foods.

- Discard without tasting any bulging, leaking, or cracked cans, or those deeply indented in the seam area.

- Rotate food stock so older items are used first. Monitor expiration dates.

- Make sure food storage areas remain reasonably clean; no obvious insect or rodent contamination should be evident.

- If home-canned foods are used, review the processing procedure to be sure it was appropriate for the pH of the food, size of bottle, and elevation above sea level. Look for mold and seals. If you suspect a home-canned food may not have been processed properly, if the lid bulges, or if the food has any bad odor or unusual characteristics after opening, **discard it**.

Thanks to Fred Hutchinson Cancer Research Center, Clinical Nutrition Department; and Swedish Medical Center, Nutrition Services Department.

Bone Marrow Transplant and Stem Cell Transplant Program
Duke University Medical Center
Box 3961
Durham NC 27710
Tel: 919-668-1002
Fax: 919-668-1091
Website: http://bmt.mc.duke.edu
E-mail: Duke_ABMT@mc.duke.edu

Chapter 39

Fatigue and Leukemia Treatment

Fatigue is described as an unusual tiredness that cannot be overcome by resting or a good night's sleep. Fatigue affects many patients with leukemia, lymphoma, Hodgkin's disease, and myeloma. These patients experience an excessive lack of energy or decreased ability to complete usual activities. Difficulty in talking, walking, concentrating, and making decisions may all be signs of fatigue.

There are reasons why many patients feel fatigue and there are ways in which patients can help themselves feel better. With the help of exercise, good nutrition, coping techniques, and a few changes in lifestyle, many patients can move from feeling fatigued to feeling more energetic or better able to deal with fatigue. This chapter answers some of the more common questions that patients may have about fatigue. Hopefully, learning about fatigue can help these patients improve energy levels and perform many of the daily activities they want and need to do.

Reasons for Fatigue

No one is exactly sure what causes fatigue. We do know it is often brought on by cancer and cancer treatments. Cancers like leukemia, lymphoma, and myeloma (blood-related cancers) can cause fatigue in the following ways.

"Understanding Fatigue," updated September 15, 2000 © The Leukemia & Lymphoma Society, Inc., reprinted with permission. For more information visit www.leukemia-lymphoma.org.

• Disease complications such as anemia (decreased red blood cells) and infections can deplete oxygen and nutrients from the body. The less oxygen or nutrition the body has, the less energy it will produce. Consequently, patients with blood-related cancers feel more tired or fatigued.

• Changes in daily routines brought about by a diagnosis of these cancers also contribute to fatigue. Working and sleeping patterns may change as patients must travel, keep up with appointments, and undergo medical exams and tests.

• The emotional stress of dealing with the diagnosis, and coping with anxiety and depression can contribute to sleeplessness, extra demands for energy, and fatigue.

• As cancer cells die, they release certain substances into the body that can cause fatigue. These substances, sometimes referred to as cytokines, can be toxic and lead to fatigue.

Feeling Fatigue after Treatment

Fatigue is often a side effect of many of the treatments for blood-related cancer. Patients say that this treatment-related fatigue is very intense, not necessarily associated with activity, and does not fully respond to rest.

• Drugs such as vincristine and vinblastine used in treatment of leukemia, lymphoma, and myeloma may cause fatigue because of their effects on the nervous system.

• Biological response modifiers (such as interferon used mostly in treatment of chronic myelogenous leukemia) can lead to severe fatigue during treatment and sometimes dosages may be limited.

• Fatigue that increases over time can result from radiation treatments for lymphoma, including Hodgkin's disease.

• Fatigue usually begins to decrease a few weeks after treatments end and will gradually go away in several months' time.

• Bone marrow transplants and peripheral stem cell transplants can take a great deal of energy from patients and their families. The treatment is long and severe and the resulting fatigue is also long-term and intense. Patients receiving these transplants experience fatigue both during and following transplants. Fatigue can extend for a long time, even years, after these treatments, although it will gradually decline over the months following the procedures.

What Can Be Done

Monitoring fatigue will give important insights into managing all of its manifestations. Patients should be alert to the signs of fatigue: tired legs, tired eyes, lack of concentration, weakness or sleepiness, irritability and impatience. Patients can keep a journal, writing down daily activities and noting energy and fatigue levels. A pattern will emerge that shows what may be contributing factors and how to tailor activities according to strengths. Do difficult tasks at times when energy is highest.

Treatment for Fatigue

One way to fight fatigue is to treat the underlying physical problems, such as anemia, infections, or treatment side effects, that cause fatigue.

If fatigue is related to anemia, for example, blood transfusions or medications designed to increase red blood cell production (Procrit) can be helpful. Patients should speak with their doctor about treatment with Procrit.

Methods to Control Fatigue

When there are no medical treatments for combating fatigue, there are methods for coping with it. These include nutrition, physical and other activities, rest, and psychological patterns. Patients should consult with their health care providers about the best type of diet and forms of exercise and activities.

Nutrition

- Eat a balanced diet including plenty of foods which supply iron and energy, such as green leafy vegetables and red meat. Maintain energy by eating more frequent, smaller meals or snacks throughout the day.

- Drink eight glasses of liquids a day to eliminate toxic substances associated with treatments that may cause fatigue.

- Get help with food preparation and shopping or contact home meal providers like Meals on Wheels to conserve energy for eating well.

Activities

- Think about things other than fatigue and illness. Listen to music, read a book, meet friends, watch a movie, go for a walk or a car ride.

- Focus on activities that can gradually build up strength and do not dramatically deplete energy. Light exercise such as walking is an activity that most people can do at some time and it actually decreases their fatigue.

- Keep an active mind and body. Do activities on a regular basis throughout the week.

Rest Patterns

- Reduce levels of activity. Many patients carry their previous energy levels in their mind. They should not feel that they must live up to this. They should learn to pace themselves and not feel guilt, stress, or anxiety when they cannot achieve certain goals.

- Rest when feeling tired. Learn to get more sleep during the night and rest for short periods during the day. Take naps, but don't let them interfere with nighttime sleep patterns.

- Ask others for help. Many family members, friends, charitable or senior citizen groups are able to help you. Ask for assistance with routine tasks such as shopping, housekeeping, laundry, and driving, and remember these other ways people can help you.

Psychological Patterns

- The negative effects of stress can be alleviated in many ways: exercise, relaxation techniques, visual imagery, meditation, spiritual practices, talking with others, and counseling.

- Many patients and their families find support groups to be very comforting. They gain answers to many questions and support for what they're going through.

Resources

Beyond Miracles: Living with Cancer. Stephen P. Hersh, M.D. Chicago: Contemporary Books, 1998.

Choices. Marion Morra and Eve Potts. New York: Avon Books, 1994.

Everyone's Guide to Cancer Therapy. Malin Dollinger, M.D., Ernest H. Rosenbaum, M.D., and Greg Cable. Kansas City: Somerville House Books Limited, 1994.

"Managing the Fatigue of Bone Marrow Transplant," Lillian M. Nail, PhD, RN, FAAN, and Carolyn W. Sutherland, MS, RN, OCN. *Home HealthCare Consultant*: Vol. 4, No. 4, April 1997, pp. 1-11.

Additional Information

The Leukemia & Lymphoma Society
1311 Mamaroneck Ave.
White Plains, NY 10605
Toll-Free: 800-955-4572
Tel: 914-949-5213
Fax: 914-949-6691
Website: www.leukemia-lymphoma.org

The Leukemia & Lymphoma Society can help with referrals to its support groups and its First Connection program which links newly diagnosed patients with similarly diagnosed survivors.

Chapter 40

Pain Control with Leukemia Treatment

Having cancer does not always mean having pain. For those with pain, there are many different kinds of medicines, ways to receive the medicine, and non-medicine methods that can relieve the pain you may have. You should not accept pain as a normal part of having cancer. When you are free of pain, you can sleep and eat better, enjoy the company of family and friends, and continue with your work and hobbies.

Important Facts about Cancer Pain Treatment

Only you know how much pain you have. Telling your doctor and nurse when you have pain is important. Not only is pain easier to treat when you first have it, but pain can be an early warning sign of the side effects of the cancer or the cancer treatment. Together—you, your nurse, and doctor—can talk about how to treat your pain. You have a right to pain relief, and you should insist on it.

Cancer Pain Can Almost Always Be Relieved.

There are many different medicines and methods available to control cancer pain. You should expect your doctor to seek all the information and resources necessary to make you as comfortable as possible. However, no one doctor can know everything about all medical problems. If you are in pain and your doctor suggests no other options,

Excerpts from "Pain Control: A Guide for People with Cancer and Their Families," National Cancer Institute (NCI), updated 11/21/2000.

ask to see a pain specialist or have your doctor consult with a pain specialist. Pain specialists may be oncologists, anesthesiologists, neurologists or neurosurgeons, other doctors, nurses, or pharmacists. A pain control team may also include psychologists and social workers.

If you have trouble locating a pain program or specialist, contact a cancer center, a hospice, or the oncology department at your local hospital or medical center. The National Cancer Institute's (NCI) Cancer Information Service (CIS) and other organizations can give you a list of pain management facilities. The American Cancer Society (ACS) and other organizations may also be able to provide names of pain specialists, pain clinics, or programs in your area.

Controlling Your Cancer Pain Is Part of the Overall Treatment for Cancer

Your doctor wants and needs to hear about what works and what doesn't work for your pain. Knowing about the pain will help your doctor better understand how the cancer and the treatment are affecting your body. Discussions about pain will not distract your doctor from treating the cancer.

Preventing Pain from Starting or Getting Worse Is the Best Way to Control It

Pain is best relieved when treated early. You may hear some people refer to this as staying on top of the pain. Do not try to hold off as long as possible between doses. Pain may get worse if you wait, and it may take longer, or require larger doses, for your medicine to give you relief.

Telling the doctor or nurse about pain is not a sign of weakness. You have a right to ask for pain relief.

Not everyone feels pain in the same way. There is no need to be stoic or brave if you have more pain than others with the same kind of cancer. In fact, as soon as you have any pain you should speak up. Remember, it is easier to control pain when it just starts rather than waiting until after it becomes severe.

People Who Take Cancer Pain Medicines, as Prescribed by the Doctor, Rarely Become Addicted to Them

Addiction is a common fear of people taking pain medicine. Such fear may prevent people from taking the medicine. Or it may cause family members to encourage you to hold off as long as possible between doses. Addiction is defined by many medical societies as uncontrollable drug craving, seeking, and use. When opioids (also known as narcotics)—the strongest pain relievers available—are taken for pain, they rarely cause addiction as defined here. When you are ready to stop taking opioids, the doctor gradually lowers the amount of medicine you are taking. By the time you stop using it completely, the body has had time to adjust. Talk to your doctor, nurse, or pharmacist about how to use pain medicines safely and about any concerns you have about addiction.

Most People Do Not Get High or Lose Control when They Take Cancer Pain Medicines as Prescribed by the Doctor

Some pain medicines can cause you to feel sleepy when you first take them. This feeling usually goes away within a few days. Sometimes you become drowsy because, with the relief of the pain, you are now able to catch up on the much needed sleep you missed when you were in pain. On occasion, people get dizzy or feel confused when they take pain medicines. Tell your doctor or nurse if this happens to you. Changing your dose or type of medicine can usually solve the problem.

Side Effects from Medicines Can Be Managed or Often Prevented

Some medicines can cause constipation, nausea and vomiting, or drowsiness. Your doctor or nurse can help you manage these side effects. These problems usually go away after a few days of taking the medicine. Many side effects can be managed by changing the medicine or the dose or times when the medicine is taken.

Your Body Does Not Become Immune to Pain Medicine

Stronger medicines should not be saved for later. Pain should be treated early. It is important to take whatever medicine is needed at the time. You do not need to save the stronger medicines for later. If your body gets used to the medicine you are taking, your medicine may not relieve the pain as well as it once did. This is called tolerance. Tolerance is not usually a problem with cancer pain treatment because the amount of medicine can be changed or other medicines can be added.

When pain is not treated properly, you may be:

- Tired

- Depressed

- Angry

- Worried

- Lonely

- Stressed

When cancer pain is managed properly, you can:

- Enjoy being active

- Sleep better

- Enjoy family and friends

- Improve your appetite

- Enjoy sexual intimacy

- Prevent depression

What Are the Different Types of Pain?

Pain may be acute or chronic. **Acute pain** is severe and lasts a relatively short time. It is usually a signal that body tissue is being injured in some way, and the pain generally disappears when the injury heals. **Chronic or persistent pain** may range from mild to severe, and it is present to some degree for long periods of time. Some people with chronic pain that is controlled by medicine can have **breakthrough pain**—this occurs when moderate to severe pain breaks through or is felt for a short time. It may occur several times a day, even when the proper dose of medicine is given for chronic and persistent pain.

What Causes Pain in People with Cancer?

The pain you feel may be from the cancer itself. Whether you have pain and the amount of pain you have may depend on the type of cancer, the stage (extent) of the disease, and your pain threshold (tolerance for pain). Most of the pain comes when a tumor presses on bones, nerves, or body organs. It can also be caused by the treatment or procedures for diagnosing cancer. Or you may have pain that has nothing to do with your illness or treatment. Like anyone, you can get headaches, muscle strains, and other aches and pains.

Pain from Procedures

Some methods used to diagnose cancer and to see how well the treatment is working are painful. If you and your doctors agree that a diagnostic procedure is necessary, concern about pain should not prevent you from having the procedure. Usually any pain you have during and after the procedure can be relieved. The needs of the person and the type of procedure to be done determine the kinds of medicine that can be given for the pain. You may be told that the pain from the procedure can't be avoided or that it won't last long. Even so, you should ask for pain medicine if you feel the need.

How Is Cancer Pain Treated?

Cancer pain is usually treated with medicine (also called analgesics) and with non-drug treatments such as relaxation techniques, biofeedback, imagery, and others. Ask your doctor, nurse, or pharmacist for advice before you take any medicine for pain. Medicines are safe when they are used properly. You can buy some effective pain relievers without a prescription or doctor's order. These medicines are also called nonprescription or over-the-counter (OTC) pain relievers. For others, a prescription from your doctor is necessary.

Developing a Plan for Pain Control

The first step in developing a plan is talking with your doctor, nurse, and pharmacist about your pain. You need to be able to describe your pain to your health professionals as well as to your family or friends. You may want to have your family or friends help you talk to your health professionals about your pain control, especially if you are too tired or in too much pain to talk to them yourself.

Using a pain scale is helpful in describing how much pain you are feeling. Try to assign a number from 0 to 10 to your pain level. If you have no pain, use a 0. As the numbers get higher, they stand for pain that is getting worse. A 10 means the pain is as bad as it can be.

You may wish to use your own pain scale using numbers from 0 to 5 or even 0 to 100. Be sure to let others know what pain scale you are using and use the same scale each time, for example, "My pain is a 7 on a scale of 0 to 10."

You can use a rating scale to describe:

- How bad your pain is at its worst.
- How bad your pain is most of the time.
- How bad your pain is at its least.
- How your pain changes with treatment.

Tell your doctor, nurse, pharmacist, and family or friends:

- Where you feel pain.
- What it feels like—sharp, dull, throbbing, steady.
- How strong the pain feels.
- How long it lasts.
- What eases the pain, what makes the pain worse.
- What medicines you are taking for the pain and how much relief you get from them.

Your doctor, nurse, and pharmacist may also need to know:

- What medicines you are taking now and what pain medicines you have taken in the past, including what has worked and not worked. You may want to record this information in a notebook.
- Any known allergies to medicines.

Questions to ask your doctor or nurse about pain medicine:

- How much medicine should I take? How often?
- If my pain is not relieved, can I take more? If the dose should be increased, by how much?
- Should I call you before increasing the dose?
- What if I forget to take it or take it too late?
- Should I take my medicine with food?
- How much liquid should I drink with the medicine?
- How long does it take the medicine to start working (called onset of action)?
- Is it safe to drink alcoholic beverages, drive, or operate machinery after I have taken pain medicine?

- What other medicines can I take with the pain medicine?

- What side effects from the medicine are possible and how can I prevent them?

Keeping Track of Details about the Pain

You may find it helpful to keep a record or a diary to track the pain and what works best to ease it. You can share this record with those caring for you. This will help them figure out what method of pain control works best for you. Your records can include:

- Words to describe the pain.

- Any activity that seems to be affected by the pain or that increases or decreases the pain.

- Any activity that you cannot do because of the pain.

- The name and the dose of the pain medicine you are taking.

- The times you take pain medicine or use another pain-relief method.

- The number from your rating scale that describes your pain at the time you use a pain-relief measure.

- Pain rating 1 to 2 hours after the pain-relief method.

- How long the pain medicine works.

- Pain rating throughout the day to record your general comfort.

- How pain interferes with your normal activities, such as sleeping, eating, sexual activity, or working.

- Any pain-relief methods other than medicine you use such as rest, relaxation techniques, distraction, skin stimulation, or imagery.

- Any side effects that occur.

What If I Need to Change My Pain Medicine?

If one medicine or treatment does not work, there is almost always another one that can be tried. Also, if a schedule or way that you are taking medicine does not work for you, changes can be made. Talk to your doctor or nurse about finding the pain medicine or method that works best for you. You may need a different pain medicine, a combination of pain medicines or a change in the dose of your pain medicines if:

471

- Your pain is not relieved.

- Your pain medicine does not start working within the time your doctor said it would.

- Your pain medicine does not work for the length of time your doctor said it would.

- You have breakthrough pain.

- You have side effects.

- You have serious side effects such as trouble breathing, dizziness, and rashes. Call your doctor right away if these occur. Side effects such as sleepiness, nausea, and itching usually go away after your body adjusts to the medication. Let your doctor know if these bother you.

- The schedule or the way you are taking the medicine does not work for you.

- Pain interferes with your normal activities, such as eating, sleeping, working, and sexual activity.

To help make the most of your pain control plan:

- Take your pain medicine on a regular schedule (by the clock) to help prevent persistent or chronic pain.

- Do not skip doses of your scheduled medicine. Once you feel the pain, it is harder to control.

- If you experience breakthrough pain, use your short-acting medicine as your doctor suggests. Don't wait for the pain to get worse—if you do, it may be harder to control.

- Be sure only one doctor prescribes your pain medicine. If another doctor changes your medicine, the two doctors should discuss your treatment with each other.

- Never take someone else's medicine. Medicines that worked for you in the past or that helped a friend or relative may not be right for you.

- Pain medicines affect different people in different ways. A very small dose may work for you, while someone else may need to take a much larger dose to obtain pain relief.

- Remember, your pain control plan can be changed at any time.

Medicines Used to Relieve Pain

The type of medicine and the method by which the medicine is given depend on the type and cause of pain. For example, constant, persistent pain is best relieved by methods that deliver a steady dose of pain medicine over a long period of time, such as a patch that is filled with medicine and placed on the skin (skin patch) or slow-release oral tablets. Following is an overview of the types of medicines used to relieve pain.

For Mild to Moderate Pain

Nonopioids: Acetaminophen and nonsteroidal anti-inflammatory drugs (NSAIDs), such as aspirin and ibuprofen. You can buy many of these over-the-counter (without a prescription). For others, you need a prescription. Check with your doctor before using these medicines. NSAIDs can slow blood clotting, especially if you are on chemotherapy.

For Moderate to Severe Pain

Opioids (also known as narcotics): Morphine, fentanyl, hydromorphone, oxycodone, and codeine. You need a prescription for these medicines. Nonopioids may be used along with opioids for moderate to severe pain.

For Breakthrough Pain

Rapid-Onset Opioids: Immediate-release oral morphine. You need a prescription for these medicines. A short-acting opioid, which relieves breakthrough pain quickly, needs to be used with a long-acting opioid for persistent pain.

For Tingling and Burning Pain

Antidepressants: Amitriptyline, nortriptyline, desipramine. You need a prescription for these medicines. Antidepressants are also prescribed to relieve some types of pain. Taking an antidepressant does not mean that you are depressed or have a mental illness.

Anticonvulsants (antiseizure medicines): Carbamazepine and phenytoin. You need a prescription for these medicines. Despite the name, anticonvulsants are used not only for convulsions, but also to control burning and tingling pain.

473

For Pain Caused by Swelling

Steroids: Prednisone, dexamethasone. A prescription is needed for these medicines. They are used to lessen swelling, which often causes pain.

How Is Pain Medicine Given?

Some people think that if their pain becomes severe, they will need to receive injections or shots. Actually, shots are rarely given to relieve cancer pain. There are many ways to get the medicine.

- **Orally**—medicine is given in a pill or capsule form.

- **Skin patch**—a bandage-like patch placed on the skin, which slowly but continuously releases the medicine through the skin for 2-3 days. One opioid medicine, fentanyl, is available as a skin patch. This form of medicine is less likely to cause nausea and vomiting.

- **Rectal suppositories**—medicine that dissolves in the rectum and is absorbed by the body.

- **Injections**
    - **Subcutaneous (SC) injection**—medicine is placed just under the skin using a small needle.

    - **Intravenous (IV) injection**—medicine goes directly into the vein through a needle.

    - **Intrathecal and epidural injections**—medicine is placed directly into the fluid around the spinal cord (intrathecal) or into the space around the spinal cord (epidural).

- **Pump: Patient-controlled analgesia (PCA)**—with this method, you can help control the amount of pain medicine you take. When you need pain relief, you can receive a preset dose of pain medicine by pressing a button on a computerized pump that is connected to a small tube in your body. The medicine is injected into the vein (intravenously), just under the skin (subcutaneously), or into the spinal area.

If your pain is not well controlled with one of the long-acting oral medicines, if you are having trouble taking pills, or if you are having irritating side effects, ask your doctor about trying one of the methods listed.

What Are the Side Effects of Pain Medicine?

Many side effects from pain medicine can be prevented. Some mild side effects that do occur, such as nausea, itching, or drowsiness, will usually go away after a few days as your body adjusts to the medicine. Let your doctor or nurse know if you are having these side effects and ask for help in controlling them.

More serious side effects of pain medicine are rare. As with the more common ones, they usually happen in the first few hours of treatment. They include trouble breathing, dizziness, and rashes. If you have any of these side effects, you should call your doctor right away.

You usually cannot take aspirin, ibuprofen, and other NSAIDs when you are on chemotherapy.

Chapter 41

Long-Term and Late Effects of Leukemia Treatments

Chapter Contents

Section 41.1

Long-Term and Late Effects of Chemotherapy and Radiation

This section describes some of the long-term and late risks associated with treatment with chemotherapy and radiation. These treatments save lives. People with blood-related cancers (such as leukemias, lymphomas, and myeloma) are among those that benefit from chemotherapy and radiation therapy use. Unfortunately, chemotherapy treatments can also cause long-term or late side effects that can complicate or delay the drug's effectiveness. As with chemotherapy, there are side effects of radiation therapy. Patients need to understand this idea of risk vs. benefit when it comes to considering treatment options.

Research is now being conducted to minimize the adverse effects for specific chemotherapy drugs and radiation doses. Studies like these can help guide changes in therapy that will maintain cure rates while improving quality of life for long-term survivors.

Long Term and Late Effects of Treatment

Long-term effects are known or expected medical problems that may occur in some persons who have received certain treatments; for example, the very low risk of infection after splenectomy. Late-effects are secondary conditions that arise as a result of having received certain cancer treatments: for example, leukemia secondary to certain chemoradiotherapy treatments for lymphoma or myeloma. Both adults and children experience long-term and late-effects of therapy for leukemia, lymphoma, and myeloma.

Children

Children may experience medical problems and secondary conditions as a result of treatment mostly for acute leukemia, chronic myelogenous leukemia, Hodgkin's disease, and non-Hodgkin's lymphoma. These include:

- *Learning Disabilities:* Intrathecal and intravenous methotrexate and/or radiation to the brain can sometimes cause damage to the central nervous system. Some children can develop learning disabilities which can start immediately or several years after treatment. Typically, poor performance is noted in mathematics, spatial relationships, problem solving, attention span, and concentration skills.

- *Problems with Growth:* It is generally believed that 2400 rads or more of cranial spinal radiation can stop or slow the growth of children. Children who receive total body irradiation prior to bone marrow transplantation may also experience delayed growth. The brain contains the hypothalamus and pituitary gland, which control many body processes including growth and reproduction. Dental abnormalities are a side effect of treatments, including radiation and bone marrow transplantation. These include failure of the teeth to develop, arrested root development, unusually small teeth, and enamel abnormalities.

- *Endocrine and Reproductive Impairment:* Some young children who receive radiation to the brain do not experience puberty at the appropriate age. A very small percentage experience premature puberty. On the other hand, puberty in some children is significantly delayed. Boys treated with Cytoxan or radiation to the testes may have abnormal testosterone levels and sperm counts. Older teenage girls are susceptible to ovarian damage from chemotherapy.

Ability to have a normal sex life is not affected. Most survivors of leukemia and other childhood cancers go on to have normal fertility and healthy offspring; however, some are unable to have children.

- *Thyroid deficiency:* Children who receive total body irradiation prior to bone marrow transplantation may have low thyroid function. An underactive thyroid can also develop in patients receiving chest and neck radiation therapy for Hodgkin's disease.

- *Cardiovascular Disorders:* Heart problems (heart muscle injury, chronic heart failure) may occur months or decades after treatment with anthracyclines (adriamycin, idarubicin or daunomycin), high doses of cyclophosphamide, or chest irradiation. The heart muscle damage is usually related to the cumulative dose of anthracyclines, many of which are used to treat acute myelogenous leukemia. High-dose cyclophosphamide, part of the preconditioning regimen for bone marrow transplantation, can contribute to chronic heart failure. Children appear to have less tolerance to doses of multiple chemotherapeutic agents than adults and when chest radiation is combined with these chemotherapeutic agents, the risk of heart failure is possible at lower doses of the drugs.

Adults

- *Heart Muscle Injury and Heart Failure:* Heart muscle damage is associated most commonly with high total doses of the anthracycline drugs. High-dose cyclophosphamide, used in transplant regimens, can contribute to heart failure.

- *Lung Tissue Injury:* Alkylating agents, methotrexate, and nitrosoureas can lead to lung scarring and to shortness of breath in some individuals. Radiation therapy for patients with Hodgkin's disease and non-Hodgkin's lymphoma can also result in lung damage. Improved techniques have been developed for shielding patients from radiation. These medical problems can also be experienced by long-term survivors of bone marrow transplants.

- *Endocrine and Reproductive Impairment:* Patients receiving radiation therapy to the head and neck region can develop an underactive thyroid. This is a particular risk in patients receiving chest and neck radiation therapy for Hodgkin's disease. Improved techniques have been developed for shielding patients from radiation.

Fertility can be impaired by certain chemotherapy agents and radiation therapy. Menopause may start earlier than usual in women.

Secondary Leukemia and Solid Tumors

- *Secondary acute myelogenous leukemia* may occur as a result of intensive therapy with radiation and chemotherapy. This type of leukemia is very resistant to treatment and cure.

Children treated with etoposide, mostly for acute lymphocytic leukemia, are at risk of developing secondary acute myelogenous leukemia.

Lymphoma survivors may develop secondary leukemia years after treatment.

* *Solid tumors:* Leukemia and lymphoma survivors treated with chemotherapy or radiation are also at risk for solid tumors. Solid tumors appear in adolescents after treatment for Hodgkin's disease. Non-Hodgkin's lymphoma has been reported as a late complication in patients treated for Hodgkin's disease or myeloma. Patients who have received radiation therapy for Hodgkin's disease have an increased risk of breast cancer, osteosarcoma, and lung cancer. Young women who received radiation to the chest as part of their Hodgkin's disease treatment should receive annual mammograms and biannual breast exams, starting a decade after their treatment.

Talk with your doctor about these possible side effects, as well as your individual concerns, whenever you consider chemotherapy or radiation therapy as a treatment option.

Additional Information

The Leukemia and Lymphoma Society
1311 Mamaroneck Ave.
White Plains, NY 10605
Toll-Free: 800-955-4572
Tel: 914-949-5213
Fax: 914-949-6691
Website: www.leukemia-lymphoma.org

Office of Cancer Survivorship
Division of Cancer Control and Population Services
National Cancer Institute
6130 Executive Blvd.
Executive Plaza North
Rockville, MD 20852
Tel: 301-594-6776
Fax: 301-594-6787
http://dccps.nci.nih.gov/ocs

Section 41.2

Long-Term Complications for Some Childhood Cancer Survivors

"Childhood Cancer Survivors: While in General Good Health, Past Treatments Result in Long-Term Complications for Some," © May 14, 2002, University of Minnesota Cancer Center, reprinted with permission.

Investigators from a national collaborative effort to study survivors of childhood cancer presented results from six separate studies at the American Society of Clinical Oncology (ASCO) meeting in Orlando, Florida on May 19, 2002. Results from the Childhood Cancer Survivor Study (CCSS) have found that the majority of survivors of childhood cancer report overall general good health, but the therapies that were used to cure some survivors may put them at increased risk for long-term complications, including pulmonary function, obesity, physical limitations, reduced quality of life, depression, and special educational needs.

"We are pleased to find that survivors are reporting general good health," said the project's principal investigator, Les Robison, Ph.D., professor of pediatrics and associate director of the University of Minnesota Cancer Center. "Identifying potential complications that can arise from childhood cancer treatments, however, gives health professionals and survivors information that can be important to their health many years after their diagnosis and treatment."

The CCSS, funded by the National Cancer Institute, consists of investigators from 25 medical centers in the United States and Canada and is coordinated by investigators at the University of Minnesota Cancer Center. CCSS investigators gathered information from more than 14,000 study participants who were diagnosed with cancer between 1970 and 1986, before reaching the age of 21. Each participant has been recruited through one of the participating centers, where he or she was diagnosed and/or treated. The study requires that all participants must have survived at least five years from their initial cancer diagnosis. The information CCSS investigators gather is being used to develop prevention strategies and assess follow-up needs.

CCSS investigator Melissa Hudson, MD, of St. Jude Children's Research Hospital presented recent results indicating that the majority of survivors over the age of 18 years reported that they considered their general health to be good, with only 11 percent reporting their general health to be fair or poor, and 12 percent reporting experiencing major medical conditions. Female survivors were found to be at higher risk of impaired health including mental health, anxiety, and physical activity. Survivors of brain tumors, Hodgkin's disease, bone tumor, and soft tissue sarcoma were at highest risk for adverse health outcomes.

Research headed by Ann Mertens, Ph.D., of the University of Minnesota Cancer Center has revealed that pulmonary complications resulting from some forms of chemotherapy and radiation used to treat childhood cancers can occur months to years after treatment. Childhood cancer survivors reported significantly higher occurrence of lung fibrosis, emphysema, pneumonia, pleurisy, and need for supplemental oxygen compared to sibling controls.

An evaluation headed by Kevin Oeffinger, MD, of the University of Texas, Southwestern, reveals that survivors of childhood acute lymphoblastic leukemia are significantly more likely to be overweight or obese when compared to siblings. Female survivors treated with cranial radiation before the age of five years were four times more likely to be obese, while male survivors were twice as likely to have a body mass index of greater than 30. These results indicate that some leukemia survivors may be at increased risk of experiencing cardiovascular and other obesity-related complications later in life.

Researchers led by Raj Nagarajan, MD, of the University of Minnesota Cancer Center have evaluated the long-term physical function and quality of life of survivors of childhood bone tumors, some of whom underwent amputation and some who had limb-sparing surgery. Among the survivors followed an average of 20 years after their diagnosis and surgery, no significant differences were observed among those treated with amputation or no amputation. Female survivors and those diagnosed and treated at older ages were found to score lower on measures of physical function and quality of life.

Brad Zebrack, Ph.D., of the UCLA School of Medicine reported the results of an investigation of psychological outcomes in long-term survivors of childhood leukemia and lymphoma. This study revealed that the majority of survivors are psychologically healthy. However, when compared to sibling controls, survivors were found to have a significantly increased risk for reporting depressive symptoms and symptoms indicating somatic distress. Increasing intensity of cancer chemotherapy was found to add to the risk of these symptoms.

Pauline Mitby, M.P.H., from the University of Minnesota Department of Pediatrics evaluated the utilization of special education services and education attainment among long-term survivors of childhood cancer. She and her colleagues report that 23 percent of childhood cancer survivors were enrolled in special education programs compared to 8 percent of siblings and that survivors treated with cranial radiation or chemotherapy directed to the central nervous system were more likely to utilize special educational services, particularly female survivors.

The University of Minnesota Cancer Center is a National Cancer Institute-designated Comprehensive Cancer Center. Awarded more than $68 million in peer-reviewed grants during fiscal year 2001, the center conducts cancer research that advances knowledge and enhances care. The center also engages community outreach and public education efforts addressing cancer.

Additional Information

University of Minnesota
Cancer Center
Mayo Mail Code 806
420 Delaware Street SE
Minneapolis, MN 55455
Toll-Free: 888-226-2376
Tel: 612-624-8484
Fax: 612-626-3069
Website: www.cancer.umn.edu
E-mail: info@cancer.umn.edu

Chapter 42

Minimal Residual Disease: Gauging the Risk of Leukemia Relapse

Measurement of Minimal Residual Disease Is the Key

Almost all children who are treated for acute lymphocytic leukemia (ALL) enter complete remission. However, nearly one-fourth of these patients subsequently experience relapse and have a poor prognosis. Many relapses may be preventable if at-risk patients can be identified early and given more intensive therapy. St. Jude physician-researcher Dario Campana and his colleagues have developed a test that sensitively monitors each patient's response to treatment and gauges the risk of impending relapse. St. Jude is the first institution to use the measurement of minimal residual disease to guide therapy on front-line leukemia protocols. This interview included Dario Campana, MD with hematologist-oncologist Torrey Sandlund, MD talking about this exciting advance in leukemia treatment.

What Is Minimal Residual Disease?

It's the presence of leukemic cells in numbers so small that they can't be detected microscopically. Although microscopic examination of the bone marrow has traditionally been used to identify remission, it can't detect levels of leukemic infiltration below 1%, or one leukemic cell in 100 normal bone marrow cells. Thus, patients may be in

"Gauging the Risk of Leukemia Relapse," *St. Jude Rounds*, Fall 1999
© St. Jude Children's Research Hospital, reprinted with permission.

remission by traditional criteria but still have a tumor burden as large as 1010 malignant cells. These patients are said to have minimal residual disease, or MRD.

Why Is Minimal Residual Disease Important?

Until recently, the significance of residual leukemic cells was controversial. However, our research (published in *Lancet*, 21 Feb, 1998) showed that residual disease is a powerful indicator of the response to therapy and the risk of relapse.

How Are Residual Leukemic Cells Detected?

We use two methods for testing bone marrow samples. One is automated flow cytometry, which distinguishes leukemic cells from normal cells by their combination of cellular antigens. The other method, polymerase chain reaction (PCR), recognizes genetic sequences that are unique to the leukemic cells. Either method can detect a leukemic infiltration as small as 0.01%, or one malignant cell among 10,000 normal cells.

How Many Patients Whose Disease Is in Remission Have Residual Leukemia?

When we measured MRD at specific points during treatment for ALL, we discovered that almost one-fourth of patients had residual disease when they entered clinical remission. The frequency of residual leukemia fell to 17% at week 14 of continuation therapy, then to 5% at week 32 and to zero at week 120, when therapy was complete.

When Is Residual Leukemia Clinically Significant?

In general, the presence of MRD at any point during remission is associated with an increased risk of subsequent relapse, regardless of other prognostic features. The higher the level of MRD, the greater the risk. For example, a high level of MRD at week 14 of continuation therapy has consistently predicted subsequent relapse, despite remission at the time of measurement. MRD that persists is also an ominous sign. Children who have residual leukemia that continues beyond month 6 of continuation therapy have an extremely poor prognosis.

Can MRD Studies Indicate a Good Prognosis as Well as a Poor One?

Definitely. Patients who have no residual leukemia at the end of remission induction therapy have a 90% chance of survival without relapse, which is very good news. Even patients who do have MRD at that point have a good chance of staying in remission if the residual leukemia disappears with continued treatment. These patients need ongoing MRD surveillance as treatment progresses, to gauge how well their residual leukemia is responding to therapy.

How Is MRD Testing Being Used to Guide Treatment?

At St. Jude, therapy is now being tailored to the risk of relapse predicted by MRD studies. For example, a child may have ALL that is classified as low-risk disease by its features at presentation. However, if the child has residual leukemia at the end of remission induction therapy, the disease is reclassified as higher-risk and a longer, much more intensive course of treatment is given. If residual disease persists after the third month of continuation therapy and there are other very high-risk features, alternative therapies such as bone marrow transplantation are then considered.

Why Has MRD Testing Not Been Used Previously to Guide Therapy?

Although MRD testing has been technically feasible for years, there were two fundamental obstacles to its use in treatment protocols. First, its clinical significance had to be proved, and we have accomplished that. Second, it had to be applicable to all patients with ALL. Flow cytometry can be used for only about 75% of patients, and PCR methods work for about 85% of patients. Once we established that the two methods could be used in tandem to reliably test all patients, MRD assays were ready for clinical use.

Will MRD Testing Help to Improve the Cure Rate for Children with ALL?

That is our expectation. The cure rate is now at an all-time high. We should be able to improve it further by using this new understanding of the relationship between residual disease and relapse to adjust therapy as needed and offset the risk of recurrence.

Other Potential Uses of Minimal Residual Disease Testing

- Detection of malignant cells in bone marrow or peripheral blood autographs

- Assessment of the efficacy of procedures used to remove malignant cells from autografts

- Detection of malignant cells that are morphologically identical to normal hematopoietic precursors

- Substantiation of CNS involvement in patients who have leukemia

Chapter 43

Support for People with Cancer and the People Who Care about Them

"A diagnosis of cancer is a powerful stimulus against procrastinating on warm and kindly or beautiful things, a reminder that many of the material things aren't all that urgent after all. Take time to watch the sunset with someone you love; there may not be another as lovely for the two of you." These are the thoughts of a woman with cancer who needed to share her feelings with someone who would care and who could understand.

This chapter is written for those affected by cancer: you, someone in your family, or someone very close to you. The main emphasis is on what the people who live with cancer in their own lives and their own homes think, feel, and do to cope with the disease.

No two people with cancer are alike as are no two relatives or friends of people with cancer. Although the material in this chapter is intended to be helpful, some sections may not apply to certain circumstances; a few might suggest responses that make you feel uncomfortable. Each person has to cope with cancer in an individual way. What follows is intended as a guide: a brief look at how some people with cancer and their loved ones feel and the ways they found to deal with those feelings.

Perhaps, if we explore together our emotions—a side of cancer that neither surgery, drugs, nor radiation can treat—we can help each other dispel some of those feelings. People with cancer, dear friends,

Excerpts from "Taking Time: Support for People with Cancer and the People Who Care about Them," National Cancer Institute (NCI).

and family members face intense fears, anxieties, and frustrations that are new to many of us, although others have taken the journey we now begin. We travel a road paved with an awesome mingling of hope and despair, courage and fear, humor and anger, and constant uncertainty.

Perhaps, sharing the experiences of those who have walked the road before will help us define our own feelings and find our own ways of coping. Our bodies and minds are not completely separate. It will help us keep our bodies strong if we also deal successfully with the emotional turmoil of cancer.

Cancer is undeniably a major illness; it is not necessarily fatal. Over 7 million Americans alive today have a history of cancer. For them cancer has become a chronic condition, somewhat like hypertension, diabetes, or a mild heart condition. As is true for others with chronic conditions, periodic health checkups will be part of their lifelong routine. They will, undeniably, be more sensitive to, and anxious about, minor signs of illness or discomfort. Unlike others with chronic disease, they most likely will not need lifelong medication or special diets to remind them daily that they once were ill. Many will live for years, grow old, and die much as they had expected to do before cancer was diagnosed. It is hard not to think about dying, but it's important to concentrate on living.

Sharing the Diagnosis

- Cancer can be unutterably lonely. No one should try to bear it alone.

- Patient, family, and friends usually learn the diagnosis sooner or later. Most people find it easier for all if everybody can share their feelings instead of hiding them. This frees people to offer each other support.

- Patients usually agree that hiding the diagnosis from them denies them the right to make important choices about their life and their treatment.

- Families say patients who try to keep the diagnosis secret rob loved ones of the chance to express that love and to offer help and support.

- Family members and intimate friends also bear great emotional burdens and should be able to share them openly with each other and the patient.

- Even children should be told. They sense when something is amiss, and they may imagine a situation worse than it really is.

- The patient might want to tell the children directly, or it may be easier to have a close friend or loving relative do so.

- The children's ages and emotional maturity should be a guide in deciding how much to tell. The goal is to let children express their feelings and ask questions about the cancer.

- By sharing the diagnosis, patient, family, and friends build foundations of mutual understanding and trust.

One question many people ask after diagnosis is "Should I tell?" Perhaps not. A family member could be too old, too young, or too emotionally fragile to accept the diagnosis, but people are surprisingly resilient. Most find ways to deal with the reality of illness and the possibility of death—even when it involves those they love most. They find the strength to bounce back from situations that seem to cause unbearable grief.

The way in which people differ is in the speed with which they bounce back. The diagnosis of cancer hits most of us with a wave of shock, of fright, of denial. Each person needs a different amount of time to pull themselves together and to deal with the reality of cancer. In reading the sections that follow, you should remember that only you really know your emotional timetable. Think about sharing at a time when you are ready to do so.

Sharing Feelings

- Some in the family are able to absorb the impact of diagnosis sooner than others. This can create clashing needs as some wish to talk and some need to be private and introspective.

- Verbal and nonverbal clues help determine when is a good time to discuss the illness and how each will learn to live with it.

- If family members cannot help each other, other emotional support systems are available in the form of support groups or professional counselors.

- The person with cancer has the primary right to set the timetable for when he or she is ready to talk. Others can encourage that readiness through their love and continued presence.

- Talking may include expressing anger, fear, and inner confusion.

- False cheeriness—the "everything will be all right" routine—denies the person with cancer the opportunity to discuss fears and anxieties.

- Emphasizing the uniqueness of each person, positive test results, or good response to treatment is true support, both valid and valuable.

- The person with cancer needs family or friends as a constant in a changing world. "I'm here," offers great reserves of support.

Sometimes, the whole family suspects the truth before the diagnosis is made. Someone recognizes the symptoms, or the family doctor seems overly concerned. Nonetheless, hearing those words, tumor... cancer... leukemia, we are stunned as we never may have been in our lives. It is often impossible to take in the diagnosis immediately. We hear it, but somehow we don't believe it. This is normal. People's minds have a wonderful capacity for absorbing information only as they are ready to accept it.

Coping within the Family

- Cancer is a blow to every family it touches. How it is handled is determined to a great extent by how the family has functioned as a unit in the past.

- Problems within the family can be the most difficult to handle; you cannot go home to escape them.

- Adjusting to role changes can cause great upheavals in the way family members interact.

- Performing too many roles at once endangers anyone's emotional well-being and ability to cope. Examine what tasks are necessary and let others slide.

- Consider hiring professional nurses or homemakers. Financial costs need to be compared with the physical and emotional cost of shouldering the load alone.

- Children may need special attention. They need comfort, reassurance, affection, guidance, and discipline at times of disruption in their routine.

Although cancer has come out of the closet, much of what we read in newspapers and magazines is about the disease itself—its probable causes or new methods of treatment. There is little information about how families deal with cancer on a day-to-day basis. This gap reinforces feelings that families coping with cancer are isolated from the rest of the world: that everyone else is managing nicely while you flounder with your feelings, hide from your spouse, and are incapable of talking to the children.

Cancer is a blow to every family it touches. How you handle it is determined to a great extent by how you have functioned as a family in the past. Families who are used to sharing their feelings with each other usually are able to talk about the disease and the changes it brings. Families in which each member solves problems alone or in which one person has played the major role in making decisions might have more difficulty coping.

The Health of the Family

The San Diego chapter of *Make Today Count*, a mutual support group for patients and families, compiled a "Bill of Rights for the Friends and Relatives of Cancer Patients." Several items address the problems of family burdens:

- The relative of a cancer patient has the right and obligation to take care of his own needs. Even though he may be accused of being selfish, he must do what he has to do to keep his own peace of mind, so that he can better minister to the needs of the patient.

- Each person will have different needs. These needs must be satisfied. The patient will benefit, too, by having a more cheerful person to care for him.

- The relative may need help from outsiders in caring for the patient. Although the patient may object to this, the relative has the right to assess his own limitations of strength and endurance and to obtain assistance when required.

- When the relative knows that he is already doing all that can reasonably be expected of anyone in caring for the patient, he can have a clear conscience in maintaining contacts with the rest of the world.

- If the patient attempts to use his illness as a weapon, the relative has the right to reject that and to do only what can reasonably be expected of him.

493

- If the cancer patient's relative responds only to the genuine needs of the moment—both his own needs and those of the patient—the stress associated with the illness can be minimized.

Increased burdens and shifting responsibilities can occur whether the patient in the household is a spouse, a child, or an elderly parent. Each family member must take care to meet his or her own needs and those of the other healthy members of the family as well as those of the patient.

When You Need Assistance

When cancer develops, many people need to learn to ask for and accept outside help for the first time. These are good ways to begin:

- Take time to ask medical questions of your doctor, nurse specialists, therapists, and technologists.

- Make lists of questions. Write or tape record the answers. Take someone else along as a second listener.

- Ask your physician to suggest other doctors if you wish a second opinion on your diagnosis before deciding on treatment.

- Ask your physician about alternative treatments if you have questions about them.

- Physicians wait for clues from their patients to determine how much to say. Let your doctor know whether you want to know everything at once or in stages.

- Remember that there is a difference between a physician who does not know that cancer need not be fatal and one who will not promise you a miracle.

- Trust and rapport between patient and physician are important; you must be able to work together to treat the cancer most effectively.

- Your physician, hospital, library, the National Cancer Institute or affiliated Cancer Information Service offices, and local chapters of the American Cancer Society are good sources of facts about cancer. Many also can provide the names of local support and service organizations established to help you cope with the emotional stresses of the disease.

- Emotional assistance takes many forms. Counseling or psychiatric therapy for individuals, for groups of patients, and for families often is available through the hospital or within the community.

- Many groups have been established by patients and their families to share practical tips and coping skills. One may be right for you.

- Your minister or rabbi, a sympathetic member of the congregation, or a specially trained pastoral counselor may be able to help you find spiritual support.

Which one of us did not feel that the world had stopped turning when cancer struck? But somehow each day goes on. During the period of active treatment a pressing number of decisions need to be made, questions must be answered, and arrangements handled.

The stress of handling such responsibilities can be enormous. A new kind of communication and acceptance becomes necessary: asking for and accepting outside help, which is an entirely new role for some. People who were raised to believe that going it alone indicated maturity and strength now might have to overcome their distaste for appearing to be in anything less than total control.

Selves and Self-Image

- Cancer treatment can extend over weeks or months; side effects may come and go.

- Side effects can make you feel rotten, even make you think the cancer has returned.

- The known is less frightening than the unknown. Learn about your cancer, its treatment, and how to treat possible side effects.

- Fears and anxieties caused by cancer can affect a sexual relationship. Remember: Cancer is not catching. Also, cancer or other chronic illnesses are rarely the cause for infidelity in a good relationship.

- Treatment might make you feel uncomfortable about your body and sexually unattractive. Open discussion of these feelings with your mate is very important.

- Intangible personal qualities make up a great part of your attraction for your mate. These have not changed with treatment.

495

- Spouses sometimes hesitate to initiate physical contact. Support, love, and affection do include hugs and caresses. These may lead the partner with cancer to feel more comfortable about sexual intimacy.

- Physical exercise improves body image and feelings of well-being.

- Taking on new hobbies and learning new skills can bolster your good feelings about yourself.

- Reconstructive surgery and well-made prostheses help some people overcome physical disabilities and emotional distress.

- If you cannot seem to regain good feelings about yourself, seek professional counseling or therapy.

- If your relationship is endangered by the stress of cancer, get professional help. You need each other at this time.

The World Outside

- Some friends will deal well with your illness and provide gratifying support.

- Some will be unable to cope with the possibility of death and will disappear from your life.

- Most will want to help but may be uncomfortable and unsure of how to go about it. Help your friends support you:

- Ask yourself, "Have friends deserted me or have I withdrawn from them?"

- Telephone those who don't call you.

- Ask for simple assistance—to run an errand, prepare a meal, or visit. These small acts bring friends back into contact and help them feel useful and needed.

- If you are alone, ask your physician, social worker, or pastor to match you with another patient. Someone else needs friendships, too.

- Groups of other cancer patients can offer new friendships, understanding, support, and companionship.

- When you return to work, coworkers, like others, may shun you, support you, or wait for your cues on how to respond.

- There are laws to protect you against job discrimination.

Anyone who has been affected intimately by cancer knows that it can change the pattern of our relationships outside the family as well as those within. Friends react as they do to other difficult situations. Some handle it well; others are unable to maintain any association at all. Casual acquaintances, and even strangers, can cause unintended pain by asking thoughtless questions about visible scars, artificial devices, or other noticeable changes in appearance.

One or two people within your circle may be gratifying in their devotion and in the sensitivity they show toward your needs. One woman said her mother-in-law found one or two close friends with whom she felt truly relaxed. They were not startled when she laughed nor ill at ease when she cried. With others she maintained an outward calm.

"I have three really good friends with whom I can talk about my cancer," explained another. "I have talked about dying with my sister, and she does understand a lot more than I thought a person without cancer could."

Living Each Day

- Each person must work through, in his or her own way, feelings of possible death, fear, and isolation. Returning to normal routines as much as possible often helps.

- Give the pleasures and responsibilities of each day the attention they deserve.

- Responsible pursuits keep life meaningful; recreation keeps it zesty. Fill your life with both.

- Remember the difference between doing and overdoing. Rest is important to both physical and emotional strength.

- It's harder to bolster one's will to live if you are alone. Yet many have acted as their own cheering squad and have found ways to lead meaningful lives.

- Family members must not make an invalid of a person with cancer who is fully capable of physical activity and responsible participation in the family.

- Family members should not equate physical incapability with mental failing. It is especially important that an ill patient feel a necessary part of the family.

- Families must guard against rehearsing how they will act if the patient dies by excluding him or her from family affairs now.

497

Whether the outlook for recovery is good or poor, the days go by, one at a time, and patient and family must learn to live each one. It's not always easy. On learning the diagnosis, some decide that death is inevitable, and there is nothing to do but give up and wait. They are not the first to feel that way.

Orville Kelly, a newspaperman, described his initial battle with the specter of death. "I began to isolate myself from the rest of the world. I spent much time in bed, even though I was physically able to walk and drive. I thought about my own impending funeral and it made me very sad."

These feelings continued from his first hospitalization through the first outpatient chemotherapy treatment. On the way home from that treatment, he was haunted by memories of the happy past, when everything was all right. Then it occurred to Kelly, "I wasn't dead yet. I was able to drive my automobile. Why couldn't I return home to barbecue ribs?"

He did, that very night. He began to talk to his wife and children about his fears and anxieties. And he became so frustrated at the feelings he had kept locked up inside himself that he wrote the newspaper article that led to the founding of "Make Today Count," the mutual help organization for cancer patients and their families.

Each person must work through individual feelings of possible death, fear, and isolation in his or her own good time. It is hard to overcome these feelings if they are never confronted head on, but it is an ongoing struggle. One day brings feelings of confidence, the next day despair. Many people find it helps considerably if they strive to return, both as individuals and as a family, to their normal lives.

Each day brings pleasures and responsibilities totally outside the realm of cancer. We should try to give each the attention it deserves. These are the threads of the fabric that enfolds our lives. They give it color and meaning.

The days can be more valuable if you can learn to enjoy common moments as well as memorable occasions. This is true whether you have weeks or years left. It is true, in fact, whether you have a life threatening disease or not. Physical well being is closely tied to emotional well being. The time you take out from attending to cancer strengthens you for the time you must devote to it.

The Years After

Cancer is not something anyone forgets. Anxieties remain as active treatment ceases and the waiting stage begins. A cold or a cramp may be cause for panic. As 6-month or annual checkups approach, you swing between hope and anxiety. As you wait for the mystical 5-year or 10-year point, you might feel more anxious rather than more secure.

These are feelings we all share. No one expects you to forget that you have had cancer or that it might recur. Each must seek individual ways of coping with the underlying insecurity of not knowing the true state of his or her health. The best prescription seems to lie in a combination of one part challenging responsibilities that command a full range of skills, a dose of activities that seek to fill the needs of others, and a generous dash of frivolity and laughter.

You still might have moments when you feel as if you live perched on the edge of a cliff. They will sneak up unbidden. But they will be fewer and farther between if you have filled your mind with thoughts other than cancer.

Cancer might rob you of that blissful ignorance that once led you to believe that tomorrow stretched forever. In exchange, you are granted the vision to see each today as precious, a gift to be used wisely and richly. No one can take that away.

Part Six

Additional Help and Information

Chapter 44

Glossary of Important Leukemia-Related Terms

Accelerated phase. The middle phase of chronic myeloid leukemia that lasts from six to 18 months. The white blood cell count increases as the disease is harder to control with conventional treatments. [1]

Acute leukemia. A rapidly progressing cancer of the bone marrow and other blood-forming tissues. [1]

Antigens. Substances that cause the immune system to make a specific immune response. [2]

Benign (beh-NINE). Not cancerous; does not invade nearby tissue or spread to other parts of the body. [2]

Biological therapy (by-o-LAHJ-i-kul). Treatment to stimulate or restore the ability of the immune system to fight infections and other diseases. Also used to lessen side effects that may be caused by some cancer treatments. Also known as immunotherapy, biotherapy, or biological response modifier (BRM) therapy. [2]

Blasts. Immature blood cells. [1]

Terms presented in this glossary were excerpted from "Living with Leukemia," *FDA Consumer* magazine, March-April 2002, U.S. Food and Drug Administration (terms marked [1] are from this document); and "Young People with Cancer: A Handbook for Parents," National Cancer Institute (NCI), NIH Publication No. 01-2378, revised January 2001 (terms marked [2] are from this document).

503

Blast crisis. The final phase of chronic myeloid leukemia, lasting about three to six months. [1]

Bone marrow. The soft, sponge-like tissue in the center of most large bones. It produces white blood cells, red blood cells, and platelets. [2]

Bone marrow aspiration (as-per-AY-shun). The removal of a small sample of bone marrow (usually from the hip) through a needle for examination under a microscope. [2]

Bone marrow transplant. A procedure to replace bone marrow that was destroyed by treatment with high doses of anticancer drugs or radiation. [1]

Catheter (KATH-i-ter). A flexible tube used to deliver fluids into or withdraw fluids from the body. [2]

Chemotherapy (kee-mo-THER-a-pee). Treatment with anticancer drugs. [2]

Child-life worker. A professional who is responsible for making a child's hospital and treatment experience less scary. [2]

Chromosome. The carrier of hereditary characteristics found in cells. [1]

Chronic leukemia. A slowly progressing cancer of the blood-forming tissues. [1]

Clinical trial. A type of research study that tests how well new medical treatments or other interventions work in people. Such studies test new methods of screening, prevention, diagnosis, or treatment of a disease. The study may be carried out in a clinic or other medical facility. Also called a clinical study. [2]

Colony-stimulating factors. Substances that stimulate the production of blood cells. Colony-stimulating factors include granulocyte colony-stimulating factors (also called G-CSF and filgrastim), granulocyte-macrophage colony-stimulating factors (also called GM-CSF and sargramostim), and promegapoietin. [2]

Combination chemotherapy. Treatment using more than one anticancer drug. [2]

Computed tomography (CT) scan. A series of detailed pictures of areas inside the body taken from different angles; the pictures are created by a computer linked to an x-ray machine. Also called computerized tomography and computerized axial tomography (CAT) scan. [2]

Cure. Five or more years of disease-free survival. [1]

Cytokines. A class of substances that are produced by cells of the immune system and can affect the immune response. Cytokines can also be produced in the laboratory by recombinant DNA technology and given to people to affect immune responses. [2]

Differentiating agents. A type of therapy that can trigger immature cells to become more mature and functional. [1]

Distraction. In medicine, a pain relief method that takes the patient's attention away from the pain. [2]

Donor. A person who donates organs, tissues, cells, or other biological material. [1]

First-line treatment. The drugs and other therapies given to a patient who is diagnosed with a disease and has not had any therapy for the disease. [1]

Graft-versus-host disease (GVHD). A reaction of donated bone marrow against a person's tissue. [1]

Hypnosis. A trance-like state in which a person becomes more aware and focused and is more open to suggestion. [2]

Imagery. A technique in which the person focuses on positive images in his or her mind. [2]

Immune system. The complex group of organs and cells that defends the body against infection or disease. [1]

Immunotherapy (IM-yoo-no-THER-a-pee). Treatment to stimulate or restore the ability of the immune system to fight infections and other diseases. Also used to lessen side effects that may be caused by some cancer treatments. Also known as biological therapy, biotherapy, or biological response modifier (BRM) therapy. [2]

Interferon (in-ter-FEER-on). A biological response modifier (a substance that can improve the body's natural response to infections and other diseases). Interferons interfere with the division of cancer cells and can slow tumor growth. There are several types of interferons, including interferon-alpha, -beta, and -gamma. The body normally produces these substances. They are also made in the laboratory to treat cancer and other diseases. [2]

Interleukins (in-ter-LOO-kins). Biological response modifiers (substances that can improve the body's natural response to infection and disease) that help the immune system fight infection and cancer. These substances are normally produced by the body. They are also made in the laboratory for use in treating cancer and other diseases. [2]

IV injection (intravenously). Injection into a vein. [1]

Leukemia (loo-KEE-mee-a). Cancer that starts in blood-forming tissue such as the bone marrow, and causes large numbers of blood cells to be produced and enter the blood stream. [2]

Lymph node (limf node). A rounded mass of lymphatic tissue that is surrounded by a capsule of connective tissue. Lymph nodes filter lymph (lymphatic fluid), and they store lymphocytes (white blood cells). They are located along lymphatic vessels. Also called a lymph gland. [2]

Lymphoid. Refers to lymphocytes, a type of white blood cell. Also refers to tissue in which lymphocytes develop. [1]

Lymphoma (lim-FO-ma). Cancer that arises in cells of the lymphatic system. [2]

Malignancy. Cancer. [1]

Malignant (ma-LIG-nant). Cancerous; a growth with a tendency to invade and destroy nearby tissue and spread to other parts of the body. [2]

Metastatic cancer. Cancer that has spread from the place in which it started to other parts of the body. [2]

Monoclonal antibodies (MAH-no-KLO-nul AN-tih-BAH-deez). Laboratory-produced substances that can locate and bind to cancer cells wherever they are in the body. Many monoclonal antibodies are used in cancer detection or therapy; each one recognizes a different protein on certain cancer cells. Monoclonal antibodies can be used alone, or they can be used to deliver drugs, toxins, or radioactive material directly to a tumor. [2]

MRI Magnetic resonance imaging (mag-NET-ik REZ-o-nans IM-a-jing). A procedure in which a magnet linked to a computer is used to create detailed pictures of areas inside the body. Also called nuclear magnetic resonance imaging (NMRI). [2]

Myeloid. Pertaining to, derived from, or manifesting certain features of the bone marrow. Also called myelogenous. [1]

Nerve block. A procedure in which medicine is injected directly into or around a nerve or into the spine to block pain. [2]

Oncologist (on-KOL-o-jist). A doctor who specializes in treating cancer. Some oncologists specialize in a particular type of cancer treatment. For example, a radiation oncologist specializes in treating cancer with radiation. [2]

Oncology nurse. A nurse who specializes in treating and caring for people who have cancer. [2]

Opioids. A family of synthetic drugs used to treat moderate to severe pain. They are similar to opiates such as morphine and codeine. [2]

Pediatric (pee-dee-AT-rik). Having to do with children. [2]

Peripheral stem cell transplantation (per-IF-er-al). A method of replacing blood-forming cells destroyed by cancer treatment. Immature blood cells (stem cells) in the circulating blood that are similar to those in the bone marrow are given to the patient after treatment. This helps the bone marrow recover and continue producing healthy blood cells. Transplantation may be autologous (an individual's own blood cells saved earlier), allogeneic (blood cells donated by someone else), or syngeneic (blood cells donated by an identical twin). Also called peripheral stem cell support. [2]

Phase I trial. The first step in testing a new treatment in humans. These studies test the best way to give a new treatment (for example, by mouth, intravenous infusion, or injection) and the best dose. The dose is usually increased a little at a time in order to find the highest dose that does not cause harmful side effects. Because little is known about the possible risks and benefits of the treatments being tested, phase I trials usually include only a small number of patients who have not been helped by other treatments. [2]

Phase II trial. A study to test whether a new treatment has an anticancer effect (for example, whether it shrinks a tumor or improves

507

blood test results) and whether it works against a certain type of cancer. [2]

Phase III trial. A study to compare the results of people taking a new treatment with the results of people taking the standard treatment (for example, which group has better survival rates or fewer side effects). In most cases, studies move into phase III only after a treatment seems to work in phases I and II. Phase III trials may include hundreds of people. [2]

Phase IV trial. After a treatment has been approved and is being marketed, it is studied in a phase IV trial to evaluate side effects that were not apparent in the phase III trial. Thousands of people are involved in a phase IV trial. [2]

Physical therapy. The use of exercises and physical activities to help condition muscles and restore strength and movement. For example, physical therapy can be used to restore arm and shoulder movement and build back strength after breast cancer surgery. [2]

Platelets (PLAYT-lets). A type of blood cell that helps prevent bleeding by causing blood clots to form. Also called thrombocytes. [2]

Prosthesis (pros-THEE-sis). An artificial replacement of a part of the body. [2]

Radiation therapy (ray-dee-AY-shun). The use of high-energy radiation from x-rays, gamma rays, neutrons, and other sources to kill cancer cells and shrink tumors. Radiation may come from a machine outside the body (external-beam radiation therapy), or from materials called radioisotopes. Radioisotopes produce radiation and can be placed in or near the tumor or in the area near cancer cells. This type of radiation treatment is called internal radiation therapy, implant radiation, interstitial radiation, or brachytherapy. Systemic radiation therapy uses a radioactive substance, such as a radiolabeled monoclonal antibody, that circulates throughout the body. Also called radiotherapy, irradiation, and x-ray therapy. [2]

Red blood cells (erythrocytes). Cells that carry oxygen to all parts of the body. [1]

Relapse. The return of signs and symptoms of cancer after a period of improvement. [1]

Relaxation techniques. Methods used to reduce tension and anxiety, and control pain. [2]

Remission. A decrease in or disappearance of signs and symptoms of cancer. In partial remission, some, but not all, signs and symptoms of cancer have disappeared. In complete remission, all signs and symptoms of cancer have disappeared, although cancer still may be in the body. [2]

Second-line treatment. The drugs and other therapies given to a patient who has a disease that has either not responded to or recurs following first-line treatment. [1]

Spinal tap. A procedure in which a needle is put into the lower part of the spinal column to collect cerebrospinal fluid or to give drugs. Also called a lumbar puncture. [2]

Spleen. An organ that is part of the lymphatic system and produces lymphocytes, filters the blood, stores blood cells, and destroys old blood cells. [1]

Standard therapy. A currently accepted and widely used treatment for a certain type of cancer, based on the results of past research. [2]

Supportive care. Care that prevents or relieves the symptoms of disease or the side effects of treatment. Supportive care does not alter the course of a disease but can improve the quality of life. It attempts to meet the physical, emotional, spiritual, and practical needs of patients by helping to relieve pain, depression, or other problems. Also known as comfort care, palliative care, and symptom management. [2]

Surgery (SERJ-uh-ree). A procedure to remove or repair a part of the body or to find out whether disease is present. An operation. [2]

Systemic therapy (sis-TEM-ik THER-a-pee). Treatment using substances that travel through the bloodstream, reaching and affecting cells all over the body. [2]

Tumor (TOO-mer). An abnormal mass of tissue that results from excessive cell division. Tumors perform no useful body function. They may be benign (not cancerous) or malignant (cancerous). [2]

White blood cells (leukocytes). A type of cell in the immune system that helps the body fight infection and disease. White blood cells include lymphocytes, granulocytes, macrophages, and others. [1]

X-ray. A type of high-energy radiation. In low doses, x-rays are used to diagnose diseases by making pictures of the inside of the body. In high doses, x-rays are used to treat cancer. [2]

Chapter 45

Directory of Additional Resources on Leukemia

American Board of Medical Specialties (ABMS)
1007 Church St.
Suite 404
Evanston, IL 60201-5913
Toll Free: 866-ASK-ABMS (275-2267)
Tel: 847-491-9091
Fax: 847-328-3596
Verification of Physician's Board Certification: 866-275-2267
Website: www.abms.org/which.asp

American Cancer Society
P.O. Box 102454
Atlanta, GA 30368-2454
Toll-Free: 800-227-2345
Website: www.cancer.org

American College of Surgeons (ACOS)
633 North Saint Clair St.
Chicago, IL 60611-3211
Tel: 312–202–5000
Fax: 312-202-5001
Website: http://web.facs.org/cpm/default.htm
E-mail: postmaster@facs.org

American Institute for Cancer Research
1759 R Street NW
Washington, DC 20009
Toll-Free: 800-843-8114
Tel: 202-328-7744
Fax: 202-328-7226
Website: www.aicr.org
E-mail: aicrweb@aicr.org

The list of resources presented in this chapter was compiled from many sources deemed reliable; contact information was verified and updated in March 2003.

American Society for Clinical Oncology

1900 Duke Street
Suite 200
Alexandria, VA 22314
Tel: 703-299-0150
Fax: 703-299-1044
Website: www.asco.org
E-mail: asco@asco.org

Association of Community Cancer Centers

11600 Nebel Street
Suite 201
Rockville, MD 20852
Tel: 301-984-9496
Fax: 301-770-1949
Website: www.accc-cancer.org/
main2001.shtml

Association of Cancer Online Resources, Inc., (ACOR)

173 Duane Street
Suite 3A
New York, NY 10013-3334
Tel: 212-226-5525
Website: www.acor.org

Blood and Bone Marrow Transplant Newsletter

2900 Skokie Valley Road
Suite B
Highland Park, IL 60035
Toll-Free: 888-597-7674
Tel: 847-433-3313
Website: www.bmtnews.org
E-mail: help@bmtinfonet.org

Bone Marrow Transplant and Stem Cell Transplant Program

Duke University Medical Center
Box 3961
Durham, NC 27710
Tel: 919-668-1002
Fax: 919-668-1091
Website: http://bmt.mc.duke.edu
E-mail:
Duke_ABMT@mc.duke.edu

Canadian Cancer Society

565 W. 10th Ave.
Vancouver, BC V5Z 4J4
Toll-Free: 888-939-3333
Tel: 604-872-4400
Website: www.bc.cancer.ca
E-mail: inquiries@bc.cancer.ca

Cancervive

11636 Chayote Street
Los Angeles, CA 90049
Toll-Free: 800-4-TO-CURE (86-2873)
Tel: 310-203-9232
Fax: 310-471-4618
Website: www.cancervive.org
E-mail: cancervivr@aol.com

Cancer Care, Inc.

275 Seventh Avenue
New York, NY 10001
Toll-Free: 800-813-HOPE (4673)
Tel: 212-712-8080
Fax: 212-712-8495
Website: www.cancercare.org
E-mail: info@cancercare.org

Candlelighters Childhood Cancer Foundation (CCCF)
P.O. Box 498
Kensington, MD 20895-0498
Toll-Free: 800-366-2223
Tel: 301-962-3520
Fax: 301-962-3521
Website: www.candlelighters.org
E-mail: info@candlelighters.org

Dana-Farber Cancer Institute
44 Binney Street
Boston, MA 02115
Tel: 866-408-3324
TDD: 617-632-5330
Website: www.dana-farber.org
E-mail: dana-farbercontactus@dfci.harvard.edu

Health Insurance Association of America
1201 F Street, NW
Suite 500
Washington, DC 2004-1204
Tel: 202-824-1600
Fax: 202-824-1722
Website: www.hiaa.org

Joint Commission on Accreditation of Healthcare Organizations (JCAHO)
One Renaissance Blvd.
Oakbrook Terrace, IL 60181-4294
Tel: 630-792-5800
Fax: 630-792-5541
Website: www.jcaho.org
E-mail: ustomerservice@jcaho.org

The Leukemia & Lymphoma Society Inc.
1311 Mamaroneck Avenue
White Plains, NY 10605
Toll-Free: 800-955-4572
Tel: 914-949-5213
Fax: 914-949-6691
Website: www.leukemia.org

M.D. Anderson Cancer Center
University of Texas
1515 Holcombe Blvd.
Houston, TX 77030
Toll-Free: 800-392-1611
Tel: 713-792-6161
Website: www.mdanderson.org/departments/cimer

National Coalition of Cancer Survivorship
1010 Wayne Avenue, Suite 770
Silver Spring, MD 20910
Toll-Free: 877-622-7937
Tel: 301-650-9127
Fax: 301-565-9670
Website: www.canceradvocacy.org
E-mail: info@cansearch.org

National Marrow Donor Program
3001 Broadway Street NE
Suite 500
Minneapolis, MN 55413-1753
Toll-Free: 800-627-7692
Tel: 612-627-5800
Website: www.marrow.org

Oncolink
University of Pennsylvania
Cancer Center
3400 Spruce Street
2 Donner
Philadelphia, PA 19104-1283
Fax: 215-349-5445
Website:
www.oncolink.upenn.edu

Oncology Nursing Society
125 Enterprise Drive
RIDC Park West
Pittsburgh, PA 15275-1214
Toll-Free: 866-257-4667
Tel: 412-859-6100
Fax: 877-369-5497
Website: www.ons.org
E-mail:
customer.service@ons.org

Patient Advocate Foundation
700 Thimble Shoals Blvd.
Suite 200
Newport News, VA 23608
Toll-Free: 800-532-5274
Fax: 757-873-8999
Website:
www.patientadvocate.org
E-mail:
help@patientadvocate.org

R.A. Bloch Cancer Foundation, Inc.
4400 Main Street
Kansas, MO 64111
Toll-Free: 800-433-0464
Tel: 816-932-8453
Fax: 816-931-7486
Website: www.blochcancer.org

University of Minnesota
Cancer Center
Mayo Mail Code 806
420 Delaware Street SE
Minneapolis, MN 55455
Toll-Free: 888-226-2376
Tel: 612-624-8484
Fax: 612-626-3069
Website: www.cancer.umn.edu
E-mail: info@cancer.umn.edu

The Wellness Community
1320 Centre Street
Suite 305
Newton Centre, MA 02459
Tel: 617-332-1919
Website:
www.wellnesscommunity.org

Government Agencies and Organizations

Agency for Healthcare Research and Quality (AHRQ)
2101 E. Jefferson
Suite 501
Rockville, MD 20852
Toll-Free: 800-358-9295
Tel: 301-594-1364
Website: www.ahrq.gov

Cancer Trials Support Unit (CTSU)
CTSU Data Operations Center
1441 W. Montgomery Ave.
Rockville, MD 20850-2062
Toll-Free: 888-823-5923
Toll-Free Fax: 888-691-8039
Website: www.ctsu.org
E-mail:
CTSUcontact@westat.com

Centers for Medicare and Medicaid Services (CMS)
7500 Security Blvd.
Baltimore, MD 21244-1850
Toll Free: 877-267-2323
Toll Free TTY: 866-226-1819
Tel: 410-786-3000
TTY: 410-786-0727
Website: www.cms.hhs.gov

National Cancer Institute
6166 Executive Boulevard
MSC 8322
Suite 3036A
Bethesda, MD 20892-8322
Toll-Free: 800-422-6237
Toll-Free TTY: 800-332-8615
Website: www.cancer.gov

National Center for Complementary and Alternative Medicine
P.O. Box 7923
Gaithersburg, MD 20898
Toll-Free: 888-644-6226
TTY: 866-464-3614
Fax: 866-464-3616
Website: http://nccam.nih.gov
E-mail: info@nccam.nih.gov

Pediatric Oncology Branch
Center for Cancer Research, NCI
6166 Executive Boulevard
MSC 8322
Suite 3036A
Bethesda, MD 20892-8322
Toll-Free: 877-624-4878
Tel: 301-496-4256
Website: www-dcs.nci.nih.gov/
branches/pedonc

Social Security Administration (SSA)
Office of Public Inquiries
Windsor Park Building
6401 Security Blvd.
Baltimore, MD 21235
Toll-Free: 800-772-1213
Toll-Free TTY: 800-325-0778
Website: www.ssa.gov

State Children's Health Insurance Program (SCHIP)
U.S. Department of Health and Human Services
200 Independence Ave., SW
Washington, DC 20201
Toll-Free: 877-543-7669
Website: www.insurekidsnow.gov

U.S. Food and Drug Administration
5600 Fishers Lane
Rockville, MD 20857-0001
Toll-Free: 888-463-6332
Website: www.fda.gov

Veterans Health Administration
Department of Veterans Affairs
810 Vermont Avenue, NW
Washington, DC 20420
Toll-Free: 877-222-VETS (8387)
Website: www.va.gov/
health_benefits

Chapter 46

Directory of Prescription Drug Assistance Programs for People with Leukemia

This directory provides contact information for companies that offer patient assistance programs for pharmaceuticals used for leukemia treatment and treatment of common side effects from leukemia treatment. For the most current information on company patient assistance programs, visit the website at www.phrma.org.

3M Pharmaceuticals
Indigent Patient Pharmaceutical Program
Medical Services Department
275-6W-13, 3M Center
St. Paul, MN 55144-1000
Toll-Free: 800-328-0255
Fax: 651-733-6068
Website: www.3m.com

Products covered by program: Most drug products sold by 3M Pharmaceuticals in the United States.

Abbott Laboratories
Patient Assistance Program
200 Abbott Park Road, D31C, J23
Abbott Park, IL 60064-6163

Excerpts from "Directory of Prescription Drug Patient Assistance Programs," © 2002 Pharmaceutical Research and Manufacturers of America, reprinted with permission.

Abbott Laboratories (continued)
Toll-Free: 847-937-6100
Website: https://abbott.com

Products covered by program: most Abbott Laboratories pharmaceutical products.

Aciphex® Patient Assistance Program
P.O. Box 220458
Charlotte, NC 28222-0458
Toll-Free: 800-523-5870
Fax: 800-526-6651
Website: www.aciphex.com/7_faq.asp

Agouron Pharmaceuticals, Inc.
Agouron Patient Assistance Program
10777 Science Center Drive
San Diego, CA 92121
Tel: 858-622-3000
Fax: 858-678-9272
Website: www.agouron.com

Products covered by program: Viracept® (nelfinavir mesylate), Rescriptor® (delavirdine mesylate).

Alza Pharmaceuticals
Indigent Patient Assistance Program
1900 Charleston Road
P.O. Box 7210
Mountain View, CA 94039-7210
Tel: 650-564-5000
Fax: 650-564-7070
Website: www.alza.com

Products covered by the program: Bicitra, Ditropan XL, Elmiron, Mycelex, Neutra-Phos, Neutra-Phos-K, Polycitra, Polycitra-K, Urispas.

Amgen, Inc.
Amgen Safety Net®
One Amgen Center Drive
Thousand Oaks, CA 91320-1799

Bristol-Myers Squibb
Patient Assistance Foundation, Inc.
P.O. Box 4500
Mail Code P25-37
Princeton, NJ 08543-4500
Toll-Free: 800-332-2056
Fax: 609-897-6859
Website: www.bms.com

Products covered by program: Many Bristol-Myers Squibb pharmaceutical products.

Foscavir® Assistance and Information on Reimbursement (F.A.I.R.)
State and Federal Associates
1101 King Street
Alexandria, VA 22314
Toll-Free: 800-488-3247
Fax: 703-683-2239

Product covered by program: Foscavir® (foscarnet sodium) injection.

Genentech, Inc.
Genentech Patient Assistance Program
1 DNA Way, MS-13A
South San Francisco, CA 94080-4990
Toll-Free: 800-530-3083
Fax: 650-225-1366
Website: www.gene.com/gene/products/patient-assist-program.jsp

Products covered by program: Activase® (Alteplase), Herceptin® (Trastuzumab), Nutropin® (somatropin), Nutropin AQ® (somatropin), Nutropin Depot®, Protropin® (somatrem), Rituxan® (Rituximab), and TNKase™ (Tenecteplase).

Gilead Sciences Reimbursement
Support and Assistance Program
333 Lakeside Drive
Foster City, CA 94404
Toll-Free: 800-445-3235
Tel: 650-574-3000
Fax: 650-578-9264
Website: www.gilead.com

Gilead Sciences Reimbursement (continued)

Products covered by program: Viread™ (tenofovir disoproxil fumarate), Vistide® (cidofovir injection), and DaunoXome® (daunorubicin citrate liposome injection).

Glaxo Wellcome, Inc.
Contact: GlaxoSmithKline Beecham
5 Moore Drive, P.O. Box 13398
Research Triangle Park, NC 27709
Toll-Free: 800-699-3806
Fax: 714-750-8513
Website: http://ipp.gsk.com/oncology

Products covered by program: All marketed Glaxo Wellcome prescription products used in an outpatient setting.

GlaxoSmithKline Beecham
The Oncology Access to Care Hotline
5 Moore Drive
P.O. Box 13398
Research Triangle Park, NC 27709
Toll-Free: 800-699-3806
Fax: 714-750-8513
Website: http://ipp.gsk.com/oncology

Product covered by program: Hycamtin (topotecan HCl).

GSK Customer Response Center
Orange Card ^{SM}
5 Moore Drive
P.O. Box 13398
Research Triangle Park, NC 27709
Toll-Free: 888-825-5249
Website http://ipp.gsk.com

Products covered by program: All outpatient GSK prescription products are included. GlaxoSmithKline's OTC products and in-patient prescription medicines are not covered.

Janssen Patient Assistance Program
P.O. Box 221857
Charlotte, NC 28222-1857

Janssen Patient Assistance Program
(continued from previous page)
Toll-Free: 800-652-6227
Toll-Free Fax: 888-526-5168

Lilly Cares
Lilly Cares Program Administrator
P.O. Box 230999
Centreville, VA 20120
Toll-Free: 800-545-6962
Website: www.lilly.com

Products covered by program: Most Lilly prescription products and insulins (except controlled substances) are covered by this program. Gemzar® is covered under a separate program.

Gemzar® Reimbursement Hotline
Toll-Free: 888-443-6927 (888-4-GEMZAR)

Product covered by program: Gemzar® (gemcitabine hydrochloride).

LillyAnswers ᔆᴹ
Toll-Free: 877-795-4559 (877-RX-LILLY)
Website: www.lillyanswers.com.

Products covered by program: All Lilly retail products will be offered, except controlled substances as well as products not distributed by retail pharmacies. The program offers many of those medications most commonly prescribed to seniors, such as Evista for osteoporosis, Humulin and Humalog for diabetes, Prozac for depression, and Zyprexa for schizophrenia.

Lovenox Patient Assistance Program (PAP)
2211 Sanders Road
NTB7
Northbrook, IL 60067
Toll-Free: 888-632-8607
Fax: 888-875-9951
Website: www.lovenox.com

Product covered by program: Lovenox (enoxaparin sodium) injection.

Merck Patient Assistance Program
One Merck Drive
P.O. Box 100
Whitehouse Station, NJ 08889-0100
Toll Free: 800-727-5400
Toll-Free: 800-994-2111 (for physicians and healthcare professionals)
Tel: 908-423-1000
Website: www.merck.com/pap/pap/consumer/index.jsp

Products covered by program: Most Merck products. Requests for vaccines and injectables are not accepted, with the exception of requests for anti-cancer injectable products.

NORD
Matulane® Patient Assistance Program
P.O. Box 8923
New Fairfield, CT 06812-8923
Toll-Free: 800-999-NORD
Website: www.rarediseases.org/programs/medication

Product covered by program: Matulane® (procarbazine hydrochloride).

Novartis Pharmaceuticals
Patient Assistance Program
P.O. Box 8609
Somerville, NJ 08876
Toll-Free: 800-277-2254
Website: www.pharm.us.novartis.com/novartis/pap/pap.jsp

Products covered by program: Certain single source and/or life-sustaining products. Controlled substances are not included.

Organon USA
Remeron Indigent Patient Program
56 Livingston Ave.
Roseland, NJ 07068
Tel: 973-325-4500
Fax: 973-325-4589
Website: www.organon-usa.com

Product covered by program: Remeron® (mirtazapine).

Ortho Biotech
Reimbursement Solutions
1250 Bayhill Drive
Suite 300
San Bruno, CA 94066
Toll-Free: 800-609-1083
Toll-Free Fax: 800-987-5572
Website: www.orthobiotech.com or www.doxil.com

Product covered: Doxil® (doxorubicin hydrochloride liposome injection).

Ortho Biotech Products, L.P.
PROCRITline™
1250 Bayhill Drive
Suite 300
San Bruno, CA 94066
Toll-Free: 800-553-3851
Toll-Free Fax: 800-987-5572
Website: www.procritline.com

Products covered by program: Procrit® (Epoetin alfa) for non-dialysis use, and Leustatin® (cladribine) injection.

Ortho-McNeil
Patient Assistance Program
P.O. Box 938
Somerville, NJ 08876
Toll-Free: 800-577-3788
Website: http://ortho-mcneil.com/frames/about.htm

Products covered by program: Prescription products prescribed according to dosage regimens.

PACT+
100 Grandview Road, Suite 210
Braintree, MA 02184
Toll-Free: 800-996-ONCO (6626)
Toll-Free Fax: 800-996-6627
Website: www.aventis-oncology.net/pact-plus.htm
E-mail: ePACT@access2health.com

Products covered by program: Anzemet, Taxotere.

Parke-Davis Patient Assistance Program
P.O. Box 1058
Somerville, NJ 08876
Contact Pfizer: 800-717-6005

Products covered by program: Accupril, Accuretic, Dilantin, Estrostep, FemHRT, Lipitor, Loestrin, Neurontin, and Zarontin.

Pfizer
Diflucan® and Zithromax® Patient Assistance Program
1101 King Street
Suite 600
Alexandria, VA 22314
Toll-Free: 800-869-9979
Website: www.Pfizer.com

Products covered by program: Diflucan® (fluconazole) and Zithromax® (azithromycin) for MAC prophylaxis and treatment.

Pfizer for Living Share Card Program
Toll-Free: 800-717-6005
Website: www.pfizerforliving.com

Products covered by program: Most Pfizer prescription medicines available at a retail pharmacy.

Pharmacia Patients in Need Foundation
P.O. Box 52059
Phoenix, AZ 85072
Toll-Free: 800-242-7014
Fax: 480-314-7163
Website: www.patientsinneed.com

Products covered by program: Numerous products.

Procter & Gamble Pharmaceuticals
Patient Assistance Program
c/o Express Scripts
P.O. Box 6553
St. Louis, MO 63166-6553
Toll-Free: 800-830-9049
Website: www.pgpharma.com

Procter & Gamble Pharmaceuticals (continued)

Products covered by program: Actonel, Asacol, Dantrium Capsules, Didronel, Macrodantin, and Macrobid.

Prograf® Patient Assistance Program
c/o Quorum Consulting, Inc.
P.O. Box 221644
Chantilly, VA 20153-1644
Toll-Free: 800-477-6472
Website: www.quorumconsulting.net

Product covered by program: Prograf® capsules (tacrolimus).

Roche Laboratories, Inc.
Roche Medical Needs Program
340 Kingsland Street
Nutley, NJ 07110
Toll-Free: 800-285-4484

Products covered by program: Kytril (granisetron), Roferon®-A (Interferon alpha-2a, recombinant), Vesanoid® (tretinoin), and Xeloda (capecitabine).

Roche Transplant Reimbursement
Toll-Free Hotline: 800-772-5790

Products covered by program: CellCept® (mycophenolate mofetil), Cytovene® (ganciclovir capsules), and Cytovene®-IV (ganciclovir sodium for injection).

Sanofi-Synthelabo
Needy Patient Program
c/o Product Information Dept.
90 Park Avenue
New York, NY 10016
Toll-Free: 800-446-6267
Tel: 212-551-4000
Website: www.sanofi-synthelabous.com

Products covered by program: Aralen, Danocrine, Drisdol, Kerlone, Mytelase, NegGram, pHisoHex, Plaquenil, Primaquine, Arixtra, Hyalgan, Primacor, and Skelid. For Avalide, Avapro, and Plavix call 800-736-0003.

Schering Laboratories/Key Pharmaceuticals
Patient Assistance Program
P.O. Box 52122
Phoenix, AZ 85072
Toll-Free: 800-656-9485
Website: www.schering-plough.com/patient.html

Products covered by program: Most Schering/Key prescription drugs. For Intron A/Eulexin: call 800-521-7157

SmithKline Beecham Foundation
Access to Care
5 Moore Drive
P.O. Box 13398
Research Triangle Park, NC 27709
Toll-Free: 800-546-0420 or 800-729-4544
Website http://ipp.gsk.com

Products covered by program: Amoxil, Augmentin, Avandia, Bactroban, Compazine, Coreg, Dyazide, Paxil, Relafen, Requip, and Tagamet.

Solvay Pharmaceuticals, Inc./Unimed Pharmaceuticals, Inc.
Patient Assistance Program
c/o Express Scripts Specialty
Distribution Services
P.O. Box 66550
St. Louis, MO 63166-6550
Toll-Free: 800-256-8918
Website: www.solvay.com

Products covered by program: **Solvay Pharmaceuticals, Inc**: Aceon® (perindopril erbumine) Tablets 2 mg, 4 mg and 8 mg; Creon® Minimicrospheres® (pancrelipase) Delayed-Release Capsules 5, 10 and 20; Estratest® (esterified estrogens, USP 1.25 mg and methyltestosterone, 2.5 mg) Tablets; Estratest® H.S. (esterified estrogens USP 0.625 mg and methyltestosterone, 1.25 mg) Tablets; Lithobid® (lithium carbonate, USP) Tablets 300 mg; Rowasa® Rectal Suspension Enema (mesalamine) 4g/60mL unit dose. **Unimed Pharmaceuticals, Inc**: Anadrol® (oxymetholone) Tablets 50 mg; AndroGel® 1% (testosterone gel) CIII 2.5 g and 5 g; Marinol® (dronabinol) Capsules 2.5 mg, 5 mg and 10 mg; and Teveten® (eprosartan mesylate) Tablets 400 mg and 600 mg.

TreatFirst ᴿᴹ

P.O. Box 2975
Phoenix, AZ 85062
Toll-Free: 877-744-5675

Products covered by program: Aromasin® (exemestane tablets), Camptosar® (irinotecan), Celebrex® (celecoxib capsules), Ellence® (epirubicin), Emcyt® (estramustine phosphate sodium capsules), Idamycin® (idarubicin), and Zinecard® (dexrazoxane).

Wyeth Pharmaceuticals

The Neumega® Access Program
5 Giralda Farms
Madison, NJ 07949
Toll-Free: 888-NEUMEGA (888-638-6342)
Website: www.wyeth.com

Product covered by program: Neumega® (oprelvekin).

Chapter 47

Financial Assistance for People with Leukemia

Organizations and Resources

American Cancer Society (ACS)
P.O. Box 102454
Atlanta, GA 30368-2454
Toll-Free: 800-227-2345
Website: www.cancer.org

The national American Cancer Society (ACS) office can provide the telephone number of the local ACS office serving your area. The ACS offers programs that help cancer patients, family members, and friends cope with the emotional challenges they face. Information on these programs is available on their website. Some materials are published in Spanish. Spanish-speaking staff are available.

Candlelighters Childhood Cancer Foundation (CCCF)
P.O. Box 498
Kensington, MD 20895-0498
Toll-Free: 800-366-2223
Tel: 301-962-3520
Fax: 301-962-3521

"Financial Assistance for Cancer Care," Fact Sheet 8.3, National Cancer Institute (NCI), reviewed 03/18/2002; and "Internet Links for Financial Assistance," © 2001 Cancer Care, Inc., reprinted with permission. Visit the Cancer Care website at www.cancercare.org for additional information.

Candlelighters Childhood Cancer Foundation (CCCF)
(continued)
Website: www.candlelighters.org
E-mail: info@candlelighters.org

The Candlelighters Childhood Cancer Foundation (CCCF) is a non-profit organization that provides information, peer support, and advocacy through publications, an information clearinghouse, and a network of local support groups. CCCF maintains a list of organizations to which eligible families may apply for financial assistance.

The Leukemia & Lymphoma Society
1311 Mamaroneck Avenue
White Plains, NY 10605
Toll-Free Information Resource Center: 800-955-4572
Tel: 914-949-5213
Fax: 914-949-6691
Website: www.leukemia-lymphoma.org

The Leukemia and Lymphoma Society (LLS) offers information and financial aid to patients who have leukemia, non-Hodgkin's lymphoma, Hodgkin's disease, or multiple myeloma. Callers may request a booklet describing LLS's Patient Aid Program or the telephone number for their local LLS office. Some publications are available in Spanish.

Hill-Burton
5600 Fishers Lane
Rockville, MD 20857
Toll-Free: 800-638-0742
Website: www.hrsa.gov/osp/dfcr/obtain/consfaq.htm

Hill-Burton is a program through which hospitals receive construction funds from the Federal Government. Hospitals that receive Hill-Burton funds are required by law to provide some services to people who cannot afford to pay for their hospitalization. Contact Hill-Burton to find which facilities are a part of this program. A brochure about the program is available in Spanish.

Centers for Medicare & Medicaid Services (CMS)
7500 Security Boulevard
Baltimore, MD 21244-1850
Toll Free: 877-267-2323
Toll Free TTY: 866-226-1819

Centers for Medicare & Medicaid Services (CMS) (continued)
Tel: 410-786-3000
TTY: 410-786-0727
Website: www.cms.hhs.gov

Medicaid (Medical Assistance) a jointly funded, Federal-State health insurance program for people who need financial assistance for medical expenses, is coordinated by the Centers for Medicare and Medicaid Services, formerly the Health Care Financing Administration. At a minimum, states must provide home care services to people who receive Federal income assistance such as Social Security Income and Aid to Families with Dependent Children. Medicaid coverage includes part-time nursing, home care aide services, and medical supplies and equipment. Information about coverage is available from local state welfare offices, state health departments, state social services agencies, or the state Medicaid office. Check the local telephone directory for the number to call. Information about specific state contacts is also available on the website. Spanish speaking staff are available in some offices.

Medicare
Toll-Free: 800-633-42227
Toll-Free TTY: 877-486-2048
Website: www.medicare.gov

Medicare is a Federal health insurance program also administered by the CMS. Eligible individuals include those who are 65 or older, people of any age with permanent kidney failure, and disabled people under age 65. Medicare may offer reimbursement for some home care services. Cancer patients who qualify for Medicare may also be eligible for coverage of hospice services if they are accepted into a Medicare-certified hospice program. To receive information on eligibility, explanations of coverage, and related publications, call Medicare or visit their website. Some publications are available in Spanish.

Patient Advocate Foundation (PAF)
700 Thimble Shoals Blvd.
Suite 200
Newport News, VA 23606
Toll-Free: 800-532-5274
Fax: 757-873-8999
Website: www.patientadvocate.org
E-mail: help@patientadvocate.org

Patient Advocate Foundation (PAF) (continued)

The Patient Advocate Foundation (PAF) is a national nonprofit organization that provides education, legal counseling, and referrals to cancer patients and survivors concerning managed care, insurance, financial issues, job discrimination, and debt crisis matters.

Social Security Administration (SSA)
Office of Public Inquiries
Windsor Park Building
6401 Security Blvd.
Baltimore, MD 21235
Toll-Free: 800-772-1213
Toll-Free TTY: 800-325-0778
Website: www.ssa.gov/SSA_Home.html

Social Security Administration (SSA) is the Government agency that oversees Social Security and Supplemental Security Income. Social Security provides a monthly income for eligible elderly and disabled individuals. Supplemental Security Income (SSI) supplements Social Security payments for individuals who have certain income and resource levels. Information on eligibility, coverage, and how to file a claim is available from the Social Security Administration.

State Children's Health Insurance Program (SCHIP)
U.S. Department of Health and Human Services
200 Independence Ave., SW
Washington, DC 20201
Toll-Free: 877-543-7669
Website: www.insurekidsnow.gov

The State Children's Health Insurance Program (SCHIP) is a Federal-State partnership that offers low-cost or free health insurance coverage to uninsured children of low-wage, working parents. Callers will be referred to the SCHIP program in their state for further information about what the program covers, who is eligible, and the minimum qualifications.

Veterans Health Administration
810 Vermont Avenue, NW
Washington, DC 20420
Toll-Free: 877-222-VETS

Veterans Health Administration (continued)
Website: www.va.gov/health_benefits

Eligible veterans and their dependents may receive cancer treatment at a Veterans Administration Medical Center. Treatment for service-connected conditions is provided, and treatment for other conditions may be available based on the veteran's financial need. Spanish-speaking staff are available in some offices.

Internet Links for Financial Assistance

Air Care Alliance
Website: www.aircareall.org

The Air Care Alliance is a nationwide league of humanitarian flying organizations dedicated to community service. This site links you to nationwide listings of organizations that provide transport for patients and sometimes family members needing to get to treatment.

American Council on Education/Health Resource Center Financial Aid for Students with Disability
Website: www.finaid.org/otheraid/disabled.phtml

This document provides information and resources for disabled students seeking financial assistance with tuition for postsecondary education.

Blood and Bone Marrow Transplant Newsletter
Website: www.bmtnews.org

If your health insurance plan has refused to pay for all or part of your treatment, BMT news can refer you to not-for-profit organizations and attorneys who may be able to help you. All the attorneys on their referral list have successfully persuaded insurers to pay for transplant-related expenses, usually without resorting to litigation.

Cancer Care
Website: www.cancercare.org/FinancialNeeds/FinancialNeedsList.cfm?c=387

The Cancer Care social workers can provide guidance on financial benefits and sources of help.

Candlelighters Childhood Cancer Foundation
Website: www.candlelighters.org

CCCF among other services provides emergency funds, summer camps, transportation for families of children with cancer.

Children's Organ Transplant Center
Website: www.cota.org

Children's Organ Transplant Association, Inc., is a voluntary health charity dedicated to providing financial and planning assistance to transplant-needy persons and their families.

Corporate Angel Network
Website: www.corpangelnetwork.org

Corporate Angel Network, a not-for-profit organization, provides free plane transportation for cancer patients going to/from recognized cancer treatment centers by using empty seats aboard corporate aircraft operating on business flights.

"Encore Plus" A YWCA Program
Website: www.ywca.org/html/B4d1.asp

The ENCOREplus® program is designed to eliminate inequalities in health care experienced by many women by removing barriers to access and promoting effective community-based outreach, education, referral to clinical services and support systems.

Internal Revenue Service
Website: www.irs.ustreas.gov

Medical costs that are not covered by insurance policies sometimes can be deducted from annual income before taxes. Your local IRS office, tax consultants, or certified public accountants can help you determine if any of such costs would be deductible. This site offers general tax information with a page to search for resources and IRS offices in your area.

National Association of Hospital Hospitality Houses, Inc.
Website: www.nahhh.org

The National Association of Hospital Hospitality Houses, Inc. is a membership organization of hospital hospitality house type programs.

These programs typically provide lodging for families of hospital patients and/or hospital outpatients.

National Cancer Institute
Website: www.cancer.org

This page provides an overview of the types of assistance that patients may be eligible for.

National Foundation for Transplants
Website: www.transplants.org

National Foundation for Transplants helps transplant patients nationwide—bone marrow, stem cell, and cord blood patients as well as solid organ transplant patients—overcome financial barriers to a second chance at life.

National Patient Air Transportation Hotline
Website: www.npath.org

The hotline provides information on free transportation for ill patients, information for health care professionals, and volunteer pilots.

Pharmaceutical Patient Assistance Programs
Website: www.needymeds.com

Many pharmaceutical manufacturers have special programs to assist people who can't afford to buy the drugs they need. This site lists available information about these programs, which vary by company.

Index

Index

Health Reference Series
COMPLETE CATALOG

Adolescent Health Sourcebook

Basic Consumer Health Information about Common Medical, Mental, and Emotional Concerns in Adolescents, Including Facts about Acne, Body Piercing, Mononucleosis, Nutrition, Eating Disorders, Stress, Depression, Behavior Problems, Peer Pressure, Violence, Gangs, Drug Use, Puberty, Sexuality, Pregnancy, Learning Disabilities, and More

Along with a Glossary of Terms and Other Resources for Further Help and Information

Edited by Chad T. Kimball. 658 pages. 2002. 0-7808-0248-9. $78.

"It is written in clear, nontechnical language aimed at general readers. . . . Recommended for public libraries, community colleges, and other agencies serving health care consumers."
— *American Reference Books Annual, 2003*

"Recommended for school and public libraries. Parents and professionals dealing with teens will appreciate the easy-to-follow format and the clearly written text. This could become a 'must have' for every high school teacher."
— *E-Streams, Jan '03*

"A good starting point for information related to common medical, mental, and emotional concerns of adolescents."
— *School Library Journal, Nov '02*

"This book provides accurate information in an easy to access format. It addresses topics that parents and caregivers might not be aware of and provides practical, useable information."
— *Doody's Health Sciences Book Review Journal, Sep-Oct '02*

"Recommended reference source."
— *Booklist, American Library Association, Sep '02*

AIDS Sourcebook, 3rd Edition

Basic Consumer Health Information about Acquired Immune Deficiency Syndrome (AIDS) and Human Immunodeficiency Virus (HIV) Infection, Including Facts about Transmission, Prevention, Diagnosis, Treatment, Opportunistic Infections, and Other Complications, with a Section for Women and Children, Including Details about Associated Gynecological Concerns, Pregnancy, and Pediatric Care

Along with Updated Statistical Information, Reports on Current Research Initiatives, a Glossary, and Directories of Internet, Hotline, and Other Resources

Edited by Dawn D. Matthews. 664 pages. 2003. 0-7808-0631-X. $78.

ALSO AVAILABLE: AIDS Sourcebook, 1st Edition. Edited by Karen Bellenir and Peter D. Dresser. 831 pages. 1995. 0-7808-0031-1. $78.

AIDS Sourcebook, 2nd Edition. Edited by Karen Bellenir. 751 pages. 1999. 0-7808-0225-X. $78.

"Highly recommended."
— *American Reference Books Annual, 2000*

"Excellent sourcebook. This continues to be a highly recommended book. There is no other book that provides as much information as this book provides."
— *AIDS Book Review Journal, Dec-Jan 2000*

"Recommended reference source."
— *Booklist, American Library Association, Dec '99*

"A solid text for college-level health libraries."
— *The Bookwatch, Aug '99*

Cited in *Reference Sources for Small and Medium-Sized Libraries, American Library Association, 1999*

Alcoholism Sourcebook

Basic Consumer Health Information about the Physical and Mental Consequences of Alcohol Abuse, Including Liver Disease, Pancreatitis, Wernicke-Korsakoff Syndrome (Alcoholic Dementia), Fetal Alcohol Syndrome, Heart Disease, Kidney Disorders, Gastrointestinal Problems, and Immune System Compromise and Featuring Facts about Addiction, Detoxification, Alcohol Withdrawal, Recovery, and the Maintenance of Sobriety

Along with a Glossary and Directories of Resources for Further Help and Information

Edited by Karen Bellenir. 613 pages. 2000. 0-7808-0325-6. $78.

"This title is one of the few reference works on alcoholism for general readers. For some readers this will be a welcome complement to the many self-help books on the market. Recommended for collections serving general readers and consumer health collections."
— *E-Streams, Mar '01*

"This book is an excellent choice for public and academic libraries."
— *American Reference Books Annual, 2001*

"Recommended reference source."
— *Booklist, American Library Association, Dec '00*

"Presents a wealth of information on alcohol use and abuse and its effects on the body and mind, treatment, and prevention."
— *SciTech Book News, Dec '00*

"Important new health guide which packs in the latest consumer information about the problems of alcoholism."
— *Reviewer's Bookwatch, Nov '00*

SEE ALSO Drug Abuse Sourcebook, Substance Abuse Sourcebook

Allergies Sourcebook, 2nd Edition

Basic Consumer Health Information about Allergic Disorders, Triggers, Reactions, and Related Symptoms, Including Anaphylaxis, Rhinitis, Sinusitis, Asthma, Dermatitis, Conjunctivitis, and Multiple Chemical Sensitivity

Along with Tips on Diagnosis, Prevention, and Treatment, Statistical Data, a Glossary, and a Directory of Sources for Further Help and Information

Edited by Annemarie S. Muth. 598 pages. 2002. 0-7808-0376-0. $78.

ALSO AVAILABLE: Allergies Sourcebook, 1st Edition. Edited by Allan R. Cook. 611 pages. 1997. 0-7808-0036-2. $78.

"This book brings a great deal of useful material together. . . . This is an excellent addition to public and consumer health library collections."
— *American Reference Books Annual, 2003*

"This second edition would be useful to laypersons with little or advanced knowledge of the subject matter. This book would also serve as a resource for nursing and other health care professions students. It would be useful in public, academic, and hospital libraries with consumer health collections." — *E-Streams, Jul '02*

Alternative Medicine Sourcebook, 2nd Edition

Basic Consumer Health Information about Alternative and Complementary Medical Practices, Including Acupuncture, Chiropractic, Herbal Medicine, Homeopathy, Naturopathic Medicine, Mind-Body Interventions, Ayurveda, and Other Non-Western Medical Traditions

Along with Facts about such Specific Therapies as Massage Therapy, Aromatherapy, Qigong, Hypnosis, Prayer, Dance, and Art Therapies, a Glossary, and Resources for Further Information

Edited by Dawn D. Matthews. 618 pages. 2002. 0-7808-0605-0. $78.

ALSO AVAILABLE: Alternative Medicine Sourcebook, 1st Edition. Edited by Allan R. Cook. 737 pages. 1999. 0-7808-0200-4. $78.

"Recommended for public, high school, and academic libraries that have consumer health collections. Hospital libraries that also serve the public will find this to be a useful resource." — *E-Streams, Feb '03*

"Recommended reference source."
— *Booklist, American Library Association, Jan '03*

"An important alternate health reference."
— *MBR Bookwatch, Oct '02*

"A great addition to the reference collection of every type of library." — *American Reference Books Annual, 2000*

Alzheimer's Disease Sourcebook, 2nd Edition

Basic Consumer Health Information about Alzheimer's Disease, Related Disorders, and Other Dementias, Including Multi-Infarct Dementia, AIDS-Related Dementia, Alcoholic Dementia, Huntington's Disease, Delirium, and Confusional States

Along with Reports Detailing Current Research Efforts in Prevention and Treatment, Long-Term Care Issues, and Listings of Sources for Additional Help and Information

Edited by Karen Bellenir. 524 pages. 1999. 0-7808-0223-3. $78.

ALSO AVAILABLE: Alzheimer's, Stroke & 29 Other Neurological Disorders Sourcebook, 1st Edition. Edited by Frank E. Bair. 579 pages. 1993. 1-55888-748-2. $78.

"Provides a wealth of useful information not otherwise available in one place. This resource is recommended for all types of libraries."
— *American Reference Books Annual, 2000*

"Recommended reference source."
— *Booklist, American Library Association, Oct '99*

SEE ALSO Brain Disorders Sourcebook

Arthritis Sourcebook

Basic Consumer Health Information about Specific Forms of Arthritis and Related Disorders, Including Rheumatoid Arthritis, Osteoarthritis, Gout, Polymyalgia Rheumatica, Psoriatic Arthritis, Spondyloarthropathies, Juvenile Rheumatoid Arthritis, and Juvenile Ankylosing Spondylitis

Along with Information about Medical, Surgical, and Alternative Treatment Options, and Including Strategies for Coping with Pain, Fatigue, and Stress

Edited by Allan R. Cook. 550 pages. 1998. 0-7808-0201-2. $78.

". . . accessible to the layperson."
— *Reference and Research Book News, Feb '99*

Asthma Sourcebook

Basic Consumer Health Information about Asthma, Including Symptoms, Traditional and Nontraditional Remedies, Treatment Advances, Quality-of-Life Aids, Medical Research Updates, and the Role of Allergies, Exercise, Age, the Environment, and Genetics in the Development of Asthma

Along with Statistical Data, a Glossary, and Directories of Support Groups, and Other Resources for Further Information

Edited by Annemarie S. Muth. 628 pages. 2000. 0-7808-0381-7. $78.

"A worthwhile reference acquisition for public libraries and academic medical libraries whose readers desire a quick introduction to the wide range of asthma information." — *Choice, Association of College & Research Libraries, Jun '01*

Attention Deficit Disorder Sourcebook

Basic Consumer Health Information about Attention Deficit/Hyperactivity Disorder in Children and Adults, Including Facts about Causes, Symptoms, Diagnostic Criteria, and Treatment Options Such as Medications, Behavior Therapy, Coaching, and Homeopathy

Along with Reports on Current Research Initiatives, Legal Issues, and Government Regulations, and Featuring a Glossary of Related Terms, Internet Resources, and a List of Additional Reading Material

Edited by Dawn D. Matthews. 470 pages. 2002. 0-7808-0624-7. $78.

Back & Neck Disorders Sourcebook

Basic Information about Disorders and Injuries of the Spinal Cord and Vertebrae, Including Facts on Chiropractic Treatment, Surgical Interventions, Paralysis, and Rehabilitation

Along with Advice for Preventing Back Trouble

Edited by Karen Bellenir. 548 pages. 1997. 0-7808-0202-0. $78.

Blood & Circulatory Disorders Sourcebook

Basic Information about Blood and Its Components, Anemias, Leukemias, Bleeding Disorders, and Circulatory Disorders, Including Aplastic Anemia, Thalassemia, Sickle-Cell Disease, Hemochromatosis, Hemophilia, Von Willebrand Disease, and Vascular Diseases

Along with a Special Section on Blood Transfusions and Blood Supply Safety, a Glossary, and Source Listings for Further Help and Information

Edited by Karen Bellenir and Linda M. Shin. 554 pages. 1998. 0-7808-0203-9. $78.

Brain Disorders Sourcebook

Basic Consumer Health Information about Strokes, Epilepsy, Amyotrophic Lateral Sclerosis (ALS/Lou Gehrig's Disease), Parkinson's Disease, Brain Tumors, Cerebral Palsy, Headache, Tourette Syndrome, and More

Along with Statistical Data, Treatment and Rehabilitation Options, Coping Strategies, Reports on Current Research Initiatives, a Glossary, and Resource Listings for Additional Help and Information

Edited by Karen Bellenir. 481 pages. 1999. 0-7808-0229-2. $78.

SEE ALSO Alzheimer's Disease Sourcebook

Breast Cancer Sourcebook

Basic Consumer Health Information about Breast Cancer, Including Diagnostic Methods, Treatment Options, Alternative Therapies, Self-Help Information, Related Health Concerns, Statistical and Demographic Data, and Facts for Men with Breast Cancer

Along with Reports on Current Research Initiatives, a Glossary of Related Medical Terms, and a Directory of Sources for Further Help and Information

Edited by Edward J. Prucha and Karen Bellenir. 580 pages. 2001. 0-7808-0244-6. $78.

"From the pros and cons of different screening methods and results to treatment options, *Breast Cancer Sourcebook* provides the latest information on the subject."
—*Library Bookwatch, Dec '01*

"This thoroughgoing, very readable reference covers all aspects of breast health and cancer. . . . Readers will find much to consider here. Recommended for all public and patient health collections."
—*Library Journal, Sep '01*

SEE ALSO *Cancer Sourcebook for Women, Women's Health Concerns Sourcebook*

■

Breastfeeding Sourcebook

Basic Consumer Health Information about the Benefits of Breastmilk, Preparing to Breastfeed, Breastfeeding as a Baby Grows, Nutrition, and More, Including Information on Special Situations and Concerns Such as Mastitis, Illness, Medications, Allergies, Multiple Births, Prematurity, Special Needs, and Adoption

Along with a Glossary and Resources for Additional Help and Information

Edited by Jenni Lynn Colson. 388 pages. 2002. 0-7808-0332-9. $78.

SEE ALSO *Pregnancy & Birth Sourcebook*

"Particularly useful is the information about professional lactation services and chapters on breastfeeding when returning to work. . . . *Breastfeeding Sourcebook* will be useful for public libraries, consumer health libraries, and technical schools offering nurse assistant training, especially in areas where Internet access is problematic."
—*American Reference Books Annual, 2003*

■

Burns Sourcebook

Basic Consumer Health Information about Various Types of Burns and Scalds, Including Flame, Heat, Cold, Electrical, Chemical, and Sun Burns

Along with Information on Short-Term and Long-Term Treatments, Tissue Reconstruction, Plastic Surgery, Prevention Suggestions, and First Aid

Edited by Allan R. Cook. 604 pages. 1999. 0-7808-0204-7. $78.

"This is an exceptional addition to the series and is highly recommended for all consumer health collections, hospital libraries, and academic medical centers."
—*E-Streams, Mar '00*

"This key reference guide is an invaluable addition to all health care and public libraries in confronting this ongoing health issue."
—*American Reference Books Annual, 2000*

"Recommended reference source."
—*Booklist, American Library Association, Dec '99*

SEE ALSO *Skin Disorders Sourcebook*

Cancer Sourcebook, 4th Edition

Basic Consumer Health Information about Major Forms and Stages of Cancer, Featuring Facts about Head and Neck Cancers, Lung Cancers, Gastrointestinal Cancers, Genitourinary Cancers, Lymphomas, Blood Cell Cancers, Endocrine Cancers, Skin Cancers, Bone Cancers, Sarcomas, and Others, and Including Information about Cancer Treatments and Therapies, Identifying and Reducing Cancer Risks, and Strategies for Coping with Cancer and the Side Effects of Treatment

Along with a Cancer Glossary, Statistical and Demographic Data, and a Directory of Sources for Additional Help and Information

Edited by Karen Bellenir. 1,119 pages. 2003. 0-7808-0633-6. $78.

ALSO AVAILABLE: *Cancer Sourcebook, 1st Edition.* Edited by Frank E. Bair. 932 pages. 1990. 1-55888-888-8. $78.

New Cancer Sourcebook, 2nd Edition. Edited by Allan R. Cook. 1,313 pages. 1996. 0-7808-0041-9. $78.

Cancer Sourcebook, 3rd Edition. Edited by Edward J. Prucha. 1,069 pages. 2000. 0-7808-0227-6. $78.

"This title is recommended for health sciences and public libraries with consumer health collections."
—*E-Streams, Feb '01*

". . . can be effectively used by cancer patients and their families who are looking for answers in a language they can understand. Public and hospital libraries should have it on their shelves."
—*American Reference Books Annual, 2001*

"Recommended reference source."
—*Booklist, American Library Association, Dec '00*

Cited in *Reference Sources for Small and Medium-Sized Libraries*, American Library Association, 1999

"The amount of factual and useful information is extensive. The writing is very clear, geared to general readers. Recommended for all levels." —*Choice, Association of College & Research Libraries, Jan '97*

SEE ALSO *Breast Cancer Sourcebook, Cancer Sourcebook for Women, Pediatric Cancer Sourcebook, Prostate Cancer Sourcebook*

■

Cancer Sourcebook for Women, 2nd Edition

Basic Consumer Health Information about Gynecologic Cancers and Related Concerns, Including Cervical Cancer, Endometrial Cancer, Gestational Trophoblastic Tumor, Ovarian Cancer, Uterine Cancer, Vaginal Cancer, Vulvar Cancer, Breast Cancer, and Common Non-Cancerous Uterine Conditions, with Facts about Cancer Risk Factors, Screening and Prevention, Treatment Options, and Reports on Current Research Initiatives

Along with a Glossary of Cancer Terms and a Directory of Resources for Additional Help and Information

Edited by Karen Bellenir. 604 pages. 2002. 0-7808-0226-8. $78.

ALSO AVAILABLE: *Cancer Sourcebook for Women, 1st Edition.* Edited by Allan R. Cook and Peter D. Dresser. 524 pages. 1996. 0-7808-0076-1. $78.

"An excellent addition to collections in public, consumer health, and women's health libraries."
— *American Reference Books Annual, 2003*

"Overall, the information is excellent, and complex topics are clearly explained. As a reference book for the consumer it is a valuable resource to assist them to make informed decisions about cancer and its treatments." — *Cancer Forum, Nov '02*

"Highly recommended for academic and medical reference collections." — *Library Bookwatch, Sep '02*

"This is a highly recommended book for any public or consumer library, being reader friendly and containing accurate and helpful information."
— *E-Streams, Aug '02*

"Recommended reference source."
— *Booklist, American Library Association, Jul '02*

SEE ALSO *Breast Cancer Sourcebook, Women's Health Concerns Sourcebook*

Cardiovascular Diseases & Disorders Sourcebook, 1st Edition

SEE *Heart Diseases & Disorders Sourcebook, 2nd Edition*

Caregiving Sourcebook

Basic Consumer Health Information for Caregivers, Including a Profile of Caregivers, Caregiving Responsibilities and Concerns, Tips for Specific Conditions, Care Environments, and the Effects of Caregiving

Along with Facts about Legal Issues, Financial Information, and Future Planning, a Glossary, and a Listing of Additional Resources

Edited by Joyce Brennfleck Shannon. 600 pages. 2001. 0-7808-0331-0. $78.

"Essential for most collections."
— *Library Journal, Apr 1, 2002*

"An ideal addition to the reference collection of any public library. Health sciences information professionals may also want to acquire the *Caregiving Sourcebook* for their hospital or academic library for use as a ready reference tool by health care workers interested in aging and caregiving." —*E-Streams, Jan '02*

"Recommended reference source."
—*Booklist, American Library Association, Oct '01*

Childhood Diseases & Disorders Sourcebook

Basic Consumer Health Information about Medical Problems Often Encountered in Pre-Adolescent Children, Including Respiratory Tract Ailments, Ear Infections, Sore Throats, Disorders of the Skin and Scalp, *Digestive and Genitourinary Diseases, Infectious Diseases, Inflammatory Disorders, Chronic Physical and Developmental Disorders, Allergies, and More*

Along with Information about Diagnostic Tests, Common Childhood Surgeries, and Frequently Used Medications, with a Glossary of Important Terms and Resource Directory

Edited by Chad T. Kimball. 662 pages. 2003. 0-7808-0458-9. $78.

Colds, Flu & Other Common Ailments Sourcebook

Basic Consumer Health Information about Common Ailments and Injuries, Including Colds, Coughs, the Flu, Sinus Problems, Headaches, Fever, Nausea and Vomiting, Menstrual Cramps, Diarrhea, Constipation, Hemorrhoids, Back Pain, Dandruff, Dry and Itchy Skin, Cuts, Scrapes, Sprains, Bruises, and More

Along with Information about Prevention, Self-Care, Choosing a Doctor, Over-the-Counter Medications, Folk Remedies, and Alternative Therapies, and Including a Glossary of Important Terms and a Directory of Resources for Further Help and Information

Edited by Chad T. Kimball. 638 pages. 2001. 0-7808-0435-X. $78.

"A good starting point for research on common illnesses. It will be a useful addition to public and consumer health library collections."
— *American Reference Books Annual 2002*

"Will prove valuable to any library seeking to maintain a current, comprehensive reference collection of health resources. . . . Excellent reference."
— *The Bookwatch, Aug '01*

"Recommended reference source."
— *Booklist, American Library Association, July '01*

Communication Disorders Sourcebook

Basic Information about Deafness and Hearing Loss, Speech and Language Disorders, Voice Disorders, Balance and Vestibular Disorders, and Disorders of Smell, Taste, and Touch

Edited by Linda M. Ross. 533 pages. 1996. 0-7808-0077-X. $78.

"This is skillfully edited and is a welcome resource for the layperson. It should be found in every public and medical library." — *Booklist Health Sciences Supplement, American Library Association, Oct '97*

Congenital Disorders Sourcebook

Basic Information about Disorders Acquired during Gestation, Including Spina Bifida, Hydrocephalus, Cerebral Palsy, Heart Defects, Craniofacial Abnormalities, Fetal Alcohol Syndrome, and More

Along with Current Treatment Options and Statistical Data

Edited by Karen Bellenir. 607 pages. 1997. 0-7808-0205-5. $78.

"Recommended reference source."
—*Booklist, American Library Association, Oct '97*

SEE ALSO *Pregnancy & Birth Sourcebook*

Consumer Issues in Health Care Sourcebook

Basic Information about Health Care Fundamentals and Related Consumer Issues, Including Exams and Screening Tests, Physician Specialties, Choosing a Doctor, Using Prescription and Over-the-Counter Medications Safely, Avoiding Health Scams, Managing Common Health Risks in the Home, Care Options for Chronically or Terminally Ill Patients, and a List of Resources for Obtaining Help and Further Information

Edited by Karen Bellenir. 618 pages. 1998. 0-7808-0221-7. $78.

"Both public and academic libraries will want to have a copy in their collection for readers who are interested in self-education on health issues."
—*American Reference Books Annual, 2000*

"The editor has researched the literature from government agencies and others, saving readers the time and effort of having to do the research themselves. Recommended for public libraries."
—*Reference and User Services Quarterly, American Library Association, Spring '99*

"Recommended reference source."
—*Booklist, American Library Association, Dec '98*

Contagious & Non-Contagious Infectious Diseases Sourcebook

Basic Information about Contagious Diseases like Measles, Polio, Hepatitis B, and Infectious Mononucleosis, and Non-Contagious Infectious Diseases like Tetanus and Toxic Shock Syndrome, and Diseases Occurring as Secondary Infections Such as Shingles and Reye Syndrome

Along with Vaccination, Prevention, and Treatment Information, and a Section Describing Emerging Infectious Disease Threats

Edited by Karen Bellenir and Peter D. Dresser. 566 pages. 1996. 0-7808-0075-3. $78.

Death & Dying Sourcebook

Basic Consumer Health Information for the Layperson about End-of-Life Care and Related Ethical and Legal Issues, Including Chief Causes of Death, Autopsies, Pain Management for the Terminally Ill, Life Support Systems, Insurance, Euthanasia, Assisted Suicide, Hospice Programs, Living Wills, Funeral Planning, Counseling, Mourning, Organ Donation, and Physician Training

Along with Statistical Data, a Glossary, and Listings of Sources for Further Help and Information

Edited by Annemarie S. Muth. 641 pages. 1999. 0-7808-0230-6. $78.

"Public libraries, medical libraries, and academic libraries will all find this sourcebook a useful addition to their collections."
—*American Reference Books Annual, 2001*

"An extremely useful resource for those concerned with death and dying in the United States."
—*Respiratory Care, Nov '00*

"Recommended reference source."
—*Booklist, American Library Association, Aug '00*

"This book is a definite must for all those involved in end-of-life care." —*Doody's Review Service, 2000*

Dental Care & Oral Health Sourcebook, 2nd Edition

Basic Consumer Health Information about Dental Care, Including Oral Hygiene, Dental Visits, Pain Management, Cavities, Crowns, Bridges, Dental Implants, and Fillings, and Other Oral Health Concerns, Such as Gum Disease, Bad Breath, Dry Mouth, Genetic and Developmental Abnormalities, Oral Cancers, Orthodontics, and Temporomandibular Disorders

Along with Updates on Current Research in Oral Health, a Glossary, a Directory of Dental and Oral Health Organizations, and Resources for People with Dental and Oral Health Disorders

Edited by Amy L. Sutton. 616 pages. 2003. 0-7808-0634-4. $78.

ALSO AVAILABLE: *Oral Health Sourcebook, 1st Edition.* Edited by Allan R. Cook. 558 pages. 1997. 0-7808-0082-6. $78.

"Unique source which will fill a gap in dental sources for patients and the lay public. A valuable reference tool even in a library with thousands of books on dentistry. Comprehensive, clear, inexpensive, and easy to read and use. It fills an enormous gap in the health care literature." —*Reference and User Services Quarterly, American Library Association, Summer '98*

"Recommended reference source."
—*Booklist, American Library Association, Dec '97*

Depression Sourcebook

Basic Consumer Health Information about Unipolar Depression, Bipolar Disorder, Postpartum Depression, Seasonal Affective Disorder, and Other Types of Depression in Children, Adolescents, Women, Men, the Elderly, and Other Selected Populations

Along with Facts about Causes, Risk Factors, Diagnostic Criteria, Treatment Options, Coping Strategies, Suicide Prevention, a Glossary, and a Directory of Sources for Additional Help and Information

Edited by Karen Belleni. 602 pages. 2002. 0-7808-0611-5. $78.

"Invaluable reference for public and school library collections alike." — Library Bookwatch, Apr '03

"Recommended for purchase."
— American Reference Books Annual, 2003

Diabetes Sourcebook, 3rd Edition

Basic Consumer Health Information about Type 1 Diabetes (Insulin-Dependent or Juvenile-Onset Diabetes), Type 2 Diabetes (Noninsulin-Dependent or Adult-Onset Diabetes), Gestational Diabetes, Impaired Glucose Tolerance (IGT), and Related Complications, Such as Amputation, Eye Disease, Gum Disease, Nerve Damage, and End-Stage Renal Disease, Including Facts about Insulin, Oral Diabetes Medications, Blood Sugar Testing, and the Role of Exercise and Nutrition in the Control of Diabetes

Along with a Glossary and Resources for Further Help and Information

Edited by Dawn D. Matthews. 622 pages. 2003. 0-7808-0629-8. $78.

ALSO AVAILABLE: *Diabetes Sourcebook, 1st Edition.* Edited by Karen Bellenir and Peter D. Dresser. 827 pages. 1994. 1-55888-751-2. $78.

Diabetes Sourcebook, 2nd Edition. Edited by Karen Bellenir. 688 pages. 1998. 0-7808-0224-1. $78.

"An invaluable reference." — Library Journal, May '00

Selected as one of the 250 "Best Health Sciences Books of 1999." — Doody's Rating Service, Mar-Apr 2000

"This comprehensive book is an excellent addition for high school, academic, medical, and public libraries. This volume is highly recommended."
— American Reference Books Annual, 2000

"Provides useful information for the general public."
— Healthlines, University of Michigan Health Management Research Center, Sep/Oct '99

". . . provides reliable mainstream medical information . . . belongs on the shelves of any library with a consumer health collection." — E-Streams, Sep '99

"Recommended reference source."
— Booklist, American Library Association, Feb '99

Diet & Nutrition Sourcebook, 2nd Edition

Basic Consumer Health Information about Dietary Guidelines, Recommended Daily Intake Values, Vitamins, Minerals, Fiber, Fat, Weight Control, Dietary Supplements, and Food Additives

Along with Special Sections on Nutrition Needs throughout Life and Nutrition for People with Such Specific Medical Concerns as Allergies, High Blood Cholesterol, Hypertension, Diabetes, Celiac Disease, Seizure Disorders, Phenylketonuria (PKU), Cancer, and

Eating Disorders, and Including Reports on Current Nutrition Research and Source Listings for Additional Help and Information

Edited by Karen Bellenir. 650 pages. 1999. 0-7808-0228-4. $78.

ALSO AVAILABLE: *Diet & Nutrition Sourcebook, 1st Edition.* Edited by Dan R. Harris. 662 pages. 1996. 0-7808-0084-2. $78.

"This book is an excellent source of basic diet and nutrition information." — Booklist Health Sciences Supplement, American Library Association, Dec '00

"This reference document should be in any public library, but it would be a very good guide for beginning students in the health sciences. If the other books in this publisher's series are as good as this, they should all be in the health sciences collections."
— American Reference Books Annual, 2000

"This book is an excellent general nutrition reference for consumers who desire to take an active role in their health care for prevention. Consumers of all ages who select this book can feel confident they are receiving current and accurate information." — Journal of Nutrition for the Elderly, Vol. 19, No. 4, '00

"Recommended reference source."
— Booklist, American Library Association, Dec '99

SEE ALSO *Digestive Diseases & Disorders Sourcebook, Eating Disorders Sourcebook, Gastrointestinal Diseases & Disorders Sourcebook, Vegetarian Sourcebook*

Digestive Diseases & Disorders Sourcebook

Basic Consumer Health Information about Diseases and Disorders that Impact the Upper and Lower Digestive System, Including Celiac Disease, Constipation, Crohn's Disease, Cyclic Vomiting Syndrome, Diarrhea, Diverticulosis and Diverticulitis, Gallstones, Heartburn, Hemorrhoids, Hernias, Indigestion (Dyspepsia), Irritable Bowel Syndrome, Lactose Intolerance, Ulcers, and More

Along with Information about Medications and Other Treatments, Tips for Maintaining a Healthy Digestive Tract, a Glossary, and Directory of Digestive Diseases Organizations

Edited by Karen Bellenir. 335 pages. 2000. 0-7808-0327-2. $78.

"This title would be an excellent addition to all public or patient-research libraries."
— American Reference Books Annual, 2001

"This title is recommended for public, hospital, and health sciences libraries with consumer health collections." — E-Streams, Jul-Aug '00

"Recommended reference source."
— Booklist, American Library Association, May '00

SEE ALSO *Diet & Nutrition Sourcebook, Eating Disorders Sourcebook, Gastrointestinal Diseases & Disorders Sourcebook*

Disabilities Sourcebook

Basic Consumer Health Information about Physical and Psychiatric Disabilities, Including Descriptions of Major Causes of Disability, Assistive and Adaptive Aids, Workplace Issues, and Accessibility Concerns

Along with Information about the Americans with Disabilities Act, a Glossary, and Resources for Additional Help and Information

Edited by Dawn D. Matthews. 616 pages. 2000. 0-7808-0389-2. $78.

"It is a must for libraries with a consumer health section." — *American Reference Books Annual 2002*

"A much needed addition to the Omnigraphics *Health Reference Series*. A current reference work to provide people with disabilities, their families, caregivers or those who work with them, a broad range of information in one volume, has not been available until now. . . . It is recommended for all public and academic library reference collections." — *E-Streams, May '01*

"An excellent source book in easy-to-read format covering many current topics; highly recommended for all libraries." — *Choice, Association of College and Research Libraries, Jan '01*

"Recommended reference source."
—*Booklist, American Library Association, Jul '00*

■

Domestic Violence & Child Abuse Sourcebook

Basic Consumer Health Information about Spousal/ Partner, Child, Sibling, Parent, and Elder Abuse, Covering Physical, Emotional, and Sexual Abuse, Teen Dating Violence, and Stalking; Includes Information about Hotlines, Safe Houses, Safety Plans, and Other Resources for Support and Assistance, Community Initiatives, and Reports on Current Directions in Research and Treatment

Along with a Glossary, Sources for Further Reading, and Governmental and Non-Governmental Organizations Contact Information

Edited by Helene Henderson. 1,064 pages. 2001. 0-7808-0235-7. $78.

"Interested lay persons should find the book extremely beneficial. . . . A copy of *Domestic Violence and Child Abuse Sourcebook* should be in every public library in the United States." — *Social Science & Medicine, No. 56, 2003*

"This is important information. The Web has many resources but this sourcebook fills an important societal need. I am not aware of any other resources of this type." — *Doody's Review Service, Sep '01*

"Recommended for all libraries, scholars, and practitioners." — *Choice, Association of College & Research Libraries, Jul '01*

"Recommended reference source."
—*Booklist, American Library Association, Apr '01*

"Important pick for college-level health reference libraries." — *The Bookwatch, Mar '01*

"Because this problem is so widespread and because this book includes a lot of issues within one volume, this work is recommended for all public libraries." — *American Reference Books Annual, 2001*

■

Drug Abuse Sourcebook

Basic Consumer Health Information about Illicit Substances of Abuse and the Diversion of Prescription Medications, Including Depressants, Hallucinogens, Inhalants, Marijuana, Narcotics, Stimulants, and Anabolic Steroids

Along with Facts about Related Health Risks, Treatment Issues, and Substance Abuse Prevention Programs, a Glossary of Terms, Statistical Data, and Directories of Hotline Services, Self-Help Groups, and Organizations Able to Provide Further Information

Edited by Karen Bellenir. 629 pages. 2000. 0-7808-0242-X. $78.

"Containing a wealth of information . . . . This resource belongs in libraries that serve a lower-division undergraduate or community college clientele as well as the general public." — *Choice, Association of College and Research Libraries, Jun '01*

"Recommended reference source."
— *Booklist, American Library Association, Feb '01*

"Highly recommended." — *The Bookwatch, Jan '01*

"Even though there is a plethora of books on drug abuse, this volume is recommended for school, public, and college libraries." —*American Reference Books Annual, 2001*

SEE ALSO Alcoholism Sourcebook, Substance Abuse Sourcebook

■

Ear, Nose & Throat Disorders Sourcebook

Basic Information about Disorders of the Ears, Nose, Sinus Cavities, Pharynx, and Larynx, Including Ear Infections, Tinnitus, Vestibular Disorders, Allergic and Non-Allergic Rhinitis, Sore Throats, Tonsillitis, and Cancers That Affect the Ears, Nose, Sinuses, and Throat

Along with Reports on Current Research Initiatives, a Glossary of Related Medical Terms, and a Directory of Sources for Further Help and Information

Edited by Karen Bellenir and Linda M. Shin. 576 pages. 1998. 0-7808-0206-3. $78.

"Overall, this sourcebook is helpful for the consumer seeking information on ENT issues. It is recommended for public libraries." —*American Reference Books Annual, 1999*

"Recommended reference source."
—*Booklist, American Library Association, Dec '98*

Eating Disorders Sourcebook

Basic Consumer Health Information about Eating Disorders, Including Information about Anorexia Nervosa, Bulimia Nervosa, Binge Eating, Body Dysmorphic Disorder, Pica, Laxative Abuse, and Night Eating Syndrome

Along with Information about Causes, Adverse Effects, and Treatment and Prevention Issues, and Featuring a Section on Concerns Specific to Children and Adolescents, a Glossary, and Resources for Further Help and Information

Edited by Dawn D. Matthews. 322 pages. 2001. 0-7808-0335-3. $78.

"Recommended for health science libraries that are open to the public, as well as hospital libraries. This book is a good resource for the consumer who is concerned about eating disorders." — *E-Streams, Mar '02*

"This volume is another convenient collection of excerpted articles. Recommended for school and public library patrons; lower-division undergraduates; and two-year technical program students." — *Choice, Association of College & Research Libraries, Jan '02*

"Recommended reference source." — *Booklist, American Library Association, Oct '01*

SEE ALSO *Diet & Nutrition Sourcebook, Digestive Diseases & Disorders Sourcebook, Gastrointestinal Diseases & Disorders Sourcebook*

Emergency Medical Services Sourcebook

Basic Consumer Health Information about Preventing, Preparing for, and Managing Emergency Situations, When and Who to Call for Help, What to Expect in the Emergency Room, the Emergency Medical Team, Patient Issues, and Current Topics in Emergency Medicine

Along with Statistical Data, a Glossary, and Sources of Additional Help and Information

Edited by Jenni Lynn Colson. 494 pages. 2002. 0-7808-0420-1. $78.

"Handy and convenient for home, public, school, and college libraries. Recommended." — *Choice, Association of College and Research Libraries, Apr '03*

"This reference can provide the consumer with answers to most questions about emergency care in the United States, or it will direct them to a resource where the answer can be found." — *American Reference Books Annual, 2003*

"Recommended reference source." — *Booklist, American Library Association, Feb '03*

Endocrine & Metabolic Disorders Sourcebook

Basic Information for the Layperson about Pancreatic and Insulin-Related Disorders Such as Pancreatitis, Diabetes, and Hypoglycemia; Adrenal Gland Disorders Such as Cushing's Syndrome, Addison's Disease, and Congenital Adrenal Hyperplasia; Pituitary Gland Disorders Such as Growth Hormone Deficiency, Acromegaly, and Pituitary Tumors; Thyroid Disorders Such as Hypothyroidism, Graves' Disease, Hashimoto's Disease, and Goiter; Hyperparathyroidism; and Other Diseases and Syndromes of Hormone Imbalance or Metabolic Dysfunction

Along with Reports on Current Research Initiatives

Edited by Linda M. Shin. 574 pages. 1998. 0-7808-0207-1. $78.

"Omnigraphics has produced another needed resource for health information consumers."
— *American Reference Books Annual, 2000*

"Recommended reference source."
— *Booklist, American Library Association, Dec '98*

Environmental Health Sourcebook, 2nd Edition

Basic Consumer Health Information about the Environment and Its Effect on Human Health, Including the Effects of Air Pollution, Water Pollution, Hazardous Chemicals, Food Hazards, Radiation Hazards, Biological Agents, Household Hazards, Such as Radon, Asbestos, Carbon Monoxide, and Mold, and Information about Associated Diseases and Disorders, Including Cancer, Allergies, Respiratory Problems, and Skin Disorders

Along with Information about Environmental Concerns for Specific Populations, a Glossary of Related Terms, and Resources for Further Help and Information

Edited by Dawn D. Matthews. 673 pages. 2003. 0-7808-0632-8. $78.

ALSO AVAILABLE: *Environmentally Induced Disorders Sourcebook, 1st Edition.* Edited by Allan R. Cook. 620 pages. 1997. 0-7808-0083-4. $78.

"Recommended reference source."
— *Booklist, American Library Association, Sep '98*

"This book will be a useful addition to anyone's library." — *Choice Health Sciences Supplement, Association of College and Research Libraries, May '98*

". . . a good survey of numerous environmentally induced physical disorders . . . a useful addition to anyone's library."
— *Doody's Health Sciences Book Reviews, Jan '98*

". . . provide[s] introductory information from the best authorities around. Since this volume covers topics that potentially affect everyone, it will surely be one of the most frequently consulted volumes in the *Health Reference Series*." — *Rettig on Reference, Nov '97*

Environmentally Induced Disorders Sourcebook, 1st Edition

SEE *Environmental Health Sourcebook, 2nd Edition*

■

Ethnic Diseases Sourcebook

Basic Consumer Health Information for Ethnic and Racial Minority Groups in the United States, Including General Health Indicators and Behaviors, Ethnic Diseases, Genetic Testing, the Impact of Chronic Diseases, Women's Health, Mental Health Issues, and Preventive Health Care Services

Along with a Glossary and a Listing of Additional Resources

Edited by Joyce Brennfleck Shannon. 664 pages. 2001. 0-7808-0336-1. $78.

"Recommended for health sciences libraries where public health programs are a priority."
— *E-Streams, Jan '02*

"Not many books have been written on this topic to date, and the *Ethnic Diseases Sourcebook* is a strong addition to the list. It will be an important introductory resource for health consumers, students, health care personnel, and social scientists. It is recommended for public, academic, and large hospital libraries."
— *American Reference Books Annual 2002*

"Recommended reference source."
— *Booklist, American Library Association, Oct '01*

"Will prove valuable to any library seeking to maintain a current, comprehensive reference collection of health resources. . . . An excellent source of health information about genetic disorders which affect particular ethnic and racial minorities in the U.S."
— *The Bookwatch, Aug '01*

■

Eye Care Sourcebook, 2nd Edition

Basic Consumer Health Information about Eye Care and Eye Disorders, Including Facts about the Diagnosis, Prevention, and Treatment of Common Refractive Problems Such as Myopia, Hyperopia, Astigmatism, and Presbyopia, and Eye Diseases, Including Glaucoma, Cataract, Age-Related Macular Degeneration, and Diabetic Retinopathy

Along with a Section on Vision Correction and Refractive Surgeries, Including LASIK and LASEK, a Glossary, and Directories of Resources for Additional Help and Information

Edited by Amy L. Sutton. 543 pages. 2003. 0-7808-0635-2. $78.

ALSO AVAILABLE: *Ophthalmic Disorders Sourcebook, 1st Edition.* Edited by Linda M. Ross. 631 pages. 1996. 0-7808-0081-8. $78.

Family Planning Sourcebook

Basic Consumer Health Information about Planning for Pregnancy and Contraception, Including Traditional Methods, Barrier Methods, Hormonal Methods, Permanent Methods, Future Methods, Emergency Contraception, and Birth Control Choices for Women at Each Stage of Life

Along with Statistics, a Glossary, and Sources of Additional Information

Edited by Amy Marcaccio Keyzer. 520 pages. 2001. 0-7808-0379-5. $78.

"Recommended for public, health, and undergraduate libraries as part of the circulating collection."
— *E-Streams, Mar '02*

"Information is presented in an unbiased, readable manner, and the sourcebook will certainly be a necessary addition to those public and high school libraries where Internet access is restricted or otherwise problematic." — *American Reference Books Annual 2002*

"Recommended reference source."
— *Booklist, American Library Association, Oct '01*

"Will prove valuable to any library seeking to maintain a current, comprehensive reference collection of health resources. . . . Excellent reference."
— *The Bookwatch, Aug '01*

SEE ALSO *Pregnancy & Birth Sourcebook*

■

Fitness & Exercise Sourcebook, 2nd Edition

Basic Consumer Health Information about the Fundamentals of Fitness and Exercise, Including How to Begin and Maintain a Fitness Program, Fitness as a Lifestyle, the Link between Fitness and Diet, Advice for Specific Groups of People, Exercise as It Relates to Specific Medical Conditions, and Recent Research in Fitness and Exercise

Along with a Glossary of Important Terms and Resources for Additional Help and Information

Edited by Kristen M. Gledhill. 646 pages. 2001. 0-7808-0334-5. $78.

ALSO AVAILABLE: *Fitness & Exercise Sourcebook, 1st Edition.* Edited by Dan R. Harris. 663 pages. 1996. 0-7808-0186-5. $78.

"This work is recommended for all general reference collections."
— *American Reference Books Annual 2002*

"Highly recommended for public, consumer, and school grades fourth through college."
— *E-Streams, Nov '01*

"Recommended reference source." — *Booklist, American Library Association, Oct '01*

"The information appears quite comprehensive and is considered reliable. . . . This second edition is a welcomed addition to the series."
— *Doody's Review Service, Sep '01*

"This reference is a valuable choice for those who desire a broad source of information on exercise, fitness, and chronic-disease prevention through a healthy lifestyle." —*American Medical Writers Association Journal, Fall '01*

"Will prove valuable to any library seeking to maintain a current, comprehensive reference collection of health resources. . . . Excellent reference."
— *The Bookwatch, Aug '01*

■

Food & Animal Borne Diseases Sourcebook

Basic Information about Diseases That Can Be Spread to Humans through the Ingestion of Contaminated Food or Water or by Contact with Infected Animals and Insects, Such as Botulism, E. Coli, Hepatitis A, Trichinosis, Lyme Disease, and Rabies

Along with Information Regarding Prevention and Treatment Methods, and Including a Special Section for International Travelers Describing Diseases Such as Cholera, Malaria, Travelers' Diarrhea, and Yellow Fever, and Offering Recommendations for Avoiding Illness

Edited by Karen Bellenir and Peter D. Dresser. 535 pages. 1995. 0-7808-0033-8. $78.

"Targeting general readers and providing them with a single, comprehensive source of information on selected topics, this book continues, with the excellent caliber of its predecessors, to catalog topical information on health matters of general interest. Readable and thorough, this valuable resource is highly recommended for all libraries."
— *Academic Library Book Review, Summer '96*

"A comprehensive collection of authoritative information." — *Emergency Medical Services, Oct '95*

■

Food Safety Sourcebook

Basic Consumer Health Information about the Safe Handling of Meat, Poultry, Seafood, Eggs, Fruit Juices, and Other Food Items, and Facts about Pesticides, Drinking Water, Food Safety Overseas, and the Onset, Duration, and Symptoms of Foodborne Illnesses, Including Types of Pathogenic Bacteria, Parasitic Protozoa, Worms, Viruses, and Natural Toxins

Along with the Role of the Consumer, the Food Handler, and the Government in Food Safety; a Glossary, and Resources for Additional Help and Information

Edited by Dawn D. Matthews. 339 pages. 1999. 0-7808-0326-4. $78.

"This book is recommended for public libraries and universities with home economic and food science programs." — *E-Streams, Nov '00*

"Recommended reference source."
—*Booklist, American Library Association, May '00*

"This book takes the complex issues of food safety and foodborne pathogens and presents them in an easily understood manner. [It does] an excellent job of covering a large and often confusing topic."
—*American Reference Books Annual, 2000*

Forensic Medicine Sourcebook

Basic Consumer Information for the Layperson about Forensic Medicine, Including Crime Scene Investigation, Evidence Collection and Analysis, Expert Testimony, Computer-Aided Criminal Identification, Digital Imaging in the Courtroom, DNA Profiling, Accident Reconstruction, Autopsies, Ballistics, Drugs and Explosives Detection, Latent Fingerprints, Product Tampering, and Questioned Document Examination

Along with Statistical Data, a Glossary of Forensics Terminology, and Listings of Sources for Further Help and Information

Edited by Annemarie S. Muth. 574 pages. 1999. 0-7808-0232-2. $78.

"Given the expected widespread interest in its content and its easy to read style, this book is recommended for most public and all college and university libraries."
— *E-Streams, Feb '01*

"Recommended for public libraries."
—*Reference & User Services Quarterly, American Library Association, Spring 2000*

"Recommended reference source."
—*Booklist, American Library Association, Feb '00*

"A wealth of information, useful statistics, references are up-to-date and extremely complete. This wonderful collection of data will help students who are interested in a career in any type of forensic field. It is a great resource for attorneys who need information about types of expert witnesses needed in a particular case. It also offers useful information for fiction and nonfiction writers whose work involves a crime. A fascinating compilation. All levels." — *Choice, Association of College and Research Libraries, Jan 2000*

"There are several items that make this book attractive to consumers who are seeking certain forensic data. . . . This is a useful current source for those seeking general forensic medical answers."
—*American Reference Books Annual, 2000*

■

Gastrointestinal Diseases & Disorders Sourcebook

Basic Information about Gastroesophageal Reflux Disease (Heartburn), Ulcers, Diverticulosis, Irritable Bowel Syndrome, Crohn's Disease, Ulcerative Colitis, Diarrhea, Constipation, Lactose Intolerance, Hemorrhoids, Hepatitis, Cirrhosis, and Other Digestive Problems, Featuring Statistics, Descriptions of Symptoms, and Current Treatment Methods of Interest for Persons Living with Upper and Lower Gastrointestinal Maladies

Edited by Linda M. Ross. 413 pages. 1996. 0-7808-0078-8. $78.

". . . very readable form. The successful editorial work that brought this material together into a useful and understandable reference makes accessible to all readers information that can help them more effectively understand and obtain help for digestive tract problems."
— *Choice, Association of College & Research Libraries, Feb '97*

SEE ALSO Diet & Nutrition Sourcebook, Digestive Diseases & Disorders, Eating Disorders Sourcebook

Genetic Disorders Sourcebook, 2nd Edition

Basic Consumer Health Information about Hereditary Diseases and Disorders, Including Cystic Fibrosis, Down Syndrome, Hemophilia, Huntington's Disease, Sickle Cell Anemia, and More; Facts about Genes, Gene Research and Therapy, Genetic Screening, Ethics of Gene Testing, Genetic Counseling, and Advice on Coping and Caring

Along with a Glossary of Genetic Terminology and a Resource List for Help, Support, and Further Information

Edited by Kathy Massimini. 768 pages. 2001. 0-7808-0241-1. $78.

ALSO AVAILABLE: Genetic Disorders Sourcebook, 1st Edition. Edited by Karen Bellenir. 642 pages. 1996. 0-7808-0034-6. $78.

"Recommended for public libraries and medical and hospital libraries with consumer health collections."
— *E-Streams, May '01*

"Recommended reference source."
— *Booklist, American Library Association, Apr '01*

"Important pick for college-level health reference libraries." — *The Bookwatch, Mar '01*

"Provides essential medical information to both the general public and those diagnosed with a serious or fatal genetic disease or disorder." — *Choice, Association of College and Research Libraries, Jan '97*

Head Trauma Sourcebook

Basic Information for the Layperson about Open-Head and Closed-Head Injuries, Treatment Advances, Recovery, and Rehabilitation

Along with Reports on Current Research Initiatives

Edited by Karen Bellenir. 414 pages. 1997. 0-7808-0208-X. $78.

Headache Sourcebook

Basic Consumer Health Information about Migraine, Tension, Cluster, Rebound and Other Types of Headaches, with Facts about the Cause and Prevention of Headaches, the Effects of Stress and the Environment, Headaches during Pregnancy and Menopause, and Childhood Headaches

Along with a Glossary and Other Resources for Additional Help and Information

Edited by Dawn D. Matthews. 362 pages. 2002. 0-7808-0337-X. $78.

"Highly recommended for academic and medical reference collections." — *Library Bookwatch, Sep '02*

Health Insurance Sourcebook

Basic Information about Managed Care Organizations, Traditional Fee-for-Service Insurance, Insurance Portability and Pre-Existing Conditions Clauses, Medicare, Medicaid, Social Security, and Military Health Care

Along with Information about Insurance Fraud

Edited by Wendy Wilcox. 530 pages. 1997. 0-7808-0222-5. $78.

"Particularly useful because it brings much of this information together in one volume. This book will be a handy reference source in the health sciences library, hospital library, college and university library, and medium to large public library."
— *Medical Reference Services Quarterly, Fall '98*

Awarded "Books of the Year Award"
— *American Journal of Nursing, 1997*

"The layout of the book is particularly helpful as it provides easy access to reference material. A most useful addition to the vast amount of information about health insurance. The use of data from U.S. government agencies is most commendable. Useful in a library or learning center for healthcare professional students."
— *Doody's Health Sciences Book Reviews, Nov '97*

Health Reference Series Cumulative Index 1999

A Comprehensive Index to the Individual Volumes of the Health Reference Series, Including a Subject Index, Name Index, Organization Index, and Publication Index

Along with a Master List of Acronyms and Abbreviations

Edited by Edward J. Prucha, Anne Holmes, and Robert Rudnick. 990 pages. 2000. 0-7808-0382-5. $78.

"This volume will be most helpful in libraries that have a relatively complete collection of the Health Reference Series." — *American Reference Books Annual, 2001*

"Essential for collections that hold any of the numerous *Health Reference Series* titles."
— *Choice, Association of College and Research Libraries, Nov '00*

Healthy Aging Sourcebook

Basic Consumer Health Information about Maintaining Health through the Aging Process, Including Advice on Nutrition, Exercise, and Sleep, Help in Making Decisions about Midlife Issues and Retirement, and Guidance Concerning Practical and Informed Choices in Health Consumerism

Along with Data Concerning the Theories of Aging, Different Experiences in Aging by Minority Groups, and Facts about Aging Now and Aging in the Future; and Featuring a Glossary, a Guide to Consumer Help, Additional Suggested Reading, and Practical Resource Directory

Edited by Jenifer Swanson. 536 pages. 1999. 0-7808-0390-6. $78.

"Recommended reference source."
—*Booklist, American Library Association, Feb '00*

SEE ALSO *Physical & Mental Issues in Aging Sourcebook*

Healthy Children Sourcebook

Basic Consumer Health Information about the Physical and Mental Development of Children between the Ages of 3 and 12, Including Routine Health Care, Preventative Health Services, Safety and First Aid, Healthy Sleep, Dental Care, Nutrition, and Fitness, and Featuring Parenting Tips on Such Topics as Bedwetting, Choosing Day Care, Monitoring TV and Other Media, and Establishing a Foundation for Substance Abuse Prevention

Along with a Glossary of Commonly Used Pediatric Terms and Resources for Additional Help and Information.

Edited by Chad T. Kimball. 648 pages. 2003. 0-7808-0247-0. $78.

Healthy Heart Sourcebook for Women

Basic Consumer Health Information about Cardiac Issues Specific to Women, Including Facts about Major Risk Factors and Prevention, Treatment and Control Strategies, and Important Dietary Issues

Along with a Special Section Regarding the Pros and Cons of Hormone Replacement Therapy and Its Impact on Heart Health, and Additional Help, Including Recipes, a Glossary, and a Directory of Resources

Edited by Dawn D. Matthews. 336 pages. 2000. 0-7808-0329-9. $78.

"**A good reference source and recommended for all public, academic, medical, and hospital libraries.**"
—*Medical Reference Services Quarterly, Summer '01*

"**Because of the lack of information specific to women on this topic, this book is recommended for public libraries and consumer libraries.**"
—*American Reference Books Annual, 2001*

"**Contains very important information about coronary artery disease that all women should know. The information is current and presented in an easy-to-read format. The book will make a good addition to any library.**"
—*American Medical Writers Association Journal, Summer '00*

"**Important, basic reference.**"
—*Reviewer's Bookwatch, Jul '00*

SEE ALSO *Heart Diseases & Disorders Sourcebook, Women's Health Concerns Sourcebook*

Heart Diseases & Disorders Sourcebook, 2nd Edition

Basic Consumer Health Information about Heart Attacks, Angina, Rhythm Disorders, Heart Failure, Valve Disease, Congenital Heart Disorders, and More,

Including Descriptions of Surgical Procedures and Other Interventions, Medications, Cardiac Rehabilitation, Risk Identification, and Prevention Tips

Along with Statistical Data, Reports on Current Research Initiatives, a Glossary of Cardiovascular Terms, and Resource Directory

Edited by Karen Bellenir. 612 pages. 2000. 0-7808-0238-1. $78.

ALSO AVAILABLE: *Cardiovascular Diseases & Disorders Sourcebook, 1st Edition.* Edited by Karen Bellenir and Peter D. Dresser. 683 pages. 1995. 0-7808-0032-X. $78.

"**This work stands out as an imminently accessible resource for the general public. It is recommended for the reference and circulating shelves of school, public, and academic libraries.**"
—*American Reference Books Annual, 2001*

"**Recommended reference source.**"
—*Booklist, American Library Association, Dec '00*

"**Provides comprehensive coverage of matters related to the heart. This title is recommended for health sciences and public libraries with consumer health collections.**"
—*E-Streams, Oct '00*

SEE ALSO *Healthy Heart Sourcebook for Women*

Household Safety Sourcebook

Basic Consumer Health Information about Household Safety, Including Information about Poisons, Chemicals, Fire, and Water Hazards in the Home

Along with Advice about the Safe Use of Home Maintenance Equipment, Choosing Toys and Nursery Furniture, Holiday and Recreation Safety, a Glossary, and Resources for Further Help and Information

Edited by Dawn D. Matthews. 606 pages. 2002. 0-7808-0338-8. $78.

"**This work will be useful in public libraries with large consumer health and wellness departments.**"
—*American Reference Books Annual, 2003*

"**As a sourcebook on household safety this book meets its mark. It is encyclopedic in scope and covers a wide range of safety issues that are commonly seen in the home.**"
—*E-Streams, Jul '02*

Immune System Disorders Sourcebook

Basic Information about Lupus, Multiple Sclerosis, Guillain-Barré Syndrome, Chronic Granulomatous Disease, and More

Along with Statistical and Demographic Data and Reports on Current Research Initiatives

Edited by Allan R. Cook. 608 pages. 1997. 0-7808-0209-8. $78.

Infant & Toddler Health Sourcebook

Basic Consumer Health Information about the Physical and Mental Development of Newborns, Infants, and Toddlers, Including Neonatal Concerns, Nutrition Recommendations, Immunization Schedules, Common Pediatric Disorders, Assessments and Milestones, Safety Tips, and Advice for Parents and Other Caregivers

Along with a Glossary of Terms and Resource Listings for Additional Help

Edited by Jenifer Swanson. 585 pages. 2000. 0-7808-0246-2. $78.

"As a reference for the general public, this would be useful in any library." —*E-Streams, May '01*

"Recommended reference source."
—*Booklist, American Library Association, Feb '01*

"This is a good source for general use."
—*American Reference Books Annual, 2001*

Injury & Trauma Sourcebook

Basic Consumer Health Information about the Impact of Injury, the Diagnosis and Treatment of Common and Traumatic Injuries, Emergency Care, and Specific Injuries Related to Home, Community, Workplace, Transportation, and Recreation

Along with Guidelines for Injury Prevention, a Glossary, and a Directory of Additional Resources

Edited by Joyce Brennfleck Shannon. 696 pages. 2002. 0-7808-0421-X. $78.

"This publication is the most comprehensive work of its kind about injury and trauma."
—*American Reference Books Annual, 2003*

"This sourcebook provides concise, easily readable, basic health information about injuries. . . . This book is well organized and an easy to use reference resource suitable for hospital, health sciences and public libraries with consumer health collections."
—*E-Streams, Nov '02*

"Practitioners should be aware of guides such as this in order to facilitate their use by patients and their families." —*Doody's Health Sciences Book Review Journal, Sep-Oct '02*

"Recommended reference source."
—*Booklist, American Library Association, Sep '02*

"Highly recommended for academic and medical reference collections." —*Library Bookwatch, Sep '02*

Kidney & Urinary Tract Diseases & Disorders Sourcebook

Basic Information about Kidney Stones, Urinary Incontinence, Bladder Disease, End Stage Renal Disease, Dialysis, and More

Along with Statistical and Demographic Data and Reports on Current Research Initiatives

Edited by Linda M. Ross. 602 pages. 1997. 0-7808-0079-6. $78.

Learning Disabilities Sourcebook, 2nd Edition

Basic Consumer Health Information about Learning Disabilities, Including Dyslexia, Developmental Speech and Language Disabilities, Non-Verbal Learning Disorders, Developmental Arithmetic Disorder, Developmental Writing Disorder, and Other Conditions That Impede Learning Such as Attention Deficit/ Hyperactivity Disorder, Brain Injury, Hearing Impairment, Klinefelter Syndrome, Dyspraxia, and Tourette Syndrome

Along with Facts about Educational Issues and Assistive Technology, Coping Strategies, a Glossary of Related Terms, and Resources for Further Help and Information

Edited by Dawn D. Matthews. 621 pages. 2003. 0-7808-0626-3. $78.

ALSO AVAILABLE: *Learning Disabilities Sourcebook, 1st Edition. Edited by Linda M. Shin. 579 pages. 1998. 0-7808-0210-1. $78.*

"Teachers as well as consumers will find this an essential guide to understanding various syndromes and their latest treatments. [An] invaluable reference for public and school library collections alike."
— *Library Bookwatch, Apr '03*

Named "Outstanding Reference Book of 1999."
—*New York Public Library, Feb 2000*

"An excellent candidate for inclusion in a public library reference section. It's a great source of information. Teachers will also find the book useful. Definitely worth reading."
—*Journal of Adolescent & Adult Literacy, Feb 2000*

"Readable . . . provides a solid base of information regarding successful techniques used with individuals who have learning disabilities, as well as practical suggestions for educators and family members. Clear language, concise descriptions, and pertinent information for contacting multiple resources add to the strength of this book as a valuable tool." —*Choice, Association of College and Research Libraries, Feb '99*

"Recommended reference source."
—*Booklist, American Library Association, Sep '98*

"A useful resource for libraries and for those who don't have the time to identify and locate the individual publications." —*Disability Resources Monthly, Sep '98*

Leukemia Sourcebook

Basic Consumer Health Information about Adult and Childhood Leukemias, Including Acute Lymphocytic Leukemia (ALL), Chronic Lymphocytic Leukemia (CLL), Acute Myelogenous Leukemia (AML), Chronic Myelogenous Leukemia (CML), and Hairy Cell Leukemia, and Treatments Such as Chemotherapy, Radiation Therapy, Peripheral Blood Stem Cell and Marrow Transplantation, and Immunotherapy

Along with Tips for Life During and After Treatment, a Glossary, and Directories of Additional Resources

Edited by Joyce Brennfleck Shannon. 587 pages. 2003. 0-7808-0627-1. $78.

Liver Disorders Sourcebook

Basic Consumer Health Information about the Liver and How It Works; Liver Diseases, Including Cancer, Cirrhosis, Hepatitis, and Toxic and Drug Related Diseases; Tips for Maintaining a Healthy Liver; Laboratory Tests, Radiology Tests, and Facts about Liver Transplantation

Along with a Section on Support Groups, a Glossary, and Resource Listings

Edited by Joyce Brennfleck Shannon. 591 pages. 2000. 0-7808-0383-3. $78.

"A valuable resource."
—American Reference Books Annual, 2001

"This title is recommended for health sciences and public libraries with consumer health collections."
—E-Streams, Oct '00

"Recommended reference source."
—Booklist, American Library Association, Jun '00

Lung Disorders Sourcebook

Basic Consumer Health Information about Emphysema, Pneumonia, Tuberculosis, Asthma, Cystic Fibrosis, and Other Lung Disorders, Including Facts about Diagnostic Procedures, Treatment Strategies, Disease Prevention Efforts, and Such Risk Factors as Smoking, Air Pollution, and Exposure to Asbestos, Radon, and Other Agents

Along with a Glossary and Resources for Additional Help and Information

Edited by Dawn D. Matthews. 678 pages. 2002. 0-7808-0339-6. $78.

"This title is a great addition for public and school libraries because it provides concise health information on the lungs."
—American Reference Books Annual, 2003

"Highly recommended for academic and medical reference collections." *—Library Bookwatch, Sep '02*

Medical Tests Sourcebook

Basic Consumer Health Information about Medical Tests, Including Periodic Health Exams, General Screening Tests, Tests You Can Do at Home, Findings of the U.S. Preventive Services Task Force, X-ray and Radiology Tests, Electrical Tests, Tests of Blood and Other Body Fluids and Tissues, Scope Tests, Lung Tests, Genetic Tests, Pregnancy Tests, Newborn Screening Tests, Sexually Transmitted Disease Tests, and Computer Aided Diagnoses

Along with a Section on Paying for Medical Tests, a Glossary, and Resource Listings

Edited by Joyce Brennfleck Shannon. 691 pages. 1999. 0-7808-0243-8. $78.

"Recommended for hospital and health sciences libraries with consumer health collections."
—E-Streams, Mar '00

"This is an overall excellent reference with a wealth of general knowledge that may aid those who are reluctant to get vital tests performed."
—Today's Librarian, Jan 2000

"A valuable reference guide."
—American Reference Books Annual, 2000

Men's Health Concerns Sourcebook

Basic Information about Health Issues That Affect Men, Featuring Facts about the Top Causes of Death in Men, Including Heart Disease, Stroke, Cancers, Prostate Disorders, Chronic Obstructive Pulmonary Disease, Pneumonia and Influenza, Human Immunodeficiency Virus and Acquired Immune Deficiency Syndrome, Diabetes Mellitus, Stress, Suicide, Accidents and Homicides; and Facts about Common Concerns for Men, Including Impotence, Contraception, Circumcision, Sleep Disorders, Snoring, Hair Loss, Diet, Nutrition, Exercise, Kidney and Urological Disorders, and Backaches

Edited by Allan R. Cook. 738 pages. 1998. 0-7808-0212-8. $78.

"This comprehensive resource and the series are highly recommended."
—American Reference Books Annual, 2000

"Recommended reference source."
—Booklist, American Library Association, Dec '98

Mental Health Disorders Sourcebook, 2nd Edition

Basic Consumer Health Information about Anxiety Disorders, Depression and Other Mood Disorders, Eating Disorders, Personality Disorders, Schizophrenia, and More, Including Disease Descriptions, Treatment Options, and Reports on Current Research Initiatives

Along with Statistical Data, Tips for Maintaining Mental Health, a Glossary, and Directory of Sources for Additional Help and Information

Edited by Karen Bellenir. 605 pages. 2000. 0-7808-0240-3. $78.

ALSO AVAILABLE: *Mental Health Disorders Sourcebook, 1st Edition.* Edited by Karen Bellenir. 548 pages. 1995. 0-7808-0040-0. $78.

"Well organized and well written."
—American Reference Books Annual, 2001

"Recommended reference source."
—Booklist, American Library Association, Jun '00

Mental Retardation Sourcebook

Basic Consumer Health Information about Mental Retardation and Its Causes, Including Down Syndrome, Fetal Alcohol Syndrome, Fragile X Syndrome, Genetic Conditions, Injury, and Environmental Sources

Along with Preventive Strategies, Parenting Issues, Educational Implications, Health Care Needs, Employment and Economic Matters, Legal Issues, a Glossary, and a Resource Listing for Additional Help and Information

Edited by Joyce Brennfleck Shannon. 642 pages. 2000. 0-7808-0377-9. $78.

"Public libraries will find the book useful for reference and as a beginning research point for students, parents, and caregivers."
—*American Reference Books Annual, 2001*

"The strength of this work is that it compiles many basic fact sheets and addresses for further information in one volume. It is intended and suitable for the general public. This sourcebook is relevant to any collection providing health information to the general public."
—*E-Streams, Nov '00*

"From preventing retardation to parenting and family challenges, this covers health, social and legal issues and will prove an invaluable overview."
—*Reviewer's Bookwatch, Jul '00*

Movement Disorders Sourcebook

Basic Consumer Health Information about Neurological Movement Disorders, Including Essential Tremor, Parkinson's Disease, Dystonia, Cerebral Palsy, Huntington's Disease, Myasthenia Gravis, Multiple Sclerosis, and Other Early-Onset and Adult-Onset Movement Disorders, Their Symptoms and Causes, Diagnostic Tests, and Treatments

Along with Mobility and Assistive Technology Information, a Glossary, and a Directory of Additional Resources

Edited by Joyce Brennfleck Shannon. 655 pages. 2003. 0-7808-0628-X. $78.

Obesity Sourcebook

Basic Consumer Health Information about Diseases and Other Problems Associated with Obesity, and Including Facts about Risk Factors, Prevention Issues, and Management Approaches

Along with Statistical and Demographic Data, Information about Special Populations, Research Updates, a Glossary, and Source Listings for Further Help and Information

Edited by Wilma Caldwell and Chad T. Kimball. 376 pages. 2001. 0-7808-0333-7. $78.

"The book synthesizes the reliable medical literature on obesity into one easy-to-read and useful resource for the general public."
—*American Reference Books Annual 2002*

"This is a very useful resource book for the lay public."
—*Doody's Review Service, Nov '01*

"Well suited for the health reference collection of a public library or an academic health science library that serves the general population." —*E-Streams, Sep '01*

"Recommended reference source."
—*Booklist, American Library Association, Apr '01*

" Recommended pick both for specialty health library collections and any general consumer health reference collection." — *The Bookwatch, Apr '01*

Ophthalmic Disorders Sourcebook, 1st Edition

SEE Eye Care Sourcebook, 2nd Edition

Oral Health Sourcebook

SEE Dental Care & Oral Health Sourcebook, 2nd Edition

Osteoporosis Sourcebook

Basic Consumer Health Information about Primary and Secondary Osteoporosis and Juvenile Osteoporosis and Related Conditions, Including Fibrous Dysplasia, Gaucher Disease, Hyperthyroidism, Hypophosphatasia, Myeloma, Osteopetrosis, Osteogenesis Imperfecta, and Paget's Disease

Along with Information about Risk Factors, Treatments, Traditional and Non-Traditional Pain Management, a Glossary of Related Terms, and a Directory of Resources

Edited by Allan R. Cook. 584 pages. 2001. 0-7808-0239-X. $78.

"This would be a book to be kept in a staff or patient library. The targeted audience is the layperson, but the therapist who needs a quick bit of information on a particular topic will also find the book useful."
—*Physical Therapy, Jan '02*

"This resource is recommended as a great reference source for public, health, and academic libraries, and is another triumph for the editors of Omnigraphics."
—*American Reference Books Annual 2002*

"Recommended for all public libraries and general health collections, especially those supporting patient education or consumer health programs."
—*E-Streams, Nov '01*

"Will prove valuable to any library seeking to maintain a current, comprehensive reference collection of health resources. . . . From prevention to treatment and associated conditions, this provides an excellent survey."
—*The Bookwatch, Aug '01*

"Recommended reference source."
—*Booklist, American Library Association, July '01*

SEE ALSO Women's Health Concerns Sourcebook

Pain Sourcebook, 2nd Edition

Basic Consumer Health Information about Specific Forms of Acute and Chronic Pain, Including Muscle and Skeletal Pain, Nerve Pain, Cancer Pain, and Disorders Characterized by Pain, Such as Fibromyalgia, Shingles, Angina, Arthritis, and Headaches

Along with Information about Pain Medications and Management Techniques, Complementary and Alternative Pain Relief Options, Tips for People Living with Chronic Pain, a Glossary, and a Directory of Sources for Further Information

Edited by Karen Bellenir. 670 pages. 2002. 0-7808-0612-3. $78.

ALSO AVAILABLE: *Pain Sourcebook, 1st Edition.* Edited by Allan R. Cook. 667 pages. 1997. 0-7808-0213-6. $78.

"A source of valuable information. . . . This book offers help to nonmedical people who need information about pain and pain management. It is also an excellent reference for those who participate in patient education."
— *Doody's Review Service, Sep '02*

"The text is readable, easily understood, and well indexed. This excellent volume belongs in all patient education libraries, consumer health sections of public libraries, and many personal collections."
— *American Reference Books Annual, 1999*

"A beneficial reference." — *Booklist Health Sciences Supplement, American Library Association, Oct '98*

"The information is basic in terms of scholarship and is appropriate for general readers. Written in journalistic style . . . intended for non-professionals. Quite thorough in its coverage of different pain conditions and summarizes the latest clinical information regarding pain treatment." — *Choice, Association of College and Research Libraries, Jun '98*

"Recommended reference source."
— *Booklist, American Library Association, Mar '98*

Pediatric Cancer Sourcebook

Basic Consumer Health Information about Leukemias, Brain Tumors, Sarcomas, Lymphomas, and Other Cancers in Infants, Children, and Adolescents, Including Descriptions of Cancers, Treatments, and Coping Strategies

Along with Suggestions for Parents, Caregivers, and Concerned Relatives, a Glossary of Cancer Terms, and Resource Listings

Edited by Edward J. Prucha. 587 pages. 1999. 0-7808-0245-4. $78.

"An excellent source of information. Recommended for public, hospital, and health science libraries with consumer health collections." — *E-Streams, Jun '00*

"Recommended reference source."
— *Booklist, American Library Association, Feb '00*

"A valuable addition to all libraries specializing in health services and many public libraries."
— *American Reference Books Annual, 2000*

Physical & Mental Issues in Aging Sourcebook

Basic Consumer Health Information on Physical and Mental Disorders Associated with the Aging Process, Including Concerns about Cardiovascular Disease, Pulmonary Disease, Oral Health, Digestive Disorders, Musculoskeletal and Skin Disorders, Metabolic Changes, Sexual and Reproductive Issues, and Changes in Vision, Hearing, and Other Senses

Along with Data about Longevity and Causes of Death, Information on Acute and Chronic Pain, Descriptions of Mental Concerns, a Glossary of Terms, and Resource Listings for Additional Help

Edited by Jenifer Swanson. 660 pages. 1999. 0-7808-0233-0. $78.

"This is a treasure of health information for the layperson." — *Choice Health Sciences Supplement, Association of College & Research Libraries, May 2000*

"Recommended for public libraries."
— *American Reference Books Annual, 2000*

"Recommended reference source."
— *Booklist, American Library Association, Oct '99*

SEE ALSO *Healthy Aging Sourcebook*

Podiatry Sourcebook

Basic Consumer Health Information about Foot Conditions, Diseases, and Injuries, Including Bunions, Corns, Calluses, Athlete's Foot, Plantar Warts, Hammertoes and Clawtoes, Clubfoot, Heel Pain, Gout, and More

Along with Facts about Foot Care, Disease Prevention, Foot Safety, Choosing a Foot Care Specialist, a Glossary of Terms, and Resource Listings for Additional Information

Edited by M. Lisa Weatherford. 380 pages. 2001. 0-7808-0215-2. $78.

"Recommended reference source."
— *Booklist, American Library Association, Feb '02*

"There is a lot of information presented here on a topic that is usually only covered sparingly in most larger comprehensive medical encyclopedias."
— *American Reference Books Annual 2002*

Pregnancy & Birth Sourcebook

Basic Information about Planning for Pregnancy, Maternal Health, Fetal Growth and Development, Labor and Delivery, Postpartum and Perinatal Care, Pregnancy in Mothers with Special Concerns, and Disorders of Pregnancy, Including Genetic Counseling, Nutrition and Exercise, Obstetrical Tests, Pregnancy Discomfort, Multiple Births, Cesarean Sections, Medical Testing of Newborns, Breastfeeding, Gestational Diabetes, and Ectopic Pregnancy

Edited by Heather E. Aldred. 737 pages. 1997. 0-7808-0216-0. $78.

Prostate Cancer Sourcebook

Basic Consumer Health Information about Prostate Cancer, Including Information about the Associated Risk Factors, Detection, Diagnosis, and Treatment of Prostate Cancer

Along with Information on Non-Malignant Prostate Conditions, and Featuring a Section Listing Support and Treatment Centers and a Glossary of Related Terms

Edited by Dawn D. Matthews. 358 pages. 2001. 0-7808-0324-8. $78.

Public Health Sourcebook

Basic Information about Government Health Agencies, Including National Health Statistics and Trends, Healthy People 2000 Program Goals and Objectives, the Centers for Disease Control and Prevention, the Food and Drug Administration, and the National Institutes of Health

Along with Full Contact Information for Each Agency

Edited by Wendy Wilcox. 698 pages. 1998. 0-7808-0220-9. $78.

Reconstructive & Cosmetic Surgery Sourcebook

Basic Consumer Health Information on Cosmetic and Reconstructive Plastic Surgery, Including Statistical Information about Different Surgical Procedures, Things to Consider Prior to Surgery, Plastic Surgery Techniques and Tools, Emotional and Psychological Considerations, and Procedure-Specific Information

Along with a Glossary of Terms and a Listing of Resources for Additional Help and Information

Edited by M. Lisa Weatherford. 374 pages. 2001. 0-7808-0214-4. $78.

Rehabilitation Sourcebook

Basic Consumer Health Information about Rehabilitation for People Recovering from Heart Surgery, Spinal Cord Injury, Stroke, Orthopedic Impairments, Amputation, Pulmonary Impairments, Traumatic Injury, and More, Including Physical Therapy, Occupational Therapy, Speech/ Language Therapy, Massage Therapy, Dance Therapy, Art Therapy, and Recreational Therapy

Along with Information on Assistive and Adaptive Devices, a Glossary, and Resources for Additional Help and Information

Edited by Dawn D. Matthews. 531 pages. 1999. 0-7808-0236-5. $78.

Respiratory Diseases & Disorders Sourcebook

Basic Information about Respiratory Diseases and Disorders, Including Asthma, Cystic Fibrosis, Pneumonia, the Common Cold, Influenza, and Others, Featuring Facts about the Respiratory System, Statistical and Demographic Data, Treatments, Self-Help Management Suggestions, and Current Research Initiatives

Edited by Allan R. Cook and Peter D. Dresser. 771 pages. 1995. 0-7808-0037-0. $78.

"A comprehensive collection of authoritative information presented in a nontechnical, humanitarian style for patients, families, and caregivers."
— *Association of Operating Room Nurses, Sep/Oct '95*

SEE ALSO *Lung Disorders Sourcebook*

Sexually Transmitted Diseases Sourcebook, 2nd Edition

Basic Consumer Health Information about Sexually Transmitted Diseases, Including Information on the Diagnosis and Treatment of Chlamydia, Gonorrhea, Hepatitis, Herpes, HIV, Mononucleosis, Syphilis, and Others

Along with Information on Prevention, Such as Condom Use, Vaccines, and STD Education; And Featuring a Section on Issues Related to Youth and Adolescents, a Glossary, and Resources for Additional Help and Information

Edited by Dawn D. Matthews. 538 pages. 2001. 0-7808-0249-7. $78.

ALSO AVAILABLE: *Sexually Transmitted Diseases Sourcebook, 1st Edition.* Edited by Linda M. Ross. 550 pages. 1997. 0-7808-0217-9. $78.

"Recommended for consumer health collections in public libraries, and secondary school and community college libraries."
— *American Reference Books Annual 2002*

"Every school and public library should have a copy of this comprehensive and user-friendly reference book."
— *Choice, Association of College & Research Libraries, Sep '01*

"This is a highly recommended book. This is an especially important book for all school and public libraries." — *AIDS Book Review Journal, Jul-Aug '01*

"Recommended reference source."
— *Booklist, American Library Association, Apr '01*

"Recommended pick both for specialty health library collections and any general consumer health reference collection." — *The Bookwatch, Apr '01*

Skin Disorders Sourcebook

Basic Information about Common Skin and Scalp Conditions Caused by Aging, Allergies, Immune Reactions, Sun Exposure, Infectious Organisms, Parasites, Cosmetics, and Skin Traumas, Including Abrasions, Cuts, and Pressure Sores

Along with Information on Prevention and Treatment

Edited by Allan R. Cook. 647 pages. 1997. 0-7808-0080-X. $78.

". . . comprehensive, easily read reference book."
— *Doody's Health Sciences Book Reviews, Oct '97*

SEE ALSO *Burns Sourcebook*

Sleep Disorders Sourcebook

Basic Consumer Health Information about Sleep and Its Disorders, Including Insomnia, Sleepwalking, Sleep Apnea, Restless Leg Syndrome, and Narcolepsy

Along with Data about Shiftwork and Its Effects, Information on the Societal Costs of Sleep Deprivation, Descriptions of Treatment Options, a Glossary of Terms, and Resource Listings for Additional Help

Edited by Jenifer Swanson. 439 pages. 1998. 0-7808-0234-9. $78.

"This text will complement any home or medical library. It is user-friendly and ideal for the adult reader."
— *American Reference Books Annual, 2000*

"A useful resource that provides accurate, relevant, and accessible information on sleep to the general public. Health care providers who deal with sleep disorders patients may also find it helpful in being prepared to answer some of the questions patients ask."
— *Respiratory Care, Jul '99*

"Recommended reference source."
— *Booklist, American Library Association, Feb '99*

Sports Injuries Sourcebook, 2nd Edition

Basic Consumer Health Information about the Diagnosis, Treatment, and Rehabilitation of Common Sports-Related Injuries in Children and Adults

Along with Suggestions for Conditioning and Training, Information and Prevention Tips for Injuries Frequently Associated with Specific Sports and Special Populations, a Glossary, and a Directory of Additional Resources

Edited by Joyce Brennfleck Shannon. 614 pages. 2002. 0-7808-0604-2. $78.

ALSO AVAILABLE: *Sports Injuries Sourcebook, 1st Edition.* Edited by Heather E. Aldred. 624 pages. 1999. 0-7808-0218-7. $78.

"This is an excellent reference for consumers and it is recommended for public, community college, and undergraduate libraries."
— *American Reference Books Annual, 2003*

"Recommended reference source."
— *Booklist, American Library Association, Feb '03*

Stress-Related Disorders Sourcebook

Basic Consumer Health Information about Stress and Stress-Related Disorders, Including Stress Origins and Signals, Environmental Stress at Work and Home, Mental and Emotional Stress Associated with Depression, Post-Traumatic Stress Disorder, Panic Disorder, Suicide, and the Physical Effects of Stress on the Cardiovascular, Immune, and Nervous Systems

Along with Stress Management Techniques, a Glossary, and a Listing of Additional Resources

Edited by Joyce Brennfleck Shannon. 610 pages. 2002. 0-7808-0560-7. $78.

"Well written for a general readership, the *Stress-Related Disorders Sourcebook* is a useful addition to the health reference literature."
— *American Reference Books Annual, 2003*

"I am impressed by the amount of information. It offers a thorough overview of the causes and consequences of stress for the layperson. . . . A well-done and thorough reference guide for professionals and nonprofessionals alike." — *Doody's Review Service, Dec '02*

◼

Stroke Sourcebook

Basic Consumer Health Information about Stroke, Including Ischemic, Hemorrhagic, Transient Ischemic Attack (TIA), and Pediatric Stroke, Stroke Triggers and Risks, Diagnostic Tests, Treatments, and Rehabilitation Information

Along with Stroke Prevention Guidelines, Legal and Financial Information, a Glossary, and a Directory of Additional Resources

Edited by Joyce Brennfleck Shannon. 606 pages. 2003. 0-7808-0630-1. $78.

◼

Substance Abuse Sourcebook

Basic Health-Related Information about the Abuse of Legal and Illegal Substances Such as Alcohol, Tobacco, Prescription Drugs, Marijuana, Cocaine, and Heroin; and Including Facts about Substance Abuse Prevention Strategies, Intervention Methods, Treatment and Recovery Programs, and a Section Addressing the Special Problems Related to Substance Abuse during Pregnancy

Edited by Karen Bellenir. 573 pages. 1996. 0-7808-0038-9. $78.

"A valuable addition to any health reference section. Highly recommended."
— *The Book Report, Mar/Apr '97*

". . . a comprehensive collection of substance abuse information that's both highly readable and compact. Families and caregivers of substance abusers will find the information enlightening and helpful, while teachers, social workers and journalists should benefit from the concise format. Recommended."
— *Drug Abuse Update, Winter '96/'97*

SEE ALSO *Alcoholism Sourcebook, Drug Abuse Sourcebook*

◼

Surgery Sourcebook

Basic Consumer Health Information about Inpatient and Outpatient Surgeries, Including Cardiac, Vascular, Orthopedic, Ocular, Reconstructive, Cosmetic, Gynecologic, and Ear, Nose, and Throat Procedures and More

Along with Information about Operating Room Policies and Instruments, Laser Surgery Techniques, Hospital Errors, Statistical Data, a Glossary, and Listings of Sources for Further Help and Information

Edited by Annemarie S. Muth and Karen Bellenir. 596 pages. 2002. 0-7808-0380-9. $78.

"Invaluable reference for public and school library collections alike." — *Library Bookwatch, Apr '03*

◼

Transplantation Sourcebook

Basic Consumer Health Information about Organ and Tissue Transplantation, Including Physical and Financial Preparations, Procedures and Issues Relating to Specific Solid Organ and Tissue Transplants, Rehabilitation, Pediatric Transplant Information, the Future of Transplantation, and Organ and Tissue Donation

Along with a Glossary and Listings of Additional Resources

Edited by Joyce Brennfleck Shannon. 628 pages. 2002. 0-7808-0322-1. $78.

"Along with these advances [in transplantation technology] have come a number of daunting questions for potential transplant patients, their families, and their health care providers. This reference text is the best single tool to address many of these questions. . . . It will be a much-needed addition to the reference collections in health care, academic, and large public libraries."
— *American Reference Books Annual, 2003*

"Recommended for libraries with an interest in offering consumer health information." — *E-Streams, Jul '02*

"This is a unique and valuable resource for patients facing transplantation and their families."
— *Doody's Review Service, Jun '02*

◼

Traveler's Health Sourcebook

Basic Consumer Health Information for Travelers, Including Physical and Medical Preparations, Transportation Health and Safety, Essential Information about Food and Water, Sun Exposure, Insect and Snake Bites, Camping and Wilderness Medicine, and Travel with Physical or Medical Disabilities

Along with International Travel Tips, Vaccination Recommendations, Geographical Health Issues, Disease Risks, a Glossary, and a Listing of Additional Resources

Edited by Joyce Brennfleck Shannon. 613 pages. 2000. 0-7808-0384-1. $78.

"Recommended reference source."
— *Booklist, American Library Association, Feb '01*

"This book is recommended for any public library, any travel collection, and especially any collection for the physically disabled."
— *American Reference Books Annual, 2001*

◼

Vegetarian Sourcebook

Basic Consumer Health Information about Vegetarian Diets, Lifestyle, and Philosophy, Including Definitions of Vegetarianism and Veganism, Tips about Adopting Vegetarianism, Creating a Vegetarian Pantry, and Meeting Nutritional Needs of Vegetarians, with Facts Regarding Vegetarianism's Effect on Pregnant and Lactat-

ing Women, Children, Athletes, and Senior Citizens

Along with a Glossary of Commonly Used Vegetarian Terms and Resources for Additional Help and Information

Edited by Chad T. Kimball. 360 pages. 2002. 0-7808-0439-2. $78.

"Organizes into one concise volume the answers to the most common questions concerning vegetarian diets and lifestyles. This title is recommended for public and secondary school libraries." —*E-Streams, Apr '03*

"Invaluable reference for public and school library collections alike." — *Library Bookwatch, Apr '03*

"The articles in this volume are easy to read and come from authoritative sources. The book does not necessarily support the vegetarian diet but instead provides the pros and cons of this important decision. The *Vegetarian Sourcebook* is recommended for public libraries and consumer health libraries."
— *American Reference Books Annual, 2003*

■

Women's Health Concerns Sourcebook

Basic Information about Health Issues That Affect Women, Featuring Facts about Menstruation and Other Gynecological Concerns, Including Endometriosis, Fibroids, Menopause, and Vaginitis; Reproductive Concerns, Including Birth Control, Infertility, and Abortion; and Facts about Additional Physical, Emotional, and Mental Health Concerns Prevalent among Women Such as Osteoporosis, Urinary Tract Disorders, Eating Disorders, and Depression

Along with Tips for Maintaining a Healthy Lifestyle

Edited by Heather E. Aldred. 567 pages. 1997. 0-7808-0219-5. $78.

"Handy compilation. There is an impressive range of diseases, devices, disorders, procedures, and other physical and emotional issues covered . . . well organized, illustrated, and indexed." — *Choice, Association of College and Research Libraries, Jan '98*

SEE ALSO *Breast Cancer Sourcebook, Cancer Sourcebook for Women, Healthy Heart Sourcebook for Women, Osteoporosis Sourcebook*

■

Workplace Health & Safety Sourcebook

Basic Consumer Health Information about Workplace Health and Safety, Including the Effect of Workplace Hazards on the Lungs, Skin, Heart, Ears, Eyes, Brain, Reproductive Organs, Musculoskeletal System, and Other Organs and Body Parts

Along with Information about Occupational Cancer, Personal Protective Equipment, Toxic and Hazardous Chemicals, Child Labor, Stress, and Workplace Violence

Edited by Chad T. Kimball. 626 pages. 2000. 0-7808-0231-4. $78.

"As a reference for the general public, this would be useful in any library." —*E-Streams, Jun '01*

"Provides helpful information for primary care physicians and other caregivers interested in occupational medicine. . . . General readers; professionals."
— *Choice, Association of College & Research Libraries, May '01*

"Recommended reference source."
— *Booklist, American Library Association, Feb '01*

"Highly recommended." — *The Bookwatch, Jan '01*

■

Worldwide Health Sourcebook

Basic Information about Global Health Issues, Including Malnutrition, Reproductive Health, Disease Dispersion and Prevention, Emerging Diseases, Risky Health Behaviors, and the Leading Causes of Death

Along with Global Health Concerns for Children, Women, and the Elderly, Mental Health Issues, Research and Technology Advancements, and Economic, Environmental, and Political Health Implications, a Glossary, and a Resource Listing for Additional Help and Information

Edited by Joyce Brennfleck Shannon. 614 pages. 2001. 0-7808-0330-2. $78.

"Named an Outstanding Academic Title."
—*Choice, Association of College & Research Libraries, Jan '02*

"Yet another handy but also unique compilation in the extensive Health Reference Series, this is a useful work because many of the international publications reprinted or excerpted are not readily available. Highly recommended." —*Choice, Association of College & Research Libraries, Nov '01*

"Recommended reference source."
—*Booklist, American Library Association, Oct '01*

Teen Health Series

Helping Young Adults Understand, Manage, and Avoid Serious Illness

Diet Information for Teens
Health Tips about Diet and Nutrition

Including Facts about Nutrients, Dietary Guidelines, Breakfasts, School Lunches, Snacks, Party Food, Weight Control, Eating Disorders, and More

Edited by Karen Bellenir. 399 pages. 2001. 0-7808-0441-4. $58.

"Full of helpful insights and facts throughout the book. ... An excellent resource to be placed in public libraries or even in personal collections."
—American Reference Books Annual 2002

"Recommended for middle and high school libraries and media centers as well as academic libraries that educate future teachers of teenagers. It is also a suitable addition to health science libraries that serve patrons who are interested in teen health promotion and education."
— E-Streams, Oct '01

"This comprehensive book would be beneficial to collections that need information about nutrition, dietary guidelines, meal planning, and weight control. . . . This reference is so easy to use that its purchase is recommended."
— The Book Report, Sep-Oct '01

"This book is written in an easy to understand format describing issues that many teens face every day, and then provides thoughtful explanations so that teens can make informed decisions. This is an interesting book that provides important facts and information for today's teens."
—Doody's Health Sciences Book Review Journal, Jul-Aug '01

"A comprehensive compendium of diet and nutrition. The information is presented in a straightforward, plain-spoken manner. This title will be useful to those working on reports on a variety of topics, as well as to general readers concerned about their dietary health."
— School Library Journal, Jun '01

Drug Information for Teens
Health Tips about the Physical and Mental Effects of Substance Abuse

Including Facts about Alcohol, Anabolic Steroids, Club Drugs, Cocaine, Depressants, Hallucinogens, Herbal Products, Inhalants, Marijuana, Narcotics, Stimulants, Tobacco, and More

Edited by Karen Bellenir. 452 pages. 2002. 0-7808-0444-9. $58.

"The chapters are quick to make a connection to their teenage reading audience. The prose is straightforward and the book lends itself to spot reading. It should be useful both for practical information and for research, and it is suitable for public and school libraries."
— American Reference Books Annual, 2003

"Recommended reference source."
— Booklist, American Library Association, Feb '03

"This is an excellent resource for teens and their parents. Education about drugs and substances is key to discouraging teen drug abuse and this book provides this much needed information in a way that is interesting and factual."   *—Doody's Review Service, Dec '02*

Mental Health Information for Teens
Health Tips about Mental Health and Mental Illness

Including Facts about Anxiety, Depression, Suicide, Eating Disorders, Obsessive-Compulsive Disorders, Panic Attacks, Phobias, Schizophrenia, and More

Edited by Karen Bellenir. 406 pages. 2001. 0-7808-0442-2. $58.

"In both language and approach, this user-friendly entry in the *Teen Health Series* is on target for teens needing information on mental health concerns."   *— Booklist, American Library Association, Jan '02*

"Readers will find the material accessible and informative, with the shaded notes, facts, and embedded glossary insets adding appropriately to the already interesting and succinct presentation."
—School Library Journal, Jan '02

"This title is highly recommended for any library that serves adolescents and parents/caregivers of adolescents."   *— E-Streams, Jan '02*

"Recommended for high school libraries and young adult collections in public libraries. Both health professionals and teenagers will find this book useful."
— American Reference Books Annual 2002

"This is a nice book written to enlighten the society, primarily teenagers, about common teen mental health issues. It is highly recommended to teachers and parents as well as adolescents."
—Doody's Review Service, Dec '01

Sexual Health Information for Teens
Health Tips about Sexual Development, Human Reproduction, and Sexually Transmitted Diseases

Including Facts about Puberty, Reproductive Health, Chlamydia, Human Papillomavirus, Pelvic Inflam-

matory Disease, Herpes, AIDS, Contraception, Pregnancy, and More

Edited by Deborah A. Stanley. 391 pages. 2003. 0-7808-0445-7. $58.

Skin Health Information For Teens

Health Tips about Dermatological Concerns and Skin Cancer Risks

Including Facts about Acne, Warts, Hives, and Other Conditions and Lifestyle Choices, Such as Tanning, Tattooing, and Piercing, That Affect the Skin, Nails, Scalp, and Hair

Edited by Robert Aquinas McNally. 430 pages. 2003. 0-7808-0446-5. $58.

Health Reference Series